Cardiac Anesthesia and Transesophageal Echocardiography

Editors

John D. Wasnick, MD, MPH, MHCM
Steven L. Berk Endowed Chair for Excellence in Medicine
Professor and Chair
Department of Anesthesiology
Texas Tech University Health Sciences Center
Lubbock, Texas

Alina Nicoara, MD
Associate Professor
Department of Anesthesiology
Duke University Medical Center
Durham, North Carolina

Contributing Editors (First Edition)

Zak Hillel, PhD, MD
Sanford Littwin, MD
David Kramer, MD

a LANGE medical book

Cardiac Anesthesia and Transesophageal Echocardiography

Second Edition

John D. Wasnick, MD, MPH, MHCM
Alina Nicoara, MD

Illustrations by
Jill K. Gregory, MFA, CMI

Electronic Media by
Alina Nicoara, MD
David Kramer, MD
Sanford Littwin, MD

New York   Chicago   San Francisco   Athens   London   Madrid   Mexico City
Milan   New Delhi   Singapore   Sydney   Toronto

Cardiac Anesthesia and Transesophageal Echocardiography

Copyright © 2019, 2011 by McGraw-Hill Education. All rights reserved. Printed in the United States of America. Except as permitted under the United States Copyright Act of 1976, no part of this publication may be reproduced or distributed in any form or by any means, or stored in a data base or retrieval system, without the prior written permission of the publisher.

1 2 3 4 5 6 7 8 9   LCR   24 23 22 21 20 19

ISBN 978-0-07-184733-9
MHID 0-07-184733-2

This book was set in Adobe Garamond Pro by Cenveo® Publisher Services.
The editors were Jason Malley and Christie Naglieri.
The production supervisor was Richard Ruzycka.
Project management was provided by Radhika Jolly, Cenveo Publisher Services.
The cover designer was W2 Design.

This book is printed on acid-free paper.

Library of Congress Cataloging-in-Publication Data

Names: Wasnick, John D., editor.
Title: Cardiac anesthesia and transesophageal echocardiography / editors,
John D. Wasnick, MD, MPH, Professor and Chair, Department of
Anesthesiology, Texas Tech Health Sciences Center School of Medicine,
Lubbock, Texas, [and four others].
Description: Second edition. | New York : McGraw-Hill Education, [2019] |
Includes bibliographical references and index.
Identifiers: LCCN 2018053664 | ISBN 9780071847339 (paperback)
Subjects: LCSH: Anesthesia in cardiology. | Transesophageal echocardiography.
| BISAC: MEDICAL / Anesthesiology.
Classification: LCC RD87.3.H43 C347 2019 | DDC 617.9/6741—dc23 LC record available at
https://na01.safelinks.protection.outlook.com/?

McGraw-Hill books are available at special quantity discounts to use as premiums and sales promotions, or for use in corporate training programs. To contact a representative please visit the Contact Us pages at www.mhprofessional.com.

Contents

Preface

This second edition of *Cardiac Anesthesia and Transesophageal Echocardiography* seeks to serve as a ready resource for learners new to the cardiac surgery operating room. Like the first edition, this text introduces the principles of cardiac anesthesia and transesophageal echocardiography concurrently much as they might be encountered in the operating room, cardiac catheterization laboratory, or intensive care unit by a student, resident, or trainee. The goal of the text is to provide a foundational introduction and review of both cardiac anesthesia practice and transesophageal echocardiography. Like the first edition, video clips present key echocardiography images essential to practice. The discussion has been updated to reflect current cardiac anesthesia practice. Likewise, the text has been expanded to provide additional management details as well as to include review of procedures that have been introduced into cardiac anesthesia practice since the first edition. We hope that learners will use this book to quickly familiarize themselves with the cardiac anesthesia environment. We believe that the foundational information presented in this book can be readily learned by newcomers to the cardiac operating room environment. The cardiac anesthesia workplace is often stressful for new learners. We believe that a strong foundational knowledge base acquired before entering the cardiac surgery operating room is the best way to enhance the experience for students and to improve their learning. Consequently, we hope learners will review this book before beginning their cardiac anesthesia rotations and that they will ultimately enjoy cardiac anesthesia practice as much as we both do.

John D. Wasnick
Alina Nicoara

Contributors to the First Edition*

Diane Anca, MD
Assistant Professor of Anesthesiology
Columbia University
Anesthesiology
St. Luke's-Roosevelt Hospital Center
New York, New York

Laura Y. Chang, MD
Fellow
Obstetrical Anesthesiology
Brigham and Women's Hospital
Boston, Massachusetts

Draginja R. Cvetkovic, MD
Assistant Professor
Anesthesiology
Montefiore Medical Center, The University
    Hospital for the Albert Einstein College
    of Medicine
Bronx, New York

Christina Delucca
Resident
Anesthesiology
St. Luke's-Roosevelt Hospital Center
New York, New York

Naomi Dong, MD
Fellow
Anesthesiology and Critical Care
Children's Hospital of Philadelphia
Philadelphia, Pennsylvania

Jeff Gadsden, MD, FRCPC, FANZCA
Assistant Professor of Clinical Anesthesiology
Anesthesiology
Columbia University College of Physicians
    and Surgeons
New York, New York

Kimberly B. Gratenstein
Regional Anesthesia Fellow
Anesthesiology
St. Luke's-Roosevelt Hospital Center
New York, New York

Zak Hillel, PhD, MD
Professor of Clinical Anesthesiology
Columbia University College of Physicians
    and Surgeons
Director, Cardiac Anesthesia
St. Luke's-Roosevelt Hospital Center
New York, New York

Shannon N. Johnson, MD
Chief Resident
Department of Anesthesiology
St. Luke's-Roosevelt Hospital Center
New York, New York

Misuzu Kameyama, DO
Chief Resident
Anesthesiology
St. Luke's Rooevelt Hospital
New York, New York

David C. Kramer, MD
Assistant Professor
Department of Anesthesiology
St. Luke's-Roosevelt Hospital Center
New York, New York

Shusmi Kurapati
Chief Resident
Department of Anesthesiology
St. Luke's-Roosevelt Hospital Center
New York, New York

Sharon Lee
Fellow
Pediatric Anesthesia
Department of Anesthesia
Washington University School of Medicine
St. Louis, Missouri

Ellen Lee
Fellow
Pain Management
Department of Anesthesiology
St. Luke's-Roosevelt Hospital Center
New York, New York

*Title at time of original contribution.

Galina Leyvi, MD
Associate Professor of Clinical Anesthesiology
Anesthesiology
Montefiore Medical Center AECOM
Bronx, New York

Sanford M. Littwin, MD
Assistant Professor
Anesthesiology
St. Luke's-Roosevelt Hospital Center
New York, New York

Alina Nicoara, MD
Assistant Professor
Department of Anesthesiology
Duke University Medical Center
Durham, North Carolina

Christy Perdue
Resident
Department of Anesthesiology
St. Luke's-Roosevelt Hospital Center
New York, New York

Nii-Ayikai Quaye
Attending Anesthesiologist
Private Practice
Silver Spring, Maryland

Shanti Raju
Resident
Department of Anesthesiology
St. Luke's-Roosevelt Hospital Center
New York, New York

Deepak Sreedharan
Resident
Department of Anesthesiology
St. Luke's-Roosevelt Hospital Center
New York, New York

John D. Wasnick, MD, MPH, MHCM
Professor and Chair
Department of Anesthesiology
Texas Tech Health Sciences Center School
    of Medicine
Lubbock, Texas

Introduction to Perioperative Echocardiography

Perioperative echocardiography is an essential tool in the anesthetic management of the cardiac surgical patient. Moreover, echocardiographic skills and knowledge can be applied to patients irrespective of the nature of surgical procedure. Consequently, this text begins with a discussion about transesophageal echocardiography (TEE) and other echocardiographic modalities. Throughout this book, TEE will be employed to illustrate various cardiac pathologies and the anesthetic manipulations required to manage patients with a variety of cardiac conditions. TEE imagery will be integrated into the discussion and explanations of perioperative management much in the way that echocardiographic images are employed in routine, daily anesthetic practice. Although it is not the authors' intention to write a definitive text of perioperative echocardiography, it is hoped that the reader will become sufficiently familiar with this valuable tool to appreciate how echocardiographic imagery can be mated with clinical knowledge and clinical experience to effectively manage the cardiac surgery patient.

WHAT CAN BE LEARNED FROM PERIOPERATIVE TRANSESOPHAGEAL ECHOCARDIOGRAPHY (TEE)?

Perioperatively, TEE is employed to help anesthesiologists, surgeons, and cardiologists answer questions about the heart's structure and function. TEE guides diagnosis and therapy in a number of ways including:

1. Identification of the source of hemodynamic instability: TEE can detect myocardial ischemia, poor ventricular function, hypovolemia, and pericardial tamponade.
2. Determination of hemodynamic parameters: TEE can be used to determine stroke volume (SV) and cardiac output (CO) and can also be used to assess pulmonary arterial and intraventricular pressures.
3. Examination and confirmation of structural diagnoses: TEE helps to detect new pathology perhaps missed on previous examinations including patent foramen ovale, atheromatous aorta, or undiagnosed valvular heart disease. More likely, however, perioperative TEE will confirm the previous cardiac diagnoses.
4. Guidance and confirmation of the adequacy of surgical interventions: TEE is used to ascertain the success of valvular repair/replacement and to detect any unexpected surgical complications.
5. Diagnosis of postoperative hemodynamic instability: Echocardiography will readily reveal causes of postoperative hemodynamic instability secondary to pericardial tamponade; left, right, or biventricular failure; pulmonary embolism; aortic dissection; and other catastrophic perioperative events.

Throughout this text, echocardiography will be integrally linked to perioperative anesthetic management and its use in each of the ways described above will be illustrated. Moreover, just as in the operating room or intensive care unit, echocardiography will inform and illustrate appropriate medical decision making.

WHAT ECHOCARDIOGRAPHIC MODALITIES ARE EMPLOYED AND HOW CAN THEY BE USED?

TEE was introduced to operating rooms in the mid- to late 1980s. By the mid-1990s it had increasingly become a "routine" part of perioperative management.[1] The National Board of Echocardiography (NBE) was subsequently established to credential and "certify" individuals in perioperative TEE. TEE is the echocardiographic modality most commonly associated with cardiac anesthesiologists. Anesthesiologists have subsequently expanded the use of TEE in noncardiac surgical suites and in the intensive care unit (ICU) (Figures Intro–1 and Intro–2 and **Video Intro–1**).

Transthoracic echocardiography (TTE), although more commonly associated with cardiology evaluations, is increasingly employed perioperatively by anesthesiologists. TTE is a noninvasive imaging modality. Although TTE is employed perioperatively in some surgical procedures, its use is awkward in the surgical suite secondary to the surgical field and drapes. On the other hand, anesthesiologists

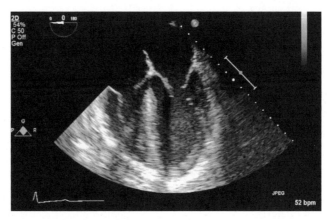

Figure Intro–1. The midesophageal four-chamber view seen here is the view most familiar to new learners of cardiac anesthesia.

and intensivists in the ICU and in preoperative evaluation frequently utilize TTE.[2] ICU physicians readily perform TTE examinations to answer basic questions about hemodynamic instability. A limited TTE examination can determine if the pumping function of the heart is adequate or not, or if the heart is sufficiently volume loaded. Such information can be invaluable in quickly determining the etiology of a patient's perioperative hypotensive episode. Noninvasive TTE can answer questions, which otherwise might require invasive hemodynamic pressure monitoring with a pulmonary artery (PA) catheter.

Goal-directed ultrasound protocols are available to assist physicians in the acute care setting make these quick hemodynamic assessments.[3] Such protocol-driven TTE exams can be completed by physicians with limited training. The Focus

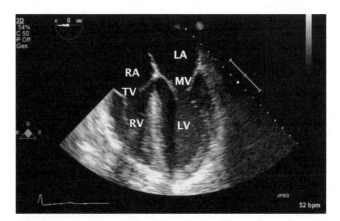

Figure Intro–2. Here the structures of the heart as seen on the previous TEE image are identified including the right atrium (RA), tricuspid valve (TV), right ventricle (RV), left atrium (LA), mitral valve (MV), and left ventricle (LV).

Assessed Transthoracic Echocardiography (FATE) protocol attempts to resolve hemodynamic questions in five steps[4] including:

1. Identify obvious pathology.
2. Assess wall thickness and chamber dimensions.
3. Assess biventricular function.
4. Visualize bilateral pleura.
5. Relate information to the clinical context.

Using TTE, four scanning positions are employed (Figure Intro–3).

Using pattern recognition, it is possible to identify various cardiac pathologies. Extended FATE views permit evaluation of the inferior vena cava (IVC) and valvular structures (Figure Intro–4A). IVC collapse/distension can be used to determine volume responsiveness in the perioperative setting (Figure Intro–4B).

Figure Intro–5 identifies common, important pathology patterns seen using the FATE protocol typical of various cardiac conditions and their potential etiologies.

There are many limited, goal-directed approaches to TTE assessment in acute care medicine. The most readily employed protocols look at left ventricular contractility and filling. More advanced limited examinations, such as the Haemodynamic Echocardiography Assessment in Real Time (HEART), provide the examiner information not just on hemodynamic function but also include evaluations of valvular structure.[5] (More information regarding the FATE protocol can be found at www.usabcd.org.)

Still, in spite of TTE's ease of use, it cannot replace transesophageal echocardiography (TEE) in the intraoperative management of the cardiac surgery patient. Consequently, this text will principally focus on TEE and the medical interventions that can be informed through its use during cardiac surgery. TEE and TTE employ different echocardiographic windows to obtain images of the heart. The FATE exam demonstrates four transthoracic windows through which cardiac images can be obtained. The esophagus is in close proximity to the left atrium and as such is likewise a window by which ultrasound images can be obtained. The challenge for the new learner of either TTE or TEE is to be able to orient the image such that the structures viewed are identified correctly irrespective of whatever window is used. Principles learned for the analysis of TEE images likewise apply when TTE images are obtained. Only the echo windows and the orientation of the images in the viewing screen are different.

Other ultrasound windows are also used perioperatively such as epiaortic ultrasound and epicardiac ultrasound. When used, an ultrasound probe robed in a sterile sheath is placed directly upon the aorta or heart to obtain echo images.

Epiaortic ultrasound (EAU) **(Video Intro–2)** and epicardiac ultrasound (Figures Intro–6 and Intro–7) are used as perioperative adjuncts to TEE but also can be used when TEE is contraindicated. EAU is useful because the ascending aorta is not completely imaged by TEE. Interposition of the airway between the TEE probe in the esophagus and the aorta prevents visualization of the distal ascending aorta and proximal aortic arch. Because aortic atherosclerosis is associated with embolic stroke during cardiac surgery,[6,7] EAU may serve to identify areas

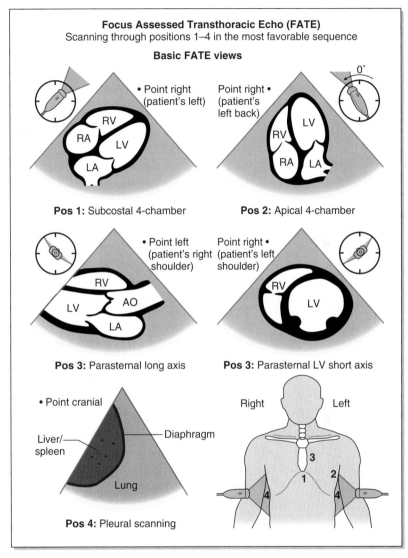

Figure Intro–3. Focus assessed transthoracic echocardiography (FATE) card with its four scanning positions. AO = aorta; LA = left atrium; LV = left ventricle; Pos = position; RA = right atrium; RV = right ventricle. [Reproduced with permission from Jørgensen MR, Juhl-Olsen P, Frederiksen CA, et al: Transthoracic echocardiography in the perioperative setting, *Curr Opin Anaesthesiol.* 2016 Feb;29(1):46-54.]

of the aorta not amenable for surgical manipulation and thus reduce the incidence of perioperative embolic stroke. Unlike TEE, the surgeon must interrupt the progress of the operation to manipulate the probe. However, if areas of aorta replete with atherosclerotic plaque are identified, then morbidity and mortality may be reduced through the use of EAU.

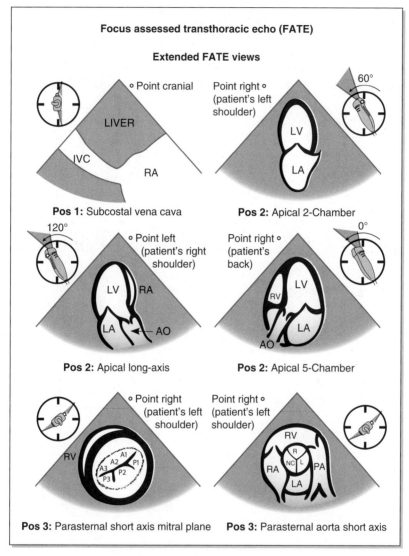

Focus assessed transthoracic echo (FATE)

Extended FATE views

Point cranial ∘
LIVER
IVC
RA
Pos 1: Subcostal vena cava

Point right ∘
(patient's left
shoulder)
60°
LV
LA
Pos 2: Apical 2-Chamber

120°
Point left ∘
(patient's right
shoulder)
LV RA
LA —AO
Pos 2: Apical long-axis

Point right ∘
(patient's
back)
0°
LV
RV
LA
AO
Pos 2: Apical 5-Chamber

Point right ∘
(patient's left
shoulder)
RV
A1
A3 A2 P1
P3 P2
Pos 3: Parasternal short axis mitral plane

Point right ∘
(patient's left
shoulder)
RV
R
RA NC L PA
LA
Pos 3: Parasternal aorta short axis

Figure Intro–4A. Focus assessed transthoracic echocardiography (FATE) protocol. Extended view. AO, aorta; IVC, inferior vena cava; LA, left atrium; LV, left ventricle; PA, pulmonary artery; RA, right atrium; RV, right ventricle. [Reproduced with permission from Jørgensen MR, Juhl-Olsen P, Frederiksen CA, et al: Transthoracic echocardiography in the perioperative setting, *Curr Opin Anaesthesiol.* 2016 Feb;29(1):46-54.]

Intraoperative 3-D echocardiography performed in real time is increasingly available and popular **(Video Intro–3)**.[8-10] The contribution of 3-D echocardiography to clinical decision making is likewise increasing. Three-dimensional echocardiography may better quantify intraventricular volumes and provide additional information regarding complex valvular structures such as the mitral valve apparatus.[11,12]

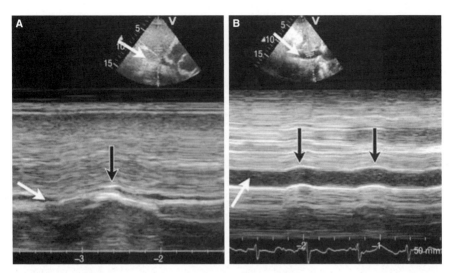

Figure Intro–4B. Examples of hemodynamic assessment by focused echocardiogra-phy. Two-dimensional and M-mode scans of the inferior vena cava. (a) Total collapse of the inferior vena cava caused by hemorrhagic shock. (b) Distended inferior vena cava, in this case caused by volume overload. Note the absence of caliber change during the respiratory cycle. White arrow, inferior vena cava; Black arrow, peak inspiration. [Repro-duced with permission from Jørgensen MR, Juhl-Olsen P, Frederiksen CA, et al: Transthoracic echocardiography in the perioperative setting, *Curr Opin Anaesthesiol.* 2016 Feb;29(1):46-54.]

However, 3-D imagery is based upon the same principles of ultrasound as 2-D echocardiography and as such is similarly subject to artifacts. Three-dimensional echo imagery both compliments and enhances 2-D TEE and will be presented where indicated to illustrate its role in the perioperative care of the cardiac surgery patient.

WHAT ARE THE INDICATIONS AND CONTRAINDICATIONS FOR PERIOPERATIVE TEE?

Studies are continually under way to demonstrate the use of perioperative TEE to improve and to positively influence surgical outcomes. However, TEE is not mandated for the management of "routine" coronary artery bypass grafting.[13] Table Intro–1 presents general indications for TEE.

Nonetheless, the so-called routine patient is somewhat of a *rara avis* in today's cardiac surgery operating room. As such, perioperative TEE has found its way into cardiac anesthesia practice to assist in the assessment and management of patients undergoing the entire spectrum of cardiac surgical procedures from "simple" coro-nary artery bypass graft surgery up to heart transplantation. Perioperative TEE can be used to:

- Assess hemodynamic instability
- Guide valvular repair

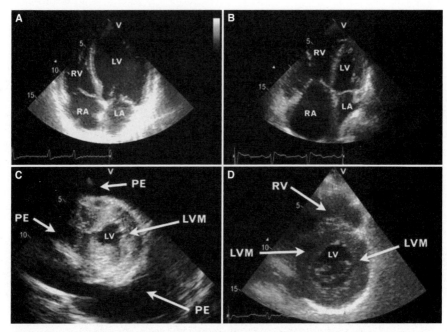

Figure Intro–5. Examples of disease of perioperative significance disclosed by focused echocardiography. (a) Dilated left ventricle, as seen in left ventricle failure. (b) Dilated right ventricle with enlarged right atrium. Typical finding if right side pressure increases, for example pulmonary embolus. (c) Pericardial effusion causing reduced left ventricular filling. The myocardium appears hypertrophic, as the left ventricle end-diastolic diameter is less than 1.5 cm. (d) Hypertrophic left ventricular myocardium. End-diastolic diameter is approximately 3.5 cm. LA, left atrium; LV, left ventricle; LVM, left ventricular myocardium; PE, pericardial effusion; RA, right atrium; RV, right ventricle. [Reproduced with permission from Jørgensen MR, Juhl-Olsen P, Frederiksen CA, et al: Transthoracic echocardiography in the perioperative setting, *Curr Opin Anaesthesiol.* 2016 Feb;29(1):46-54.]

- Guide congenital heart disease repair
- Assess resections of myocardial tissue during hypertrophic obstructive cardiomyopathy surgery or ventricular aneurysmectomy
- Detect atrial and ventricular septal defects
- Diagnose pericardial tamponade
- Detect myocardial ischemia
- Monitor responses to inotropic therapy
- Evaluate aortic diseases such as aortic atherosclerosis and aortic dissections
- Determine correct placement of ventricular assist device cannulas
- Confirm correct placement of an intra-aortic balloon pump
- Provide perioperative hemodynamic measurements in place of a pulmonary artery (PA) catheter

In other words, TEE provides much information to the anesthesiologist and the surgeon during cardiac surgical procedures that can influence patient outcomes assuming the images are correctly interpreted by the echocardiographer. Diagnoses that alter or influence surgical procedures should be made only by those individuals capable of performing TEE at an advanced level. The cognitive and technical skills required to perform perioperative TEE at an advanced level or at a basic level are presented in Table Intro–2.

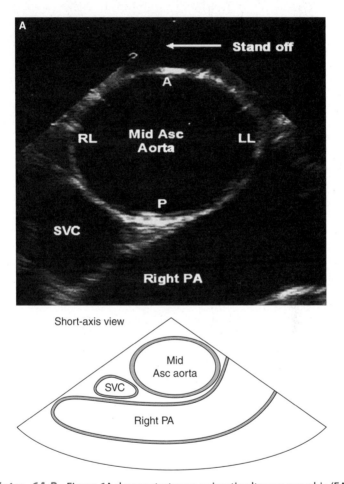

Figure Intro–6A,B. Figure 6A demonstrates an epiaortic ultrasonographic (EAU) image of the normal ascending (Asc) aorta in the short-axis view. Seen are the anterior (A), posterior (P), right lateral (RL), and left lateral (LL) walls of the aorta. The right pulmonary artery (PA) and superior vena cava are also seen. The "standoff" is that area of fluid between the handheld EAU probe and the aorta. Figure 6B presents the long-axis view. TEE cannot visualize the ascending aorta due to the presence of the airway. [Reproduced with permission from Glas KE, Swaminathan M, Reeves ST, et al: Guidelines for the performance of a comprehensive intraoperative epiaortic ultrasonographic examination: recommendations of the American Society of Echocardiography and the Society of Cardiovascular Anesthesiologists; endorsed by the Society of Thoracic Surgeons, *Anesth Analg.* 2008 May;106(5):1376-1384.]

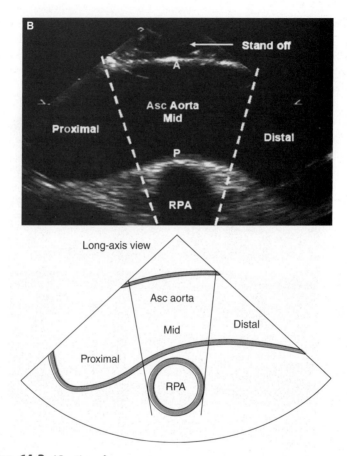

Figure Intro–6A,B. (Continued)

TEE can also be used at a basic level to assist in the diagnosis and management of hemodynamic instability, but TEE is contraindicated in patients with overt esophageal pathology (Table Intro–3).

Esophageal cancer, esophageal strictures, and other esophageal problems are absolute contraindications to TEE. TEE is relatively contraindicated in patients with previous mediastinal irradiation, among other conditions. The risks and benefits of TEE probe placement should also be considered in patients with gastric pathology such as ulcers and hiatal hernias. Perforation of the esophagus can be a life-threatening complication associated with a high mortality and morbidity. During preoperative assessment, the anesthesiologist contemplating use of TEE should elicit a history of any esophageal pathology or swallowing difficulties. Risks associated with the use of TEE include endotracheal tube dislodgement, dental injury, esophageal abrasions, and esophageal perforation. As with most things in anesthesiology, it is *never* wise to apply force to place the TEE probe. A laryngoscope often facilitates probe placement. The TEE probe should pass easily and

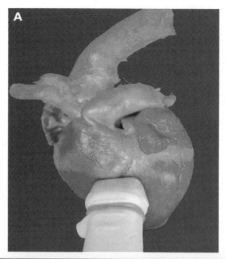

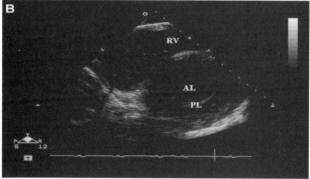

Figure Intro-7. An epicardial left ventricle (LV) basal short-axis view (SAX) seen here reveals the right ventricle (RV) and the anterior (AL) and posterior (PL) leaflets of the mitral valve. The orientation of the handheld probe against the heart is demonstrated in panel A. [Reproduced with permission from Reeves ST, Glas KE, Eltzschig H, et al: Guidelines for performing a comprehensive epicardial echocardiography examination: recommendations of the American Society of Echocardiography and the Society of Cardiovascular Anesthesiologists, *Anesth Analg.* 2007 Jul;105(1):22-28.]

be freely manipulated. Should resistance be encountered, it is best to forgo TEE examination. Although the information is far less complete, the handheld EAU probe can be used by the surgeon to provide intermittent epicardial and epiaortic echo imagery from the surgical field.

TEE generates heat that could in theory produce a thermal injury. TEE machines will generally shut down to permit cooling when the probe reaches a preset elevated temperature.

Finally, it is important to note that correct interpretation of TEE images takes much time, practice, and rigorous credentialing. Simply put, TEE cannot be learned in a day—but, some basic TEE imagery can be mastered and some

Table Intro-1. Indications for Perioperative Transesophageal Echocardiography

General indication	Specific examples
1. Evaluation of cardiac and aortic structure and function in situations where the findings will alter management and TTE is nondiagnostic or TTE is deferred because there is a high probability that it will be nondiagnostic.	a. Detailed evaluation of the abnormalities in structures that are typically in the far field such as the aorta and the left atrial appendage. b. Evaluation of prosthetic heart valves. c. Evaluation of paravalvular abscesses (both native and prosthetic valves). d. Patients on ventilators. e. Patients with chest wall injuries. f. Patients with body habitus preventing adequate TTE imaging. g. Patients unable to move into left lateral decubitis position.
2. Intraoperative TEE.	a. All open heart (i.e., valvular) and thoracic aortic surgical procedures. b. Use in some coronary artery bypass graft surgeries. c. Noncardiac surgery when patients have known or suspected cardiovascular pathology which may impact outcomes.
3. Guidance of transcatheter procedures.	a. Guiding management of catheter-based intracardiac procedures (including septal defect closure or atrial appendage obliteration, and transcatheter valve procedures).
4. Critically ill patients.	a. Patients in whom diagnostic information is not obtainable by TTE and this information is expected to alter management.

essential diagnoses made similar to the FATE examination previously described. Of course, TTE has virtually no potential for complications outside of misreading the images, whereas TEE always is associated with an element of patient risk from the procedure.

BRIEFLY, HOW DOES ECHOCARDIOGRAPHY WORK?

Echocardiography relies upon the principles of ultrasound. Ultrasound is sound at a frequency greater than normal hearing. It is mechanical energy transmitted by pressure waves in a medium.[14] In TEE, a piezoelectrode in the esophageal probe transducer converts electrical energy delivered to the probe into ultrasound waves by vibration and, reciprocally, reflected ultrasound waves into electrical energy. Typical ultrasound waves used in echocardiography range in frequency from 2 to 10 MHz. Frequency is the number of cycles that occur per second. The higher the ultrasound frequency, the greater the resolution of the image. The lower the frequency, the

Table Intro–2. Cognitive and Technical Skills Required to Perform Perioperative Transesophageal Echocardiography

Panel A. Cognitive Skills Needed to Perform Perioperative Echocardiography at a Basic Level

- Basic knowledge for echocardiography.
- Knowledge of the equipment handling, infection control, and electrical safety recommendations associated with the use of TEE.
- Knowledge of the indications and the absolute and relative contraindications to the use of TEE.
- General knowledge of appropriate alternative diagnostic modalities, especially transthoracic, and epicardial echocardiography.
- Knowledge of the normal cardiovascular anatomy as visualized by TEE.
- Knowledge of commonly encountered blood flow velocity profiles as measured by Doppler echocardiography.
- Detailed knowledge of the echocardiographic presentations of myocardial ischemia and infarction.
- Detailed knowledge of the echocardiographic presentations of normal and abnormal ventricular function.
- Detailed knowledge of the physiology and TEE presentation of air embolization.
- Knowledge of native valvular anatomy and function, as displayed by TEE.
- Knowledge of the major TEE manifestations of valve lesions and of the TEE techniques available for assessing lesion severity.
- Knowledge of the principal TEE manifestations of cardiac masses, thrombi, and emboli; cardiomyopathies; pericardial effusions and lesions of the great vessels.

Panel B. Technical Skills Needed to Perform Perioperative Echocardiography at a Basic Level

- Ability to operate the ultrasound machine, including controls affecting the quality of the displayed data.
- Ability to perform a TEE probe insertion safely in the anesthetized, intubated patient.

- Ability to perform a basic TEE examination.
- Ability to recognize major echocardiographic changes associated with myocardial ischemia and infarction.
- Ability to detect qualitative changes in ventricular function and hemodynamic status.
- Ability to recognize echocardiographic manifestations of air embolization.
- Ability to visualize cardiac valves in multiple views and recognize gross valvular lesions and dysfunction.
- Ability to recognize large intracardiac masses and thrombi.
- Ability to detect large pericardial effusions.
- Ability to recognize common artifacts and pitfalls in TEE examinations.
- Ability to communicate the results of a TEE examination to patients and other health care professionals and to summarize these results cogently in the medical record.

Panel C. Cognitive Skills Needed to Perform Perioperative Echocardiography at the Advanced Level

- All the cognitive skills defined for the basic level.
- Knowledge of the principles and methodology of quantitative echocardiography.
- Detailed knowledge of native valvular anatomy and function. Knowledge of prosthetic valvular structure and function. Detailed knowledge of the echocardiographic manifestations of valve lesions and dysfunction.
- Knowledge of the echocardiographic manifestations of CHD.
- Detailed knowledge of echocardiographic manifestations of pathologic conditions of the heart and great vessels (such as cardiac aneurysms, hypertrophic cardiomyopathy, endocarditis, intracardiac masses, cardioembolic sources, aortic aneurysms and dissections, pericardial disorders, and post-surgical changes).
- Detailed knowledge of other cardiovascular diagnostic methods for correlation with TEE findings.

(Continued)

Table Intro-2. Cognitive and Technical Skills Required to Perform Perioperative Transesophageal Echocardiography (*Continued*)

Panel D. Technical Skills Needed to Perform Perioperative Echocardiography at the Advanced Level	
• All the technical skills defined for the basic level. • Ability to perform a complete TEE examination. • Ability to quantify subtle echocardiographic changes associated with myocardial ischemia and infarction. • Ability to utilize TEE to quantify ventricular function and hemodynamics. • Ability to utilize TEE to evaluate and quantify the function of all cardiac valves including prosthetic valves (e.g., measurement of pressure gradients and valve areas, regurgitant jet area, effective regurgitant orifice area). Ability to assess surgical intervention on cardiac valvular function.	• Ability to utilize TEE to evaluate congenital heart lesions. Ability to assess surgical intervention in CHD. • Ability to detect and assess the functional consequences of pathologic conditions of the heart and great vessels (such as cardiac aneurysms, hypertrophic cardiomyopathy, endocarditis, intracardiac masses, cardioembolic sources, aortic aneurysms and dissections, and pericardial disorders). Ability to evaluate surgical intervention in these conditions if applicable. • Ability to monitor placement and function of mechanical circulatory assistance devices.

CHD, Coronary heart disease.

Panel A lists the cognitive skills required for competence in perioperative echocardiography at the basic level. Panel B lists the technical skills required for competence in perioperative echocardiography at the basic level. Panel C lists the cognitive skills required for competence in perioperative echocardiography at the advanced level. Panel D lists the technical skills required for competence in perioperative echocardiography at the advanced level.

Reproduced with permission from Hahn RT, Abraham T, Adams MS, et al: Guidelines for performing a comprehensive transesophageal echocardiographic examination: recommendations from the American Society of Echocardiography and the Society of Cardiovascular Anesthesiologists, *J Am Soc Echocardiogr.* 2013 Sep;26(9):921-964.

greater the depth of ultrasound penetration. The ultrasound image is created because blood and tissue have different acoustic impedance. That is, when sound travels through several media of the same acoustic impedance, it travels without difficulty. However, when ultrasound travels though media of different acoustic impedances, the sound wave is affected by its interaction with these various tissues resulting in reflection, refraction, and scattering of the sound wave. Specular reflection occurs when the sound wave encounters a smooth surface and the wave is reflected back to the transducer. Irregular surfaces produce scattering of the sound wave resulting in far less reflection of the sound to the transducer. Refraction of the sound wave results in the direction of the sound wave being changed, often resulting in reflections to the transducer producing unexpected artifact images. The reflected sound wave (the echo) interacts with the transducer, which records the time delay between the transmitted and the reflected wave. Knowing the time delay and the speed of the ultrasound wave through soft tissues (1540 m/s), the location of various cardiac structures can be displayed with accuracy, and therefore images can be constructed. Obviously, this is a very rudimentary explanation and there are numerous resources available that describe the physics of ultrasound in greater detail.

Table Intro–3. Absolute and Relative Contraindications to Transesophageal Echocardiography

Absolute	Relative
• Perforated viscus	• History of radiation to neck and mediastinum
• Esophageal stricture	• History of GI surgery
• Esophageal tumor	• Recent upper GI bleed
• Esophageal perforation, laceration	• Barrett's esophagus
• Esophageal diverticulum	• History of dysphagia
• Active upper GI bleed	• Restriction of neck mobility (severe cervical arthritis, atlantoaxial joint disease)
	• Symptomatic hiatal hernia
	• Esophageal varices
	• Coagulopathy, thrombocytopenia
	• Active esophagitis
	• Active peptic ulcer disease

GI, Gastrointestinal.
Reproduced with permission from Hahn RT, Abraham T, Adams MS, et al: Guidelines for performing a comprehensive transesophageal echocardiographic examination: recommendations from the American Society of Echocardiography and the Society of Cardiovascular Anesthesiologists, *J Am Soc Echocardiogr.* 2013 Sep;26(9):921-964.

Resolution determines the accuracy of imaging, and it can be spatial or temporal. Spatial resolution of the image is the ability to correctly discriminate two structures that are very close together. Spatial resolution is axial (the structures are parallel to the sound beam's main axis) and lateral (the structures are side by side or perpendicular to the sound beam). Short pulses of higher-frequency ultrasound have better axial resolution. When an ultrasound wave is generated at the transducer, the sound beam gradually narrows in the focal zone and then diverges. Lateral resolution is best in the focal zone (Figure Intro–8).

Figure Intro–9 demonstrates that sound of shorter wavelength and thus higher frequency (Velocity = Wavelength × Frequency) improves axial resolution. Figure Intro–10 similarly demonstrates that imaging within the focal zone improves lateral resolution.

Temporal resolution is the ability to precisely position moving structures and is essential during cardiac imaging. Temporal resolution is determined by frame rate. The frame rate is the frequency at which an imaging sector is scanned. Increasing the imaging sector size and depth increases the time necessary for the ultrasound beam to travel from the transducer to the tissues and therefore decreases the frame rate and reduces temporal resolution.

Echocardiography also makes use of the Doppler effect. The Doppler effect is the result of the apparent change in frequency of sound waves when the source of the wave and the observer of the wave are in relative motion. Observer and source moving toward one another results in the sound wave being compressed, whereas

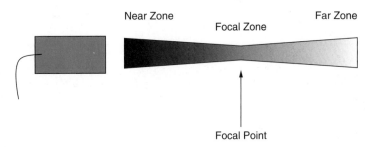

Figure Intro-8. The focal point is demonstrated. The anatomy of a sound beam. The transducer (red) is on the left. The near field (near zone) is closest to the transducer. The far field (far zone) is furthest. The narrowest point of the beam is the focal point. The beam diameter at the beginning of the near zone is the same diameter as the transducer lens. [Reproduced with permission from Shriki J: Ultrasound physics, *Crit Care Clin*. 2014 Jan; 30(1):1-24.]

the source and the observer moving apart from one another results in the sound wave being elongated. For example, the blood in the heart is in motion either away from the transducer in the esophagus or toward it. As they travel, red blood cells reflect ultrasound resulting in a change of the frequency emitted by the transducer based on the direction of flow. When blood flows toward the transducer (i.e., blood ejected out from the left ventricle into the ascending aorta), the reflected signal will

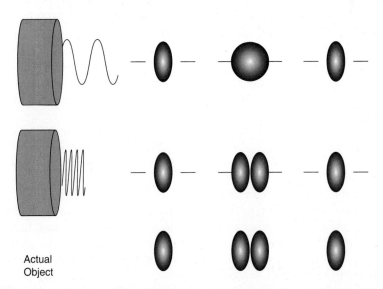

Figure Intro-9. Axial resolution. The bottom dots represent the actual objects in the space. The top transducer has a longer pulse. The lower transducer has a shorter pulse. Shorter pulses can resolve images that are closer together. [Reproduced with permission from Shriki J: Ultrasound physics, *Crit Care Clin*. 2014 Jan;30(1):1-24.]

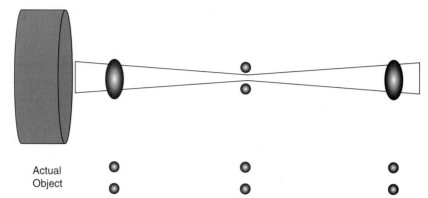

Figure Intro-10. Lateral resolution. The bottom dots represent the actual objects in space. The sound beam narrows until the focal point and then widens again. It is in this narrowest part of the beam that the transducer can most accurately resolve images. [Reproduced with permission from Shriki J: Ultrasound physics, *Crit Care Clin.* 2014 Jan; 30(1):1-24.]

be compressed resulting in a signal with a higher frequency. When blood flows away from the transducer (blood flowing in diastole through the mitral valve from the left atrium to the left ventricle), the frequency of the reflected signal received by the transducer is going to be lower than the original frequency transmitted by the transducer. The change in the transmitted frequency is known as the Doppler frequency shift. Using the Doppler equation, the velocity of the blood flow is calculated from the Doppler frequency shift.

Doppler equation:

$$V = (F_R - F_T/\cos \theta)(1540 \text{ m/s}/2F_T)$$

where:

V = blood velocity
F_T = transmitted Doppler frequency
F_R = received Doppler frequency
1540 m/s = speed of sound in tissue
$\cos \theta$ = cosine of the angle of incidence between the Doppler beam and the blood flow
$\cos 90° = 0 \cos 0° = 1$

Therefore, velocity determinations are best made when there is no angulation between the Doppler beam and the flow of blood. The velocity of blood cannot be determined when the Doppler beam is perpendicular to the blood flow.

As shall be seen in later chapters, alterations of both the direction of blood flow in the heart and the velocity of that flow are used by echocardiographers to discern defects in cardiac structure and function. The echo machine has the ability to determine and display a range of velocities of blood flow in the heart using either continuous wave (CW) or pulsed wave (PW) Doppler. When using CW Doppler, the echo machine sends a sound wave from one ultrasound emitting crystal and receives the returned signal using a second crystal. In PW Doppler, the machine uses the same ultrasound emitting crystal to send and receive the reflected sound wave. The ultrasound machine will wait a specific time to listen for echoes to return to the crystal. Because the speed of sound is constant in soft tissue, the time it takes for the echo to return relates directly to the distance that the sound must travel to the point of interest and back to the ultrasound probe. Thus, PW Doppler can determine the velocity and direction of blood flow at a specific point. However, PW Doppler is limited to measuring slower blood velocities in the heart because the single emitter has to wait for the reflected echo before sending another burst of ultrasound. The rate at which the transducer emits ultrasound bursts is known as the pulse repetition frequency (PRF). PW Doppler observations occur when the crystal receives a returning echo. The machine must wait to listen for the echo from the point selected. The longer the machine must wait, the more PRF is reduced. With a lower PRF, the machine makes fewer observations at the point of interest. If flow velocity is less than ½ PRF, the Nyquist limit, the machine correctly assesses the velocity and directionality of blood flow. However, when the Doppler frequency shifts and velocities exceed the Nyquist limit, PW Doppler can no longer determine the directionality of flow. The apparent direction of flow becomes confused, and the machine interprets this fast flow as going in a direction opposite to that in which blood is actually flowing. This phenomenon is called "aliasing" and is very useful in perioperative TEE as shall be seen.

CW Doppler uses two crystals: one to send a signal and the other to receive the reflected echo. CW Doppler is therefore useful to determine both the direction of flow and the velocity of blood flow at higher velocities. Normal blood flow velocity in the heart is less than 1 m/s. In areas of cardiac pathology (i.e., valvular stenosis or regurgitation), flow velocity can become greatly increased confusing PW Doppler measurements. In this instance CW Doppler can be used to measure the velocity of rapid blood flow. However, since two crystals are employed in CW Doppler, echoes are received from any point along the ultrasound beam path. Unlike PW Doppler this eliminates the ability to time gate the returning signal to discern flow at a specific point. Rather, CW Doppler reflects the highest velocities along the echo beam and is not subject to aliasing.

Lastly, color flow Doppler (CFD) (**Video Intro–4**) creates a visual picture of blood flow by color coding Doppler velocities to enable a visual estimation of the direction and velocity of blood flow in the heart. CFD is a form of PW Doppler in which more commonly flow toward the transducer is depicted arbitrarily as red and flow away from the transducer is blue with various color hues assigned to turbulent, high-velocity blood flow. Because it uses PW Doppler for velocity measurements, CFD is subject to aliasing. At velocities higher than the Nyquist limit, although the blood flow is directed toward the transducer (i.e., red), it will be displayed as flow directed away from the transducer (i.e., blue). CFD is useful to identify areas of pathological blood flow. Tissue Doppler uses Doppler to color code the myocardium as it moves toward and away from the esophageal probe during the cardiac cycle. Tissue Doppler is very useful for the assessment of diastolic dysfunction. Tissue Doppler, speckle tracking, strain, and strain rate will be discussed in Chapter 5.

WHAT CONSTITUTES THE STANDARD PERIOPERATIVE TEE EXAMINATION?

The American Society of Echocardiography (ASE) and the Society of Cardio-vascular Anesthesiologists (SCA) in 1999 published guidelines for the performance of a perioperative TEE examination (Figures Intro–11 and Intro–12). At that time, 20 transesophageal echocardiographic views were identified to provide consistency and standardization of the perioperative TEE examination. In 2013, revised guidelines expanded the suggested views to 28 to include multiple long- and short-axis views of the four cardiac valves, the four heart chambers, and the great vessels.[13] Table Intro–4 summarizes these suggested views along with the structures imaged.

At times in a busy cardiac operating room, it may not be possible to obtain all 28 views. Figure Intro–12 identifies common structures seen in the most routinely acquired 20 views.

The cardiac anesthesiologist usually places the TEE probe after induction of general anesthesia and placement of the endotracheal tube. General anesthesia is not necessary per se for a TEE examination as cardiologists routinely perform this procedure with sedation and topicalization of the oropharynx. At times anesthesiologists may be called upon to provide sedation for the TEE examination performed by the cardiologist.

The probe is introduced into the esophagus and advanced until the heart and great vessels are visualized. Generally, the four-chamber view is identified and from this point the examination commences.

The TEE machine can be rather overwhelming when first encountered. There are many, many controls that are described in great detail in the technical manuals. For the purposes of this introduction, the key settings and controls are those that help provide the best view of the structures of interest. For example, the frequency of the probe can be adjusted to provide for higher resolution (at higher frequency) or greater imaging depth (at lower frequency). Recall, a higher frequency provides better resolution, while a lower frequency penetrates farther. The depth knob helps to center the image in the center of the screen. This is important since the greater the depth, the longer that sound must travel, which decreases the frame rate impeding temporal resolution of the image. The gain control augments the signal returning to the transducer. Too much gain and the image is unclear and too bright. Too little gain and the image is too dark. Usually the cardiac structures appear as grayish white structures and the blood appears dark. CFD gain can also be changed; too high or too low gain can exaggerate or minimize flow patterns. CFD gain should be optimally set below the level that results in the appearance of unexpected color speckles originating from the tissue.

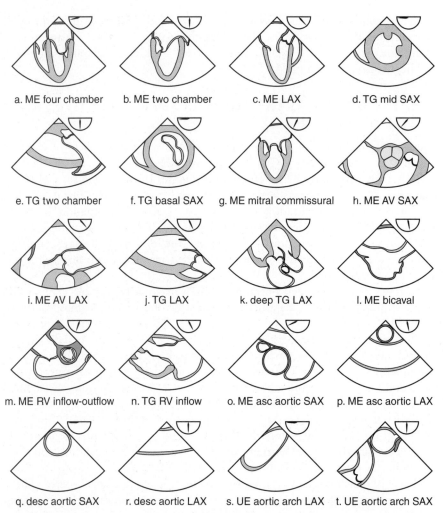

a. ME four chamber   b. ME two chamber   c. ME LAX   d. TG mid SAX

e. TG two chamber   f. TG basal SAX   g. ME mitral commissural   h. ME AV SAX

i. ME AV LAX   j. TG LAX   k. deep TG LAX   l. ME bicaval

m. ME RV inflow-outflow   n. TG RV inflow   o. ME asc aortic SAX   p. ME asc aortic LAX

q. desc aortic SAX   r. desc aortic LAX   s. UE aortic arch LAX   t. UE aortic arch SAX

Figure Intro–11. The American Society of Echocardiography (ASE) and Society of Cardiovascular Anesthesiologists (SCA) 20 recommended views for a comprehensive TEE examination. The compass in the right upper corner of each view approximates the angle of the ultrasound sector. Views are designated as: Asc = ascending, AV = aortic valve, Desc = descending, LAX = long axis, ME = midesophageal, RV = right ventricle, SAX = short axis, TG = transgastric, UE = upper esophageal. These standard views provide two-dimensional windows to examine the three-dimensional heart. [Reproduced with permission from Shanewise JS, Cheung AT, Aronson S, et al: ASE/SCA guidelines for performing a comprehensive intraoperative multiplane transesophageal echocardiography examination: recommendations of the American Society of Echocardiography Council for Intraoperative Echocardiography and the Society of Cardiovascular Anesthesiologists Task Force for Certification in Perioperative Transesophageal Echocardiography, *Anesth Analg.* 1999 Oct;89(4):870-884.]

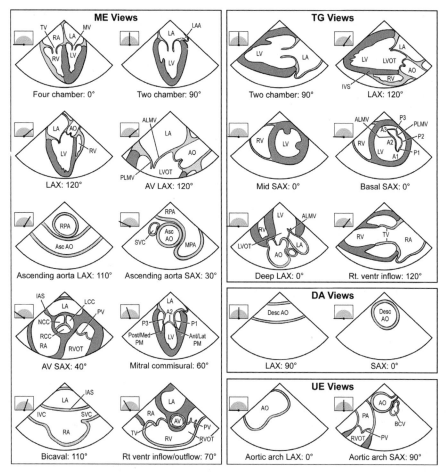

Figure Intro–12. The 20 original suggested views have now been grouped together based upon the location in the esophagus where they are obtained, upper esophageal (UE), middle esophageal (ME), transgastric (TG), and descending aortic (DA). Major cardiac structures are labeled including:

right atrium (RA)
left atrium (LA)
mitral valve (MV)
tricuspid valve (TV)
right ventricle (RV)
left ventricle (LV)
left atrial appendage (LAA)
aorta (AO)
anterior leaflet of the mitral valve (ALMV)
posterior leaflet of the mitral valve (PLMV)
ascending aorta (Asc AO)
right pulmonary artery (RPA)
superior vena cava (SVC)
main pulmonary artery (MPA)

inter atrial septum (IAS)
pulmonic valve (PV)
right ventricular outflow tract (RVOT)
noncoronary cusp of the aortic valve (NCC)
right coronary cusp of the aortic valve (RCC)
left coronary cusp of the aortic valve (LCC)
posterior scallops of the mitral valve P1, P2, P3
anterior scallops of the mitral valve A1, A2, A3
posterior medial papillary muscle (Post/Med PM)
anterolateral papillary muscle (Ant/Lat PM)
inferior vena cava (IVC)
descending aorta (Desc AO)
left brachiocephalic vein (BCV)

Table Intro–4. Comprehensive Transesophageal Echocardiographic Examination. The Table Lists the Suggested 28 Views in a Comprehensive Transesophageal Echocardiographic Examination. Each View is Shown as a 3-D Image, the Corresponding Imaging Plane, and a 2-D Image. The Acquisition Protocol and the Structures Imaged in each View are Listed in the Subsequent Column

Imaging plane	3-D model	2-D TEE image	Acquisition protocol	Structures imaged
Midesophageal Views				
1. ME 5-Chamber View			**Transducer Angle:** ~0 - 10° **Level:** Midesophageal **Maneuver** (from prior image): NA	Aortic valve LOVT Left atrium/Right atrium Left ventricle/ Right ventricle/ IVS Mitral valve (A₂A₁-P₁) Tricuspid valve
2. ME 4-Chamber View			**Transducer Angle:** ~0-10° **Level:** Midesophageal **Maneuver** (from prior image): Advance ± Retroflex	Left atrium/Right atrium IAS Left ventricle/ Right ventricle/ IVS Mitral valve (A₃A₂-P₂P₁) Tricuspid valve
3. ME Mitral Commissural View			**Transducer Angle:** ~50 - 70° **Level:** Midesophageal **Maneuver** (from prior image): NA	Left atrium Coronary Sinus Left ventricle Mitral valve (P₃-A₃A₂A₁-P₁) Papillary muscles Chordae tendinae
4. ME 2-Chamber View			**Transducer Angle:** ~80 - 100° **Level:** Midesophageal **Maneuver** (from prior image): NA	Left atrium Coronary sinus Left atrial appendage Left ventricle Mitral valve (P₃-A₃A₂A₁)
5. ME Long Axis View			**Transducer Angle:** ~120 - 140° **Level:** Midesophageal **Maneuver** (from prior image): NA	Left atrium Left ventricle LVOT RVOT Mitral valve (P₂-A₂) Aortic valve Proximal ascending aorta

Mitral valve subscripts rendered: $(A_2A_1\text{-}P_1)$, $(A_3A_2\text{-}P_2P_1)$, $(P_3\text{-}A_3A_2A_1\text{-}P_1)$, $(P_3\text{-}A_3A_2A_1)$, $(P_2\text{-}A_2)$.

(Continued)

Table Intro–4. Comprehensive Transesophageal Echocardiographic Examination. The Table Lists the Suggested 28 Views in a Comprehensive Transesophageal Echocardiographic Examination. Each View is Shown as a 3-D Image, the Corresponding Imaging Plane, and a 2-D Image. The Acquisition Protocol and the Structures Imaged in each View are Listed in the Subsequent Column (*Continued*)

Imaging plane	3-D model	2-D TEE image	Acquisition protocol	Structures imaged
6. ME AV LAX View			**Transducer Angle:** ~120 - 140° **Level:** Midesophageal **Maneuver** (from prior image): Withdraw ± anteflex	Left atrium LVOT RVOT Mitral valve (A₂-P₂) Aortic valve Proximal ascending aorta
7. ME Ascending Aorta LAX View			**Transducer Angle:** ~90 - 110° **Level:** Upper-Esophageal **Maneuver** (from prior image): Withdraw	Mid-ascending aorta Right pulmonary artery
8. ME Ascending Aorta SAX View			**Transducer Angle:** ~0 - 30° **Level:** Upper-Esophageal **Maneuver** (from prior image): CW	Mid-ascending aorta (SAX) Main/bifurcation pulmonary artery Superior vena cava
9. ME Right Pulmonary Vein View			**Transducer Angle:** ~0 - 30° **Level:** Upper-esophageal **Maneuver** (from prior image): CW, Advance	Mid-ascending aorta Superior vena cava Right pulmonary veins
10. ME AV SAX View			**Transducer Angle:** ~25 - 45° **Level:** Midesophageal **Maneuver** (from prior image): CCW, Advance, Anteflex	Aortic valve Right atrium Left atrium Superior IAS RVOT Pulmonary valve
11. ME RV Inflow-Outflow View			**Transducer Angle:** ~50 - 70° **Level:** Midesophageal **Maneuver** (from prior image): CW, Advance	Aortic valve Right atrium Left atrium Superior IAS Tricuspid valve RVOT Pulmonary valve

Table Intro–4. Comprehensive Transesophageal Echocardiographic Examination. The Table Lists the Suggested 28 Views in a Comprehensive Transesophageal Echocardiographic Examination. Each View is Shown as a 3-D Image, the Corresponding Imaging Plane, and a 2-D Image. The Acquisition Protocol and the Structures Imaged in each View are Listed in the Subsequent Column (*Continued*)

Imaging plane	3-D model	2-D TEE image	Acquisition protocol	Structures imaged
12. ME Modified Bicaval TV View			**Transducer Angle:** ~50 - 70° **Level:** Midesophageal **Maneuver** (from prior image): CW	Right atrium Left atrium Mid-IAS Tricuspid valve Superior vena cava Inferior vena cava/coronary sinus
13. ME Bicaval View			**Transducer Angle:** ~90 - 110° **Level:** Midesophageal **Maneuver** (from prior image): CW	Left atrium Right atrium/appendage IAS Superior vena cava Inferior vena cava
14. UE Right and Left Pulmonary Veins View			**Transducer Angle:** ~90 - 110° **Level:** Upper-esophageal **Maneuver** (from prior image): Withdraw, CW for the right veins, CCW for the left veins	Pulmonary vein (upper and lower) Pulmonary artery
15. ME Left Atrial Appendage View			**Transducer Angle:** ~90 - 110° **Level:** Midesophageal **Maneuver** (from prior image): Advance	Left artrial appendage Left upper pulmonary vein
Transgastric Views				
16. TG Basal SAX View			**Transducer Angle:** ~0 - 20° **Level:** Transgastric **Maneuver** (from prior image): Advance ± Anteflex	Left ventricle (base) Right ventricle (base) Mitral valve (SAX) Tricuspid valve (short axis)

(*Continued*)

Table Intro–4. Comprehensive Transesophageal Echocardiographic Examination. The Table Lists the Suggested 28 Views in a Comprehensive Transesophageal Echocardiographic Examination. Each View is Shown as a 3-D Image, the Corresponding Imaging Plane, and a 2-D Image. The Acquisition Protocol and the Structures Imaged in each View are Listed in the Subsequent Column (*Continued*)

Imaging plane	3-D model	2-D TEE image	Acquisition protocol	Structures imaged
17. TG Mid Papillary SAX View			**Transducer Angle:** ~0 - 20° **Level:** Transgastric **Maneuver** (from prior image): Advance ± Anteflex	Left ventricle (mid) Papillary muscles Right ventricle (mid)
18. TG Apical SAX View			**Transducer Angle:** ~0 - 20° **Level:** Transgastric **Maneuver** (from prior image): Advance ± Anteflex	Left ventricle (apex) Right ventricle (apex)
19. TG RV Basal View			**Transducer Angle:** ~0 - 20° **Lavel:** Transgastric **Maneuver** (from prior image): Anteflex	Left ventricle (mid) Right ventricle (mid) Right ventricular outflow tract Tricuspid valve (SAX) Pulmonary valve
20. TG RV Inflow-Outflow View			**Transducer Angle:** ~0 - 20° **Lavel:** Transgastric **Maneuver** (from prior image): Right-flex	Right atrium Right ventriclar Right ventricular outflow tract Pulmonary valve Tricuspid valve
21. Deep TG 5-Chamber View			**Transducer Angle:** ~0 - 20° **Level:** Transgastric **Maneuver** (from prior image): Left-flex, Advance, Anteflex	Left ventricle Left ventricular outflow tract Right ventricle Aortic valve Aortic root Mitral valve
22. TG 2-Chamber View			**Transducer Angle:** ~90 - 110° **Level:** Transgastric **Maneuver** (from prior image): Neutral flexion, Withdraw	Left ventricle Left atrium/ appendage Mitral valve

(*Continued*)

Table Intro–4. Comprehensive Transesophageal Echocardiographic Examination. The Table Lists the Suggested 28 Views in a Comprehensive Transesophageal Echocardiographic Examination. Each View is Shown as a 3-D Image, the Corresponding Imaging Plane, and a 2-D Image. The Acquisition Protocol and the Structures Imaged in each View are Listed in the Subsequent Column (*Continued*)

Imaging plane	3-D model	2-D TEE image	Acquisition protocol	Structures imaged
23. TG RV Inflow View			**Transducer Angle:** ~90 - 110° **Level:** Transgastric **Maneuver** (from prior image): CW	Right ventricle Right atrium Tricuspid valve
24. TG LAX View			**Transducer Angle:** ~120 - 140° **Level:** Transgastric **Maneuver** (from prior image): CCW	Left ventricle Left ventricular outflow tract Right ventricle Aortic valve Aortic root Mitral valve
Aortic Views				
25. Descending Aorta SAX View			**Transducer Angle:** ~0 - 10° **Level:** Transgastric to Midesophageal **Maneuver** (from prior image): Neutral flexion	Descending aorta Left thorax Hemiazygous and azygous veins Intercostal arteries
26. Descending Aorta LAX View			**Transducer Angle:** ~90 - 100° **Level:** Transgastric to Midesophageal **Maneuver** (from prior image): Neutral flexion	Descending aorta Left thorax
27. UE Aortic Arch LAX View			**Transducer Angle:** ~0 - 10° **Level:** Upper Esophageal **Maneuver** (from prior image): Withdrawl	Aortic arch Innominate vein Mediastinal tissue
28. UE Aortic Arch SAX View			**Transducer Angle:** ~70 - 90° **Level:** Transgastric to Midesophageal **Maneuver** (from prior image): NA	Aortic arch Innominate vein Pulmonary artery Pulmonary valve Mediastinal tissue

CW = clockwise rotation; CCW = counterclockwise rotation.
Reproduced with permission from Hahn RT, Abraham T, Adams MS, et al: Guidelines for performing a comprehensive transesophageal echocardiographic examination: recommendations from the American Society of Echocardiography and the Society of Cardiovascular Anesthesiologists, *J Am Soc Echocardiogr.* 2013 Sep;26(9):921-964.

The Nyquist limit is set by adjusting the color scale, which determines the velocity at which aliasing will occur.

The probe has a number of dials that mechanically turn the probe from left to right and from anterior to posterior (Figure Intro–13). The probe also has a locking feature that locks the probe in a certain position. Manipulating the probe when locked in a certain position may cause patient injury. TEE probes also have a button, which rotates the ultrasound beam through 180 degrees permitting a multiplane examination. Depending upon the position of the probe and the orientation of the ultrasound beam, the two-dimensional image will change, permitting different views of the three-dimensional structure of the heart (Figure Intro–14). With time and practice, anesthesiologists can readily obtain the 28 views, which constitute the standard echocardiography examination as recommended by the guidelines established by the ASE and SCA. Each of these views has their own nomenclature depending if they are originated from the midesophageal (ME), upper esophageal (UE), transgastric (TG), or deep transgastric (deep TG) positions.

HOW IS TEE ROUTINELY USED PERIOPERATIVELY?

TEE is a very sensitive monitor of myocardial ischemia and function. The left ventricle is supplied by the two main coronary arteries, the right coronary artery and the left coronary artery, which in turn divides into two main branches, the left circumflex and the left anterior descending arteries (Figure Intro–15A and B). The left ventricle is divided into 16 segments, which can be visualized during echocardiographic examination. Figure Intro–15 provides the classical distribution of the coronary supply to the myocardium. More recently, it has been discerned that this diagram is an oversimplification and that much myocardium supplied by the circumflex artery may also receive distribution from either the left anterior descending artery or the right coronary artery. Using echocardiographic imaging it is possible to determine if ventricular wall motion is normal (30% thickened during contraction), hypokinetic, akinetic, or dyskinetic. Segmental wall motion should be judged based on the percentage of myocardial thickening and inward endocardial border excursion in systole. Akinetic wall motion means that the myocardium does not thicken during systole. Dyskinetic wall motion implies that the wall does not contract during systole but rather moves outwardly. A normally contracting LV is easy to identify **(Video Intro–5)**. Likewise, the LV of the patient with severe systolic heart failure is not easily missed **(Video Intro–6)**. On the other hand, areas with segmental wall motion abnormalities can be somewhat subtler to identify. **(Video Intro–7)**.

The right ventricle (RV) is a much thinner structure than the LV. It does not have the same descriptive system to identify wall motion abnormalities as does the LV. Nonetheless, the normal RV is contractile, in the shape of a crescent hugging the LV when seen in a transgastric view **(Video Intro–8)**. When the RV becomes dysfunctional, it becomes more dilated and rounded **(Video Intro–9)**.

The valves of the heart are visualized in multiple views during the routine examination.

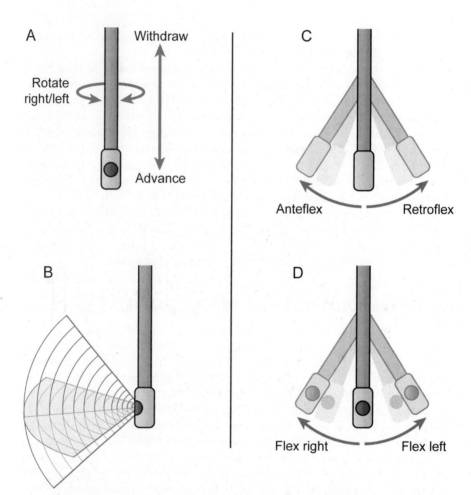

Figure Intro-13. The echo probe is manipulated by the examiner in multiple ways to create the standard images that constitute the comprehensive perioperative TEE examination. Never force the probe. If resistance is encountered, abandon the examination. Echocardiographic information can be provided by intraoperative epicardial and epiaortic examination. Advancing the probe in the esophagus permits the upper, mid, and transgastric examinations (A). The probe can be turned in the esophagus from left to right to examine both left- and right-sided structures (A). Using the button located on the probe permits the echocardiographer to rotate the scan beam through 180 degrees, thereby creating various two-dimensional imaging slices of the three-dimensional heart (B). Lastly, panels C and D demonstrate manipulation of the tip of the probe to permit the beam to be directed to best visualize the image. [Reproduced with permission from Shanewise JS, Cheung AT, Aronson S, et al: ASE/SCA guidelines for performing a comprehensive intraoperative multiplane transesophageal echocardiography examination: recommendations of the American Society of Echocardiography Council for Intraoperative Echocardiography and the Society of Cardiovascular Anesthesiologists Task Force for Certification in Perioperative Transesophageal Echocardiography, *Anesth Analg.* 1999 Oct;89(4):870-884.]

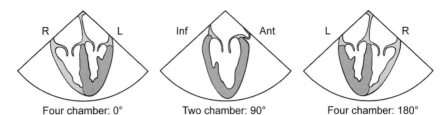

Four chamber: 0°   Two chamber: 90°   Four chamber: 180°

Figure Intro-14. As the sector beam is rotated from 0 to 180 degrees, the two-dimensional image changes orientation. At 0 degrees, the four-chamber view is seen with the patient's right heart structures seen on the left of the screen. The left heart (shaded darker red) occupies the full screen in the two-chamber views obtained at 90 degrees displaying anterior and inferior structures. Completing the arc to 180 degrees mirrors the image obtained at 0 degrees. One of the first tasks of the echocardiographer when viewing an image is to take note of the angle of the sector beam since that determines the image. [Reproduced with permission from Shanewise JS, Cheung AT, Aronson S, et al: ASE/SCA guidelines for performing a comprehensive intraoperative multiplane transesophageal echocardiography examination: recommendations of the American Society of Echocardiography Council for Intraoperative Echocardiography and the Society of Cardiovascular Anesthesiologists Task Force for Certification in Perioperative Transesophageal Echocardiography, *Anesth Analg.* 1999 Oct;89(4):870-884.]

The aortic valve normally consists of three leaflets. The left coronary artery can often be seen as it takes off from the aorta above the aortic valve (**Video Intro–10**). The two-leaflet mitral valve is likewise seen in many different images (Figure Intro–16). The mitral valve has two leaflets, anterior and posterior. The sections of these leaflets have their own descriptive code to help identify areas of the valve that might be in need of surgical repair and facilitate communication among cardiologists, anesthesiologists, and surgeons.

The tricuspid valve is readily examined by TEE (**Video Intro–11**). The pulmonic valve is the farthest valve from the esophagus and is not as easily visualized.

The routine TEE examination also includes a thorough examination of the aorta. Examination of the aorta can identify areas of intimal thickening or calcification that could create arterial emboli if manipulated during surgery. Use of TEE and EAU can help guide surgeons away from areas of calcification or atherosclerosis to minimize the incidence of emboli[15] (**Video Intro–12**).

The interatrial septum is examined (**Video Intro–13**) to rule out the presence of a patent foramen ovale (PFO). In the presence of a PFO, right-heart pressures higher than left-heart pressures may result in shunting of the blood across the PFO from right to left leading to a reduction in arterial saturation. Emboli could also cross from the right to the left side of the heart with potentially injurious results if thrown in the systemic circulation. Roughly, 20% of the population may have a PFO.

In the following chapters, the above disease states and others will be encountered in the context of their anesthesia management. Perioperative echocardiography will be illustrated both in its ability to identify cardiac pathologies but also to inform intraoperative clinical decision making.

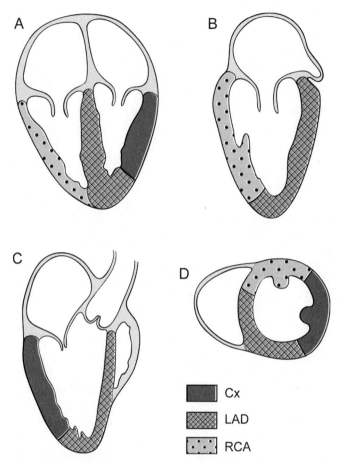

Figure Intro–15A. The above graphic demonstrates the midesophageal four-chamber view (A), the midesophageal two-chamber view (B), the midesophageal long-axis view (C), and the transgastric mid short-axis view (D). The different views provide the opportunity to observe the myocardium supplied by each of the three main coronary vessels, the left circumflex (Cx), the left anterior descending (LAD), and the right coronary artery (RCA). Areas of impaired myocardial perfusion are suggested by the inability of the myocardium to both thicken and move inwardly during systole. Image D is very useful for monitoring in the operating room because left ventricular myocardium supplied by each of the three vessels can be seen in one image. [Reproduced with permission from Shanewise JS, Cheung AT, Aronson S, et al: ASE/SCA guidelines for performing a comprehensive intraoperative multiplane transesophageal echocardiography examination: recommendations of the American Society of Echocardiography Council for Intraoperative Echocardiography and the Society of Cardiovascular Anesthesiologists Task Force for Certification in Perioperative Transesophageal Echocardiography, *Anesth Analg.* 1999 Oct; 89(4):870-884.]

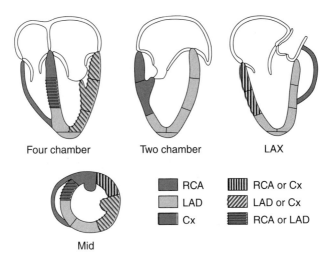

Four chamber   Two chamber   LAX

	RCA		RCA or Cx
	LAD		LAD or Cx
	Cx		RCA or LAD

Mid

Figure Intro–15B. Typical distributions of the RCA, the LAD coronary artery, and the circumflex (CX) coronary artery from transesophageal views of the left ventricle. The arterial distribution varies among patients. Some segments have variable coronary perfusion. [Reproduced with permission from Lang RM, Bierig M, Devereux RB, Flachskampf FA, Foster E, Pellikka PA, et al. Recommendations for chamber quantification: a report from the American Society of Echocardiography's Guidelines and Standards Committee and the Chamber Quantification Writing Group, developed in conjunction with the European Association of Echocardiography, a branch of the European Society of Cardiology. *J Am Soc Echocardiogr.* 2005 Dec;18(12):1440-1463.]

WHAT IS THE ROLE OF THREE-DIMENSIONAL ECHOCARDIOGRAPHY IN PERIOPERATIVE MANAGEMENT?

Real time three-dimensional echocardiography[16,17] is now increasingly employed as the probes and technology become more available to practitioners. Recall that routine TEE provides a two-dimensional image of a three-dimensional structure—the heart. The echo beam is rotated through 180 degrees creating images of the heart in various two-dimensional orientations. Real-time 3-D TEE employs matrix array transducers containing many imaging elements that scan a pyramid-shaped volume (Figure Intro–17). Table Intro–5 presents advantages of 3-D over 2-D imaging.

Three-dimensional echocardiography may provide better imaging for volume analysis of the heart as well as additional information regarding valvular structure and function. Computer software permits construction of models of valvular and ventricular function, which can aid in perioperative assessment. Three-dimensional TEE complements two-dimensional imaging and is now routinely incorporated in perioperative examinations. Table Intro–6 presents 3-D TEE images that should be acquired perioperatively.

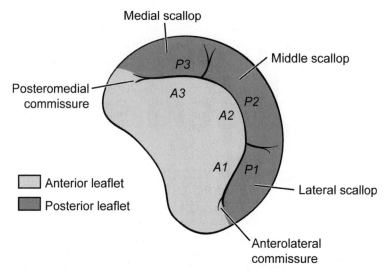

Figure Intro–16. The Carpentier system for identifying the leaflets of the mitral valve is presented in this schematic. The anterior leaflet occupies the greatest area of the mitral valve. The posterior leaflet, however, covers the greater circumference. The posterior leaflet is divided into three scallops extending from the anterolateral to the posteromedial commissures. The anterior leaflet is continuous with fibrous attachment of the aortic valve known as the crux of the heart. The mitral annulus is a fibrous ring that provides the valve its shape. [Reproduced with permission from Shanewise JS, Cheung AT, Aronson S, et al: ASE/SCA guidelines for performing a comprehensive intraoperative multiplane transesophageal echocardiography examination: recommendations of the American Society of Echocardiography Council for Intraoperative Echocardiography and the Society of Cardiovascular Anesthesiologists Task Force for Certification in Perioperative Transesophageal Echocardiography, *Anesth Analg.* 1999 Oct;89(4):870-884.]

HOW CAN ECHOCARDIOGRAPHY BE USED TO DETERMINE CARDIAC OUTPUT, PRESSURE GRADIENTS, AND OTHER HEMODYNAMIC MEASURES FORMERLY DONE WITH A PULMONARY ARTERY (PA) CATHETER?

The PA catheter has long been used as an aid in the clinical management of patients at risk for or experiencing hemodynamic instability. Using measures of cardiac output (CO), pulmonary capillary occlusion pressure (PCOP), and central venous pressure (CVP), anesthesiologists and intensivists attempt to discern why patients are hemodynamically unstable. Many of these questions can be answered with TTE as previously described or using TEE. A poorly contracting heart is obvious even to the most inexperienced observer. Likewise, a contractile but underfilled heart is easily identified (**Video Intro–14**). Often perioperatively, visual determinations ("eyeballing") supply all the information that the anesthesiologist wants or needs to initiate appropriate treatment.

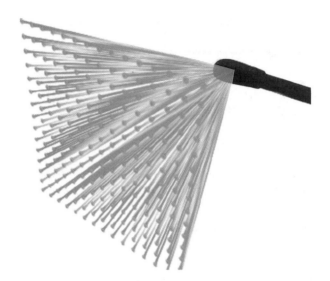

Figure Intro–17. A 2-D matrix array with a pyramidal scanning volume. This represents the basis for instantaneous 3-D image acquisition. [Modified with permission from Fischer GW, Salgo IS, Adams DH: Real-time three-dimensional transesophageal echocardiography: the matrix revolution, *J Cardiothorac Vasc Anesth.* 2008 Dec;22(6):904-912.]

Table Intro–5. Clinical Applications in which 3-D Echocardiography Presents an Advantage Over a 2-D Approach

Cardiac structure	Characteristics of 3-D echocardiographic approach and utility
LV function and volumes	Full volume acquisition avoids foreshortened views and permits complete (infinite number of views) and dynamic (function) LV assessment Improved accuracy and reliability compared with 2-D Quantitative software, semiautomated analysis
RV function and volumes	Utility of 3-D approach needs to be established
MV anatomy and function	En face view offers accurate identification of pathology in surgical orientation and facilitates perioperative communication 3-D color Doppler allows precise determination of vena contracta Accurate measure of stenotic valve opening Growing role in percutaneous procedures
AV, TV, PV	Inconsistent quality of 3-D images, will benefit from further technologic advances Potential role in percutaneous procedures
Atria and LAA	Guide during surgical and percutaneous procedures Accurate structural display Further study required

AV = aortic valve; LAA = left atrial appendage; LV = left ventricle; MV = mitral valve; PV = pulmonic valve; RV = right ventricle; TV = tricuspid valve.

Reproduced with permission from Mackensen GB, Swaminathan M, Mathew JP: PRO editorial: PRO: three-dimensional transesophageal echocardiography is a major advance for intraoperative clinical management of patients undergoing cardiac surgery, *Anesth Analg.* 2010 Jun 1;110(6):1574-1578.

Table Intro–6. Protocol for Three-Dimensional Transesophageal Echocardiography Image Acquisition

Left Ventricle	1. Obtain a view of the left ventricle from the 0°, 60°, or 120° midesophageal positions 2. Use the biplane mode to check that the left ventricle is centered in a second view 90° to the original. 3. Acquire using wide-angle, multi-beat mode	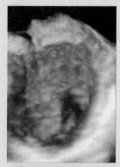
Right Ventricle	1. Obtain a view of the right ventricle from the 0° midesophageal position with the right ventricle tilted so that it is in the center of the image 2. Acquire using wide-angle, multi-beat mode	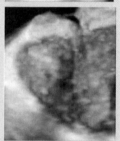
Interatrial Septum	1. 0° with the probe rotated to the interatrial septum 2. Acquire using narrow-angle, single-beat or wide-angle, multi-beat modes	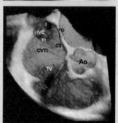
Aortic Valve	1. Obtain a view of the aortic valve from either the 60° midesophageal, short-axis view or the 120° midesophageal, long-axis view 2. Acquire using either the narrow-angle, single-beat or the wide-angle, multi-beat modes	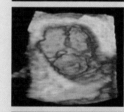
Mitral Valve	1. Obtain a view of the mitral valve from the 0°, 60°, 90°, or 120° midesophageal views 2. Use the biplane mode to check that the mitral valve annulus is centered with the acquisition plane in a second view 90° to the original. 3. Acquire using narrow-angle, single-beat mode	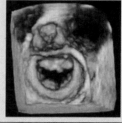

(Continued)

Table Intro–6. Protocol for Three-Dimensional Transesophageal Echocardiography Image Acquisition (*Continued*)

Pulmonic Valve	1. Obtain a view of the pulmonic valve from either the 90° high-esophageal view or the 120° midesophageal, three-chamber view rotated to center the pulmonic valve 2. Acquire using narrow-angle, single-beat mode	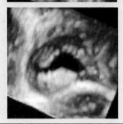
Tricuspid Valve	1. Obtain a view of the tricuspid valve from either the 0° to 30° midesophageal, four-chamber view tilted so that the valve is centered in the imaging plane or the 40° transgastric view with anteflexion 2. Acquire using a narrow-angle, single-beat mode	

Reproduced with permission from Hahn RT, Abraham T, Adams MS, et al: Guidelines for performing a comprehensive transesophageal echocardiographic examination: recommendations from the American Society of Echocardiography and the Society of Cardiovascular Anesthesiologists, *J Am Soc Echocardiogr.* 2013 Sep;26(9):921-964.

However, should the anesthesiologist desire more quantitative assessments, echocardiography can be employed to this end. Echocardiography machines incorporate software that facilitates the calculation of cardiac output, valve areas, and pressure gradients. These calculations will be illustrated during the course of the text as they apply to different cardiac conditions. Most of these measurements depend upon either the continuity equation or the Bernoulli equation.

The continuity equation is based upon the principle of the conservation of mass. In other words, as blood flows through the heart, its mass is conserved. The blood that flows through one point (left ventricular outflow tract) is the same as the volume of blood that flows through another point (aortic valve) in the absence of shunts (ventricular septal defect). The flow of water down a river is often used to illustrate this principle. When the river is wide, the water flows leisurely; however, when it narrows—watch out for *the rapids* (Figure Intro–18). The heart is no different. When blood flows through areas of pathology, the flow is often accelerated.

Recall, Doppler measures blood flow speed and direction either toward (+) or away (–) from the TEE probe in the esophagus. Because of the Doppler equation, the Doppler beam needs to be as parallel with the blood flow as possible to provide for an accurate measurement.

For example, when the PW Doppler sampling gate is placed in the left ventricular outflow track (LVOT), the machine measures the velocities in cm/s passing through that point in the LVOT (Figure Intro–19). The LVOT shape can be approximated with a cylinder and the cross-sectional area of the LVOT to a circle. Therefore, the cross-sectional area of the LVOT can be calculated by measuring

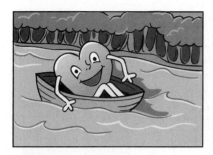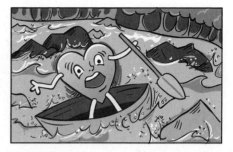

Figure Intro–18. The healthy heart free from abnormal structures permits the blood to flow at lower velocities (< 100 cm/s). Often when the heart has structural abnormalities the blood flows much more swiftly (> 400 cm/s). Continuous wave (CW) Doppler can be used to detect these regions of accelerated blood flow.

the diameter of the LVOT. Using TEE, the LVOT diameter can be measured (Figure Intro–20) in the ME long-axis view or the ME aortic valve long-axis view.

What is not yet known is the volume of blood that is moving in the heart with each beat. Fortunately, the machine provides a Doppler measurement by which the stroke volume (SV) can be determined (Figure Intro–21). Not all blood flows at the same speed as it passes through the LVOT, so there are numerous velocities captured on the PW Doppler. These collected velocities are displayed as a spectral envelope on the PW Doppler image. By tracing this wave, the machine can mathematically integrate the velocities and generate the velocity-time integral (VTI), which represents a measurement of the distance that the blood has traveled in the

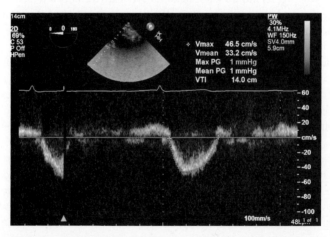

Figure Intro–19. PW Doppler is employed in this deep transgastric view interrogation of the left ventricular outflow track (LVOT). Blood is flowing in the LVOT away from the esophagus. Therefore, the flow velocities appear below the baseline. Flow velocity through the LVOT is 46.5 cm/s. This is as expected when there is no pathology noted as blood is ejected along the LVOT. Tracing the flow envelope (dotted lines) identifies the time-velocity integral (TVI). In this example the TVI is 14 cm.

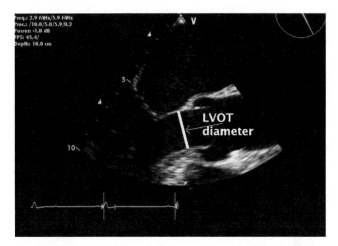

Figure Intro–20. The midesophageal long-axis view is employed in this image to identify and to measure the diameter of the LVOT. Knowing the diameter of the LVOT permits calculation of the LVOT area ($D^2 \times 0.785$ = LVOT area).

LVOT during any particular heartbeat. This distance is commonly known as stroke distance.

$$Area \times Length = Volume$$

where:

$$Area = (LVOT\ diameter)^2 \times 0.785\ \text{[the number comes from the formula}$$
for area of a circle ($\pi \times D^2/2$) where D = diameter of the circle]

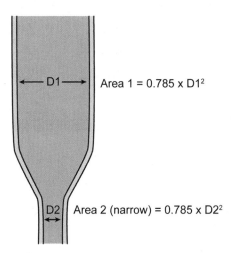

Figure Intro–21A. The continuity principle; all the volume in Area 1 must pass through Area 2. Since Area 2 is narrower than Area 1, the velocity of flow through Area 2 is greater than Area 1.

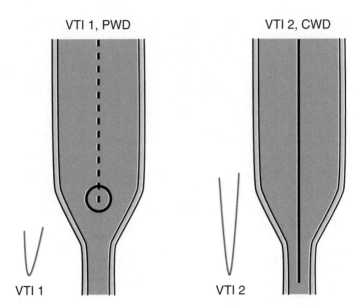

VTI 1, PWD   VTI 2, CWD

VTI 1   VTI 2

Figure Intro–21B. The time-velocity integral can be determined for Area 1 and Area 2. The PW Doppler sampling gate allows determination of the VTI 1 where the area is wide and velocity is less than 100 cm/s. VTI 2 is determined using CW Doppler. Unlike pulse wave Doppler, continuous wave Doppler detects signals over the entire length of the beam because it has no specific sampling gate. However, since velocity is swiftest at the narrowing of Area 2, the VTI from CW Doppler will reflect this maximal velocity.

> Length = the measurement of the trace from the Doppler spectral enve-
> lope known as the velocity-time integral (VTI)

Therefore,

$$SV = (LVOT\ diameter)^2 \times 0.785 \times LVOT\ VTI$$
$$Cardiac\ output\ (CO) = SV \times Heart\ rate\ (HR)$$

Consequently, TEE can provide a measurement of cardiac output.

Because blood mass is conserved based upon the continuity equation (assuming there are no shunts or regurgitant lesions), it is possible to compare the SV calculation at different points in the heart.

For example, SV1 (Area$_1$ × VTI$_1$) must equal SV2 (Area$_2$ × VTI$_2$). Generally, Area$_1$, VTI$_1$, and VTI$_2$ can be measured and are used to calculate Area$_2$. These calculations will be demonstrated in detail when discussing evaluation of valvular heart disease.

The PA catheter is also used for the measurement of intracardiac pressures. Physicians have traditionally used these pressures to estimate the volume loading conditions of the heart. The relationship between volume and pressure in the heart is determined by compliance. Healthy hearts tend to be more compliant and as such can accommodate volume with relatively minimal increases in pressure. Unhealthy hearts tend to be less compliant, and consequently small increases in volume can cause great increases in intracardiac pressures. The PA catheter has been used to identify poor compliance by estimates of PA pressures, PCOP, and CVP. Echocardiography can estimate intracardiac pressures using the Bernoulli equation.

The simplified Bernoulli equation states:

Pressure gradient = $4 \times V^2$, where V is the maximal flow velocity in m/s measured.

The gradient is always directed from areas of high pressure to areas of low pressure. Pressure gradients are used to estimate intracardiac pressures when both the gradient and the pressure in one of the two chambers are known.

Left Atrial Pressure (LAP)

The pulmonary capillary occlusion pressure (PCOP) is an estimate of left atrial pressure and by extension of the left ventricular end-diastolic pressure (LVEDP). Increased LVEDP can be reflective of poor ventricular compliance as might be encountered in a patient with diastolic heart failure. (See Chapter 5.)

The pressure gradient between the left ventricle (LV) and the left atrium (LA) can be measured using echocardiography. The left ventricle generates increased pressure during systole. Assuming there is no aortic valve disease, the systolic blood pressure is the same as LV systolic pressure. If the patient has any degree of mitral regurgitation, flow occurs during systole not only from the LV through the aortic valve into the ascending aorta but also somewhat from the LV into the LA. The maximal velocity of the flow from the LV into the LA can be measured echocardiographically using Doppler, and the pressure gradient between the two chambers can be calculated using the Bernoulli equation:

$$\text{Pressure gradient} = 4 \times V^2_{max}$$
$$\text{Pressure gradient} = \text{LV systolic pressure} - \text{Left atrial pressure}$$
$$\text{Left atrial pressure} = \text{LV systolic pressure} - (4 \times V^2_{max})$$

Similar calculations can be done to obtain estimates of pressures in other heart chambers.

Pulmonary Artery Pressures

Routinely, cardiologists estimate systolic PA pressure in patients with tricuspid regurgitation (TR) by using the same principle as discussed above. In the absence of pulmonic valve disease, the pressure in the right ventricle during systole is equal with the PA systolic pressure. Assuming that the right atrial pressure (i.e., CVP) is known, one can estimate the PA systolic pressure by measuring the velocity of the tricuspid regurgitant jet.

$$4 \times V^2 = \text{RV systolic pressure} - \text{Right atrial pressure (CVP)}$$

where:

RV systolic pressure = PA systolic pressure

PA systolic pressure = $4V^2$ (TR) + CVP

Left Ventricular End-Diastolic Pressure (LVEDP)

Likewise, LVEDP can be estimated in the presence of aortic insufficiency (AI) using the patient's diastolic blood pressure (DBP) and the velocity at end diastole of the aortic insufficiency jet.

LVEDP = DBP − $4V^2$ (end − AI velocity)

As can be seen, intracavitary pressure estimates require a pressure gradient between two chambers where the pressure in one chamber is known and there is flow from high pressure to lower pressure (the regurgitant jet), which can be interrogated by Doppler. By determining the velocity (V) of regurgitant flow (m/s), the Bernoulli equation ($4V^2$) is used to determine the pressure gradient in mm Hg (Figure Intro–22).

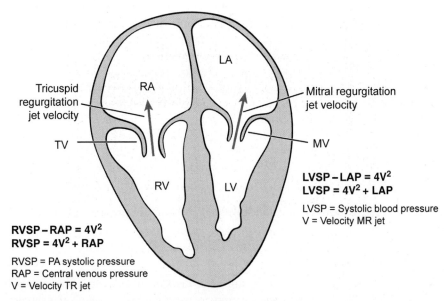

Figure Intro–22. Intracavitary pressures can be calculated using known pressures and the Bernoulli equation when regurgitant jets are present. The PA systolic pressure is obtained when tricuspid regurgitation is present and the right atrial pressure known. Assuming no pulmonic valve disease, the right ventricular systolic pressure and the pulmonary systolic pressure are the same. The left atrial pressure can be similarly calculated if mitral regurgitation is present. Again, assuming no valvular disease, LV systolic pressure should equal systemic systolic blood pressure. Subtracting $4V^2$ from the LVSP estimates the left atrial pressure.

Learning Cardiac Anesthesia and TEE

The purpose of this text is to concurrently introduce both basic perioperative echocardiography and cardiac anesthesia management. This is appropriate for the anesthetist new to the cardiac operating room as echocardiography is essential to effective cardiac anesthesia practice. That said, echocardiography can be distracting to the trainee in cardiac anesthesia. It is not the intention of the authors to present a detailed review or text of perioperative echocardiography—there are countless such works available. Rather, as cardiac anesthesia principles are introduced, TEE imagery and techniques will be employed much as in current practice where TEE informs and influences decision making during the conduct of cardiac anesthesia.

To start, it is important to review the standard images of the heart presented in this introductory chapter. The most recent guidelines offered by the American Society of Echocardiography and the Society of Cardiovascular Anesthesiologists should be studied.[18] The following image and video atlas further introduces and labels the cardiac structures visualized using the most frequently obtained perioperative TEE views.

IMAGE AND VIDEO ATLAS

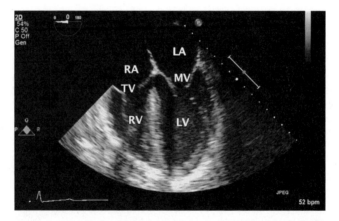

Figure A1. The midesophageal four-chamber view seen here permits imaging of the right atrium (RA), left atrium (LA), right ventricle (RV), left ventricle (LV), tricuspid valve (TV), and mitral valve (MV). Note the sector angle of 0 degrees in the upper right-hand corner. Always identify the sector angle to help to identify right from left and anterior from inferior **(Video A1)**.

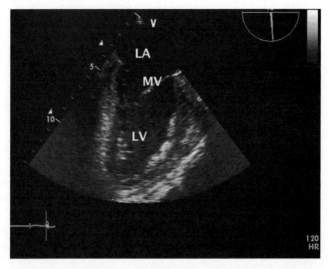

Figure A2. The midesophageal two-chamber view seen here reveals the mitral valve (MV), left atrium (LA), and left ventricle (LV) **(Video A2)**.

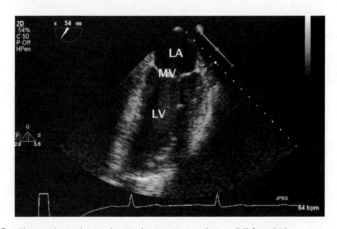

Figure A3. The midesophageal mitral commissural view **(Video A3)**.

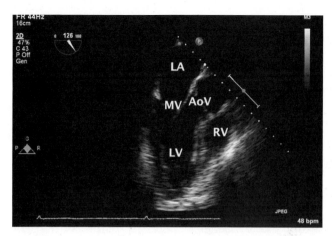

Figure A4. The midesophageal long-axis view provides excellent images of the anterior leaflet of the mitral valve (MV) and the aortic valve (AoV). The right ventricle (RV) is also seen **(Video A4)**.

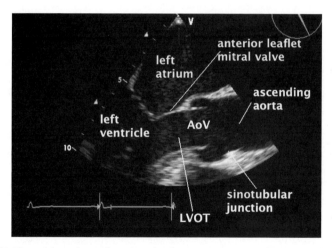

Figure A5. The midesophageal aortic valve long-axis view seen here provides a close examination of the AoV, sinotubular junction (STJ), ascending aorta, and anterior leaflet of the mitral valve **(Video A5)**.

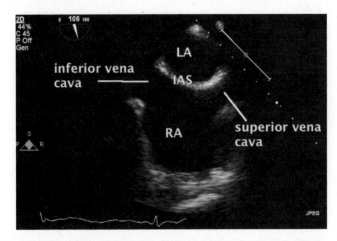

Figure A6. The midesophageal bicaval view demonstrating the superior vena cava, inferior vena cava, and intra-atrial septum **(Video A6)**.

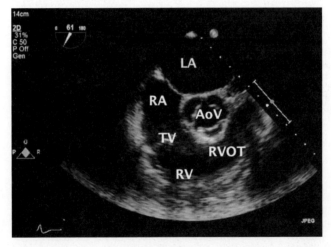

Figure A7. The midesophageal right ventricular inflow-outflow view is presented here. The right atrium (RA), left atrium (LA), tricuspid valve (TV), and right ventricular outflow track (RVOT) are seen. A short-axis view of the aortic valve (AoV) is likewise seen **(Video A7)**.

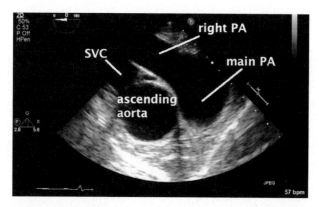

Figure A8. The midesophageal ascending aorta short-axis view provides images of the ascending aorta, main and right pulmonary artery, as well as the superior vena cava (SVC). The entire ascending aorta cannot be examined using TEE secondary to interference from the airway **(Video A8)**.

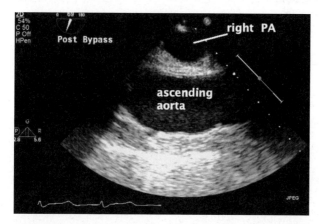

Figure A9. The midesophageal ascending aorta long-axis view is presented here. Both the ascending aorta and the right pulmonary artery (in cross section) can be seen **(Video A9)**.

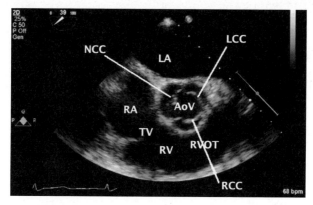

Figure A10. The midesophageal aortic valve short-axis view permits close examination of the three leaflets of the aortic valve. The right coronary cusp (RCC), left coronary cusp (LCC), and the noncoronary cusp (NCC) **(Video A10)**.

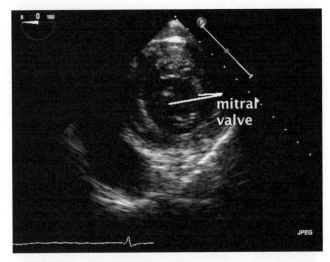

Figure A11. The transgastric basal short-axis view is seen in this image. The leaflets of the mitral valve appear as a fish's mouth when examined in this view **(Video A11).**

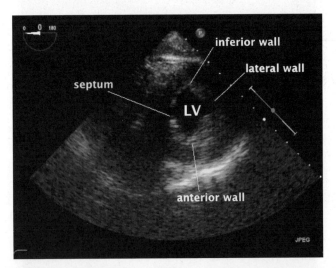

Figure A12. The transgastric midpapillary short-axis view is seen here. This image provides an opportunity to observe the contractility of the left ventricle as the anterior, inferior, lateral, and septal walls are seen. Areas of myocardium supplied by the left anterior descending artery, right coronary artery, and circumflex artery are concurrently seen making this a useful view for perioperative monitoring of the heart's function and loading conditions **(Video A12).**

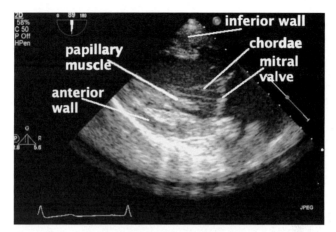

Figure A13. The transgastric two-chamber view is seen in this image. The mitral apparatus, papillary muscles, and chordae are seen **(Video A13)**.

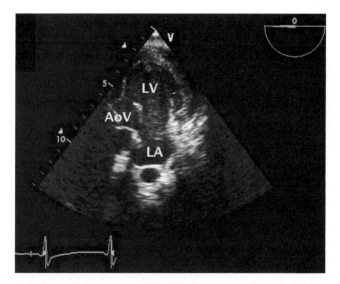

Figure A14. The deep transgastric long-axis view seen here is routinely employed in Doppler flow measurements in the left ventricular outflow track. This view aligns the Doppler beam parallel to the flow of blood in the LVOT, thus minimizing measurement errors that occur when the Doppler signal is not oriented parallel to flow **(Video A14)**.

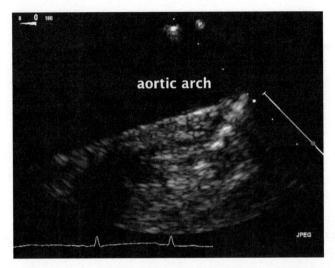

Figure A15. The upper esophageal aortic arch long-axis view is seen in this image. This image can be used to search for aortic dissections as well as atheromatous deposits.

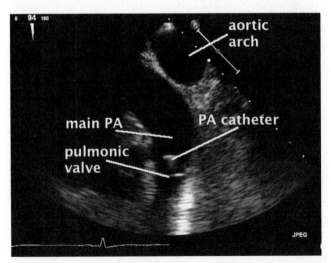

Figure A16. The upper esophageal aortic arch short-axis view is seen in this image. A pulmonary artery catheter is visible in the main pulmonary artery. Much like the deep transgastric long-axis view, this image facilitates Doppler interrogation of flow because the Doppler beam can be aligned in parallel with blood flow. In this case, flow in the pulmonary artery can be aligned with the Doppler beam (**Video A16**).

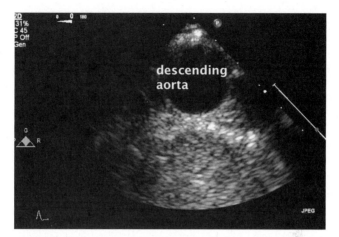

Figure A17. Rotating the probe provides this short-axis view of the descending aorta (**Video A17**).

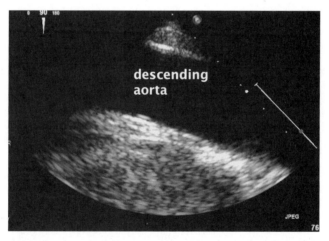

Figure A18. Rotating the sector plane provides the descending aorta long-axis view. Aortic pathology and dissections can be seen with this window.

REFERENCES

1. Shanewise JS, Cheung AT, Aronson S, et al. ASE/SCA Guidelines for performing a comprehensive intraoperative multiplane transesophageal echocardiography examination: recommendations of the American Society of Echocardiography and the Society of Cardiovascular Anesthesiologists Task Force for Certification in Perioperative Transesophageal Echocardiography. *J Am Soc Echocardiogr.* 1999;12:884-900.
2. Price S, Via G, Sloth E, et al. World Interactive Network Focused on Critical UltraSound ECHO-ICU Group. Echocardiography practice, training, and accreditation in the intensive care: document for the World Interactive Network Focused on Critical Ultrasound (WINFOCUS). *Cardiovasc Ultrasound.* 2008;6:49.

3. Royse C, Canty D, Faris J, et al. Core review: physician-performed ultrasound: the time has come for routine use in acute care medicine. *Anesth Analg.* 2012;115:1007-1028.

4. Holm J, Frederiksen C, Juhl-Olsen P, Sloth E. Perioperative use of focus assessed transthoracic echocardiography (FATE). *Anesth Analg.* 2012;115:1029-1032.

5. Faris J, Veltman M, Royse C. Limited transthoracic echocardiography assessment in anaesthesia and critical care. *Best Pract Res Clin Anaesthesiol.* 2009;23:285-298.

6. Glas KE, Swaminathan M, Reeves ST, et al. The Council for Intraoperative Echocardiography of the American Society of Echocardiography; Society of Cardiovascular Anesthesiologists. Guidelines for the performance of a comprehensive intraoperative epiaortic ultrasonographic examination: recommendations of the American Society of Echocardiography and the Society of Cardiovascular Anesthesiologists; endorsed by the Society of Thoracic Surgeons. *J Am Soc Echocardiogr.* 2007;20(11):1227-1235.

7. Reeves ST, Glas KE, Eltzshig H, et al. American Society of Echocardiography; Society of Cardiovascular Anesthesiologists. Guidelines for performing a comprehensive epicardial echocardiography examination; recommendations of the American Society of Echocardiography and the Society of Cardiovascular Anesthesiologists. *J Am Soc Echocardiogr.* 2007;20:427-437.

8. Sugeng L, Shernan SK, Salgo IS, et al. Live 3-dimensional transesophageal echocardiography: initial experience using the fully-sampled matrix array probe. *JACC.* 2008;52(6):446-449.

9. Jungwirth B, Mackensen GB. Real-time 3-dimensional echocardiography in the operating room. *Semin Cardiothorac Vasc Anesth.* 2008;12(4):248-264.

10. Lang RM, Mor-Avi V, Sugeng L, Nieman PS, Sahn DJ. Three-dimensional echocardiography: the benefits of the additional dimension. *JACC.* 2006;48(10):2053-2069.

11. Ashikhmina E, Shook D, Cobey F, et al. Three-dimensional versus two-dimensional echocardiographic assessment of functional mitral regurgitation proximal isovelocity surface area. *Anesth Analg.* 2015;120(3):534-542.

12. Jiang L, Montealegre-Gallegos M, Mahmood F. Three-dimensional echocardiography: another dimension of imaging or complexity. *J CardioThorac Vasc Anesth.* 2013;27(5):1064.

13. Hahn R, Abraham T, Adams M, et al. Guidelines for performing a comprehensive transesophageal echocardiographic examination: recommendations from the American Society of Echocardiography and the Society of Cardiovascular Anesthesiologists. *J Am Soc Echocardiogr.* 2013;26:921-964.

14. Shriki J. Ultrasound physics. *Crit Care Clin* 2014;30:1-24.

15. Gold JP, Torres KE, Maldarelli W, Zhuravlev I, Condit D, Wasnick J. Improving outcomes in coronary surgery: the impact of echo directed aortic cannulation and perioperative hemodynamic management in 500 patients. *Ann Thorac Surg.* 2004;78:1579-1585.

16. Vegas A, Meineri M. Three-dimensional transesophageal echocardiography is a major advance for intraoperative clinical management of patients undergoing cardiac surgery: a core review. *Anesth Analg* 2010;110:1548-1573.

17. Mackensen G, Swaminathan M, Mathew J. Three-dimensional transesophageal echocardiography is a major advance for intraoperative clinical management of patients undergoing cardiac surgery. *Anesth Analg.* 2010;110(6):1574-1578.

18. Reeves ST, Finley AC, Skubas NJ, et al. Basic perioperative transesophageal echocardiography examination: a consensus statement of the American Society of Echocardiography and the Society of Cardiovascular Anesthesiologists. *J Am Soc Echocardiogr.* 2013;26(5):443-456.

Preoperative Evaluation of the Heart Surgery Patient

1

TOPICS

It is often said that the anesthesiologist is the internist of the operating room (OR). By extension, the cardiac anesthesiologist becomes the cardiologist of the OR. Even though it is certainly true that anesthesiologists have knowledge of medicine in general and cardiology in particular, the practice of cardiac anesthesia is a unique discipline unto itself. Although cardiac anesthesiologists must understand why someone is being taken to cardiac surgery, they will not be the ones to decide if surgery is or is not indicated. Rather, cardiac anesthesiologists must review the totality of the patient's cardiac and medical history to determine the best approaches to manage these often very sick patients throughout the perioperative period.

This chapter will briefly examine how someone is referred for cardiac surgery and the essential elements of preoperative evaluation necessary for patient management. Frequent visitation to the American Heart Association website (www.my.americanheart.org) is suggested as a starting place to find the latest guidelines on the medical management of cardiovascular disease. Although these statements are generally directed to patient care outside of the cardiothoracic operating room, cardiac anesthesiologists should review the current guidelines for cardiovascular disease management.

CONSENT FOR CARDIAC ANESTHESIA

From the smallest hypoxemic infant with congenital heart disease to the 90-year-old patient with aortic stenosis, the cardiac anesthesiologist is called upon to care for a wide range of patients. Patients undergoing the same type of surgery can vary greatly depending upon their preoperative comorbidities and the impact their disease has had upon their cardiac function. A patient with well-preserved ventricular function presents far different challenges than an individual with reduced ejection fraction and heart failure. Likewise, the patient who has intact kidney function and is free of diabetes and lung disease is potentially less problematic than the person afflicted with these comorbidities. In this regard the conduct of cardiac anesthesia parallels that of any anesthetic. A patient's comorbidities are considered as the anesthetist determines the appropriate anesthetic technique, monitoring, and plan for postoperative management. What is perhaps unique about cardiac anesthesia is that so many of these comorbidities are regularly present; the "routine" cardiac surgery patient is incredibly sick both as a consequence of having primary heart disease as well as the associated illnesses that occur frequently in this patient population.

Generally, the "routine" cardiac surgery patient is designated as an American Society of Anesthesiologists (ASA) class 3 or 4. All patients are informed of the inherent risk of death, stroke, neurological dysfunction, and/or kidney injury. The risks and benefits of transesophageal echocardiography (TEE) should likewise be discussed with the patient preoperatively. Although the risk of stroke following bypass surgery is low (3%)[1] and that of death even lower, cardiac surgery is associated with multiple postoperative morbidities including cognitive dysfunction, kidney injury, gut ischemia, blood product transfusion, and potentially prolonged treatment in the intensive care unit (ICU). Because both the surgeon and the anesthesia team influence the patient's hemodynamic performance, it is often difficult to discern whether surgery or anesthesia is responsible for any adverse outcome. Anesthesiologists entering into cardiac anesthesia practice should be aware that outcomes may be disappointing and there is the ever-present risk of litigation even if the anesthesiologist has practiced according to all possible standards of care. Unfortunately, adverse events happen to people during cardiac surgery as a consequence of both patient illness and the numerous techniques necessary to repair the dysfunctional heart. Careful documentation and frank, honest discussions with patients and their families are essential in cardiac anesthesia practice.

CARDIAC SURGERY AND TEAMWORK

Equally important to understanding the patient's primary illness and comorbidities is understanding the steps of the surgical procedure and complications associated with each step, as well as their anesthetic implications. Recent studies in patient safety in cardiac surgery have shown that breakdowns in teamwork lead to operative flow disruption and technical errors. Even if they are minor, disruptions may impact the ability of the team to manage major events and may lead to adverse events and compromise patient safety.[2]

The American Heart Association (AHA) recently released a scientific statement on patient safety in the cardiac operating room. It summarizes the critical components of teamwork as the six "C's": "communication, cooperation, coordination, cognition (collective knowledge and shared understanding), conflict resolution, and coaching."[3] Also, in a review of litigated surgical outcomes, communication failure between caregivers accounted for 87% of system failures that led to an indemnity payment.[4]

Recently, interventions designed to improve teamwork, such as team training, structured communication tools, and protocols, have been implemented in the cardiac operating room. In addition to timeouts and checklists, communication tools such as surgical briefings and debriefings provide an opportunity for the entire operating room staff to engage in a dialogue focused on the unique aspects and requirements of the procedure to be performed. A growing body of literature supports the use of surgical briefings and debriefings in cardiac operating rooms and suggests that they may result in decreased mortality and morbidity.

CORONARY STENTS OR CORONARY ARTERY BYPASS?

The increased use of angioplasty and stents to treat coronary artery disease (CAD) has changed the profile of the patient presenting for coronary artery bypass graft (CABG) surgery. The otherwise healthy patient with preserved ventricular function and angina in need of a two-vessel bypass is increasingly rare in the cardiac surgery OR. Many patients undergo various percutaneous coronary interventions (PCIs) as first-line therapy upon presentation with anginal pain. Many studies have tried to highlight the risks and benefits of CABG versus medical therapy (MT) versus bare metal stents versus drug-eluting stents for the definitive treatment of CAD. As catheter-mediated valve replacement becomes ever more perfected, debate will likely follow on the benefits and risks of valve surgery versus catheter-mediated valve replacement.

An important trial in elucidating an answer to the question of CABG versus PCI was the Synergy Between PCI with Taxus and Cardiac Surgery (SYNTAX) trial, which randomly assigned patients with either three-vessel or left main CAD to either CABG or PCI.[5] The SYNTAX score is used to classify the complexity of CAD as low ($\leq$ 22), intermediate (23-32) or high ($\geq$ 33). The American College of Cardiology Foundation (ACCF) and the AHA provided in 2011 guidelines outlining best practices and indications for patients undergoing CABG surgery.[6] The writing committee for this summary notes that the goals for revascularization are to improve patient survival and reduce symptoms. Revascularization can be achieved through PCI or CABG, and the ACCF/AHA recommends a "heart team" approach to revascularization for patients with complex CAD. These guidelines also suggest calculation of the SYNTAX score to discern appropriate revascularization strategies.[7] The ACCF/AHA guidelines note that it is reasonable to choose CABG over PCI with complex three-vessel coronary disease in patients with a SYNTAX score greater than 22. Moreover, the writing committee reports that CABG to improve survival is reasonable in patients with significant (> 70% diameter) stenosis in two major coronary arteries with severe or extensive myocardial ischemia on stress and myocardial perfusion testing.

Serruys et al. prospectively randomized 1800 patients with severe three-vessel or left main CAD to cardiac surgery or PCI assuming that both techniques in the opinion of the patient's cardiologist and cardiac surgeon could achieve equivalent anatomical revascularization.[8] They demonstrated that the rates of adverse cardiac or cerebrovascular events at 1 year were higher in the PCI group secondary to the increased need for repeat revascularization efforts in those patients treated with stents as opposed to surgery. The medicine, angioplasty, or surgery study (MASS) II trial randomized 611 patients with coronary disease to surgery, PCI, or MT.[9] At 5 years the three approaches resulted in similarly low death rates. However, patients undergoing surgery required fewer additional procedures during the study period. A meta-analysis looking at four trials comparing stent versus bypass surgery revealed that the overall incidence of adverse cardiac or cerebrovascular events was lower in the surgery group secondary to the reduced need in operated patients to perform repeat revascularization procedures.[10] However, survival at 5 years was not found to be different between the groups.

Deb et al.[11] have systematically reviewed revascularization for patients with unprotected left main disease (ULMD), multivessel CAD, diabetes mellitus, and left ventricular dysfunction. ULMD is left main coronary disease with luminal narrowing greater than 50% without bypass grafting to the left main coronary artery's branches. Deb et al. note that current evidence suggests that 1- and 5-year mortality is similar in patients with ULMD treated with either CABG or PCI; however, they recommend that CABG be performed for stable patients. If the patient is considered too high risk for surgery, then PCI is an alternative. PCI should be avoided in those patients with a SYNTAX score greater than or equal to 33. Deb et al. likewise agree with ACCF/AHA that CAD patients are best served when cared for by a multidisciplinary team. Patients with multivessel CAD are best treated according to the SYNTAX score where PCI is appropriate for patients with a lower SYNTAX score and CABG for higher-scoring patients. CABG is strongly suggested as preferable revascularization for patients with multivessel coronary disease and diabetes. Lastly, Deb et al. note that in patients with left ventricular dysfunction evidence is limited as to which approach to revascularization is preferable.

Many patients present for cardiac surgery following previous PCIs. The risk of stent thrombosis with both bare metal and drug-eluting stents is well known.[12] Patients following stent placement are treated with various antiplatelet regimens to prevent stent thrombosis. The anesthesia staff should not take it upon themselves alone to discontinue antithrombotic or antiplatelet medication perioperatively in patients treated with stents. A team (cardiologist, surgeon, cardiac anesthesiologist) discussion should determine if and when antiplatelet medications should be discontinued preoperatively and if surgery is to be considered in a patient with prior stent placement. However, patients requiring antiplatelet therapy preoperatively are likely to require large amounts of blood products during surgery, and the anesthesiologist should be prepared for this situation.

Frequently, the cardiac patient coming for revascularization will have undergone PCI at some point in the past. Surgery is elected when lesions are not amenable to PCI or the patient has combined coronary arterial and valvular heart disease. Such patients may have presented with recurrent myocardial infarctions prior to each stent placement. Over time, patients can develop ventricular dysfunction.

CARDIOLOGY EVALUATION

Patients with cardiac angina, positive stress tests, nuclear medicine scans suggestive of myocardial ischemia, valvular heart disease, and ventricular dysfunction are routinely taken to the cardiac catheterization laboratory for diagnostic purposes. Catheterization demonstrates the coronary vasculature and pathology. PCI is usually performed at the time of diagnosis or the patient is referred for surgery. Figure 1–1 demonstrates the normal left and right coronary anatomy. Figure 1–2 reveals occlusions in both the left and right circulations. Coronary artery lesions are frequently

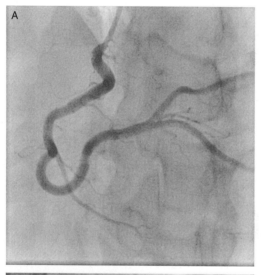

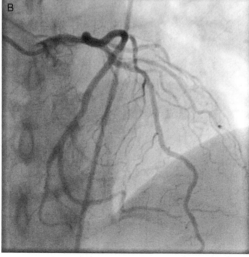

Figure 1–1. Normal right (A) and left (B) coronary anatomy.

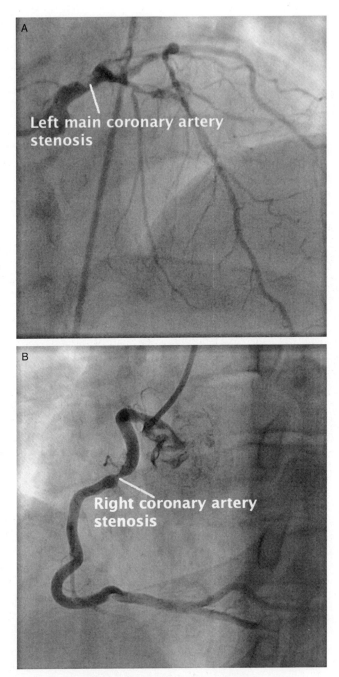

Figure 1-2. Occluded left (A) and right (B) coronary arteries.

treated with percutaneously placed stents. When the patient's anatomy does not favor PCI, patients are referred for surgery. Newer technologies using magnetic resonance imaging and computed tomography have been employed to visualize the coronary arteries.[13,14] The role of these technologies in the diagnosis and treatment of CAD is likely to increase. However, at present, cardiac catheterization remains the most common pathway by which patients find their way to surgery.

Patients present with cardiac disease to the cardiologist either electively or emergently. Increasingly, patients are being treated with emergency catheterization and PCI rather than with systemic thrombolytic therapy (an alternative emergency therapy for acute myocardial ischemia refractory to antianginal drugs). From time to time patients will present directly from the catheterization laboratory after emergency cardiac interventions when PCI is not considered feasible or when PCI has failed to restore blood flow. Such patients usually have been administered antiplatelet drugs such as glycoprotein IIb/IIIa inhibitors and/or anticoagulants (heparin or direct thrombin inhibitors). These patients when taken to surgery emergently are at very high risk for protracted bleeding. Intra-aortic balloon counterpulsation or percutaneous left ventricular assist devices can support patients during and after PCI (see Chapter 11).

Patients presenting for elective surgery, generally have the benefit of a more thorough cardiology workup. Transthoracic echocardiography (TTE) has usually been performed preoperatively to provide an estimate of valvular integrity and cardiac function.

Occasionally there are significant differences between the preoperative TTE and the intraoperative TTE examination. Therefore, the cardiac anesthesiologist should perform an independent assessment through a comprehensive and thorough intraoperative TEE examination.

Ultimately the choice of the therapeutic modality (surgery versus PCI) is the decision of the surgeon and the cardiologist. However, the anesthesiologist should inform both surgeon and cardiologist regarding specific anesthesia-related concerns (airway difficulties, malignant hyperthermia risk, etc.) that might increase the patient's risk of surgery versus catheter-mediated therapies. In this way, they may factor those anesthesia-specific concerns into the overall risk/benefit calculations and discussions with the patient. The cardiac anesthesiologist should participate with the cardiac surgeon as a part of a "heart team" such that patients receive the optimal approach to coronary revascularization.

PREOPERATIVE ASSESSMENT

Although patients of all ages, races, and genders present for cardiac anesthesia and surgery, access by all demographic groups to cardiac surgery therapies may not be equal.[15]

Patients presenting for heart surgery, whether electively or emergently, require the routine preoperative assessment that is incumbent with general anesthesiology practice. Obviously, the patient undergoing cardiopulmonary resuscitation (CPR) arriving from the catheterization laboratory in cardiac arrest precludes the usual anesthesia routine. Fortunately, such patients are indeed quite rare, and even most patients who are "urgent" can have a complete anesthesia assessment in a matter of moments. The cardiac anesthesia workup should focus upon:

a. Identification and hospital protocols: All patients *must* be identified by at least two separate patient identifiers. Before anything else, the patient must be correctly identified and any hospital flow protocols carefully followed such as the World Health Organization checklist. Perioperative antibiotic orders should be confirmed. Increasingly, electronic order sets are employed to ensure that routine but essential items such as antibiotics and deep venous thrombosis prophylaxis measures are not overlooked in the cardiac surgery patient.

b. Routine anesthesia evaluation: All patients are asked the routine anesthesia questions regarding past personal and family anesthesia history, last oral intake, routine medications, allergies, etc.

c. Assessment of cardiac function: The patient's chart likely contains extensive information from catheterization and echocardiographic studies. These should be carefully reviewed. Many patients coming for heart surgery are undergoing treatment for heart failure (HF) according to the ACCF/AHA guidelines.[16] Elements of diastolic and systolic HF are present in most patients manifesting HF. Many patients with HF have a reduced ejection fraction (HFrEF) that is less than 40%. Other patients with HF have a preserved ejection fraction (HFpEF) yet still manifest dyspnea and fatigue associated with HF. Hypertension, diabetes mellitus, and atherosclerosis contribute to the development of HF along with genetic, inflammatory, infectious, ischemic, and toxic causes. Many of these conditions present in cardiac surgery patients. As such, many patients taken to surgery have both systolic and diastolic HF. The perioperative management of these conditions will be discussed in detail in Chapter 5. Preoperative assessment necessitates that the extent of HF be recognized, as patients with HFrEF are at risk of severe hemodynamic instability at the time of anesthetic induction. HFpEF patients are subject to pulmonary venous congestion secondary to diastolic dysfunction. Natriuretic peptide measurements (BNP) provide a guide as to the severity or acuity of HF. Patients are routinely treated with angiotensin converting enzyme (ACE) inhibitors or angiotensin receptor blockers (ARBs) along with diuretics, aldosterone antagonists, appropriate beta-blockers, and statins (if indicated for other reasons). In patients with HFpEF, blood pressure control and diuretics for the relief of symptoms are class 1 recommendations of the ACCF/AHA. Cardiac resynchronization therapy devices are often also employed in the management of patients with reduced ejection fraction (see Chapter 14). Some patients with advanced HF require treatment with mechanical assist devices (see Chapter 11). Medical history of arrhythmias and anti-arrhythmic therapies (see Chapter 3) should also be reviewed. Lastly, the anesthetist following the chart review should have detailed knowledge of the surgical procedure to be performed.

d. TEE: TEE is used routinely in most cardiac cases. The anesthesiologist should clearly discuss the risk and benefits of TEE with the patient and ascertain if the patient manifests any absolute or relative contraindications to TEE examination.

e. Pulmonary history: Many patients presenting for cardiac surgery have a long history of lung disease usually secondary to smoking. Dyspnea in the cardiac surgery patient can be secondary to either, or both, cardiac and pulmonary dysfunction. The patient's history regarding the use of oral corticosteroids and bronchodilators should be reviewed. Patients taking baseline steroids require stress dose corticosteroids perioperatively. Bronchodilators are given perioperatively to decrease bronchospasm. Patients with severe lung disease may have pulmonary hypertension and impaired right ventricular function. Right ventricular dysfunction (see Chapter 8) may be associated with or independent of left ventricular dysfunction and can contribute to perioperative hemodynamic instability.

f. Kidney history: Patients with impaired kidney function are at increased risk perioperatively. Hypertension, acid-base imbalances, and hyperkalemia may all complicate the perioperative management of the kidney failure patient undergoing heart surgery. Dialysis-dependent patients are frequently dialyzed preoperatively rendering them relatively hypovolemic at the time of anesthesia induction. Postoperatively, dialysis is often needed to remove excessive fluid and potassium acquired during cardioplegia administration. Close communication with nephrology and dialysis staff before going to surgery will provide early renal replacement therapy in those patients with impaired kidney function taken to heart surgery. Hypotension, hypovolemia, and kidney hypoperfusion all contribute to the development of acute kidney injury perioperatively (see Chapter 14).

g. Hepatic disease: The patient's history of alcohol abuse and other substance abuse is obtained to determine both the possibility of cross-tolerance to anesthetic agents or postoperative alcohol withdrawal syndrome. Patients with a history of hepatic failure are at risk for coagulopathy, ascites, portal hypertension with varices, encephalopathy, arteriovenous shunting, and hepatorenal syndrome. The diseased liver may be sensitive to perioperative hypoperfusion leading to "shock" liver postoperatively and coagulopathy.

h. Hematological disorders: There are a variety of hematological conditions that can complicate cardiac surgery. Close coordination with the patient's hematologist in the preoperative period is critical to minimize the impact of these conditions on the patient's perioperative course. Hemophilia A is an X-linked recessive disorder leading to reduced factor VIII pro-coagulant. Hemophilia B is similarly an X-linked recessive disorder leading to decreased factor IX. The hematologist through perioperative factor replacement manages these conditions. Von Willebrand disease is associated with a decrease in von Willebrand factor and decreased platelet adhesion. DDAVP (1-deamino-8-D-arginine vasopressin) in a dose of 0.3 μg/kg can be administered to increase circulating von Willebrand factor perioperatively. Patients with severe aortic stenosis or with left ventricular assist devices may present with an acquired form of von Willebrand disease. Patients taking warfarin undergoing emergency cardiac surgery are likely to bleed perioperatively. Fresh frozen plasma, prothrombin complex concentrates, and vitamin K can be administered to attempt to correct the patient's international normalized ratio (INR). Deficiencies in protein S and protein C as well as the presence of factor V Leiden put the patient at risk for hypercoagulability (see Chapter 16.)

Heparin-induced thrombocytopenia prevents the use of heparin perioperatively complicating the management of cardiopulmonary bypass (see Chapter 17). Sickle cell disease places the patient at risk of a sickling crisis during hypothermia and periods of hypoxemia. Exchange transfusion is necessary to reduce the amount of hemoglobin S in the blood perioperatively, and consultation with the patient's hematologist is advised. Irrespective of the nature of the patient's hematological condition, close coordination between the anesthesiologist, surgeon, and hematologist is critical. Lastly, patients for a variety of reasons often refuse blood product transfusion. Such refusal must be clearly documented prior to taking the patient to surgery, and alternative modalities of blood salvage should be discussed.

i. Neurological history: Many patients have combined carotid and CAD or a history of previous strokes or other neurological injuries. It is imperative to document the patient's mental status, motor function, and pupil size preoperatively as a baseline to be compared against any postoperative deterioration. Regrettably, there are many sources of postoperative neurological dysfunction including embolization, hypoperfusion, and inflammation that can lead to both overt stroke and cognitive dysfunction.

j. Physical examination: A routine anesthesia examination is performed. The airway is assessed and locations for vascular access and invasive monitoring examined. The lungs are auscultated to identify any new wheezing or HF. The carotids are examined for signs of bruits.

k. Laboratory/ECG review: Routine labs are reviewed. In particular, the patient's blood glucose is noted. Blood glucose control by regular insulin infusion is routinely employed perioperatively to optimize patient outcomes (see Chapter 5). Baseline electrolytes especially potassium, calcium, and magnesium are noted. Patients on diuretic therapy may have hypokalemia; however, often at the end of surgery the potassium concentration is increased secondary to the delivery of potassium-rich cardioplegia solutions during cardiopulmonary bypass. Serum calcium measures are dependent upon the patient's albumin concentration and are of limited use. Ionized calcium concentrations are measured perioperatively. Ionized calcium concentration may decrease transiently during cardiopulmonary bypass only to return to baseline following the bypass run. Magnesium replacement is often needed postoperatively, and its baseline concentration should be noted. Other routine lab values are screened relating to platelet count, coagulation status, hemoglobin concentration, and liver and kidney function. The baseline ECG is reviewed, and the patient's baseline rhythm noted.

PREOPERATIVE PATIENT CARE AND COMFORT

Patients presenting for any type of cardiac surgery by their very nature are potentially unstable. As such they can deteriorate, arrest, or stroke at any point in the time up to the induction of anesthesia (and certainly afterward—see Chapter 4). It is critically important that such patients be carefully monitored during the entire time they are under the care of the anesthesia team. Consequently, the authors do not routinely administer oral premedications to patients awaiting surgery. It is often said that the best premedication is a caring anesthetist at the patient's bedside answering their questions and allaying their fears. When that does not work, small amounts of intravenous midazolam can be employed (0.5-2.0 mg IV) in the holding area assuming the patient is monitored and the anesthetist is present at the patient's bedside. Patients with critical aortic stenosis as well as those with severely impaired ventricular function are best not medicated at all until such time as the induction of anesthesia. Whenever any premedication is given, a plan for monitoring and resuscitating the patient should be in place in the event of unexpected patient instability.

Anxious patients may develop tachycardia leading to myocardial ischemia. Most patients are treated with beta-blockers as a part of their medical regimen, thus reducing the incidence of sinus tachycardia preoperatively. Should beta blockade be inadequate, small doses of short-acting beta-blockers (e.g., esmolol) can be administered. Supplemental oxygen should be provided to all patients preoperatively.

REFERENCES

1. Roach G, Kanchuger M, Mora Mangano C, et al. Adverse cerebral outcomes after coronary bypass surgery. *NEJM*. 1996;335(25):1857-1863.

2. ElBardissi AW, Wiegmann DA, Henrickson S, et al. Identifying methods to improve heart surgery: an operative approach and strategy for implementation on an organizational level. *Eur J Cardiothorac Surg*. 2008;34(5):1027-1033.

3. Wahr JA, Prager RL, Abernathy JH, et al. Patient safety in the cardiac operating room: human factors and teamwork: a scientific statement from the American Heart Association. *Circulation*. 2013;128(10):1139-1169.

4. Morris JA, Carrillo Y, Jenkins JM. Surgical adverse events, risk management, and malpractice outcome: morbidity and mortality review is not enough. *Ann Surg*. 2003;237:844-851.

5. Ong AT, Serruys PW, Mohr PW, et al. The SYNergy between percutaneous coronary intervention with TAXus and cardiac surgery (SYNTAX) study: design, rationale, and run-in phase. *Am Heart J* 2006;151:1194-1204.

6. Hillis LD, Smith PK, Anderson JL, et al. 2011 ACCF/AHA guideline for coronary artery bypass graft surgery: executive summary: a report of the American College of Cardiology Foundation/American Heart Association Task Force on Practice Guidelines. Developed in collaboration with the American Association for Thoracic Surgery, Society of Cardiovascular Anesthesiologists, and Society of Thoracic Surgeons. *J Am Coll Cardiol*. 2011;58:e123-210.

7. Sianos G, Morel MA, Kappetein AP. The SYNTAX Score: an angiographic tool grading the complexity of coronary artery disease. *EuroInterv*. 2005;1:219-227.

8. Serruys P, Morice M, Kappetein AP, et al. Percutaneous coronary intervention versus coronary artery bypass grafting for severe coronary artery disease. *NEJM*. 2009;360(10):961-972.

9. Hueb W, Lopes N, Gersh B, et al. Five year follow-up of the medicine, angioplasty, or surgery study (MASSII): a randomized controlled clinical trial of 3 therapeutic strategies for multivessel coronary artery disease. *Circulation*. 2007;115:1082-1089.

10. Daemen J, Boersma E, Flather M, et al. Long term safety and efficacy of percutaneous coronary intervention with stenting and coronary artery bypass surgery for multivessel coronary artery disease: a meta-analysis with 5 year patient level data from the ARTS, ERACI-II, MASS-II and SoS trials. *Circulation*. 2008;118:1146-1154.

11. Deb S, Wijeysundera H, Ko D, et al. Coronary artery bypass graft surgery vs. percutaneous interventions in coronary revascularization: a systematic review. *JAMA*. 2013;310(19):2086-2095.

12. Kim H, Park K, Kwak J, et al. Stent related cardiac events after non-cardiac surgery: drug eluting stent vs. bare metal stent. *Int J Cardiology*. 2008;123:353-354.

13. Yokoyama K, Nitatori T, Kanke N, et al. Efficacy of cardiac MRI in the evaluation of ischemic heart disease. *Magn Reson Med Sci.* 2006;5(1):33-40.

14. Stehning C, Boernert P, Nehkre K. Advances in coronary MRA from vessel wall to whole heart imaging. *Magn Reson Med Sci.* 2007;6(3):157-170.

15. Jones J. The question of racial bias in thoracic surgery: appearances and realities. *Ann Thorac Surg.* 2001;72:6-8.

16. Yancy C, Jessup M, Bozkurt B, et al. 2013 ACCF/AHA guideline for the management of heart failure: a report of the American College of Cardiology Foundation/American Heart Association Task Force on Practice Guidelines. *J Am Coll Cardiol.* 2013;62:e147-239.

Hemodynamics and Cardiac Anesthesia

2

Understanding hemodynamic principles helps cardiac anesthesiologists determine the mechanisms underlying hemodynamic instability and guides treatment. Fortunately, the same basic physiologic principles apply in both the healthy patient undergoing laparoscopic cholecystectomy as well as in the patient with low ejection fraction undergoing multiple valve replacements. Unfortunately, the patient undergoing cardiac surgery is more likely to decompensate severely when faced with the hemodynamic roller coaster sometimes associated with general anesthesia induction (Figure 2–1).

HEMODYNAMIC CALCULATIONS AND INVASIVE MONITORS: WHY ARE THEY IMPORTANT AND HOW DOES ONE DETERMINE THEM?

Blood Pressure

Although the absolute definition of hypotension is somewhat clouded in the literature,[1] a patient is considered hypotensive when the systolic blood pressure is reduced by 20% or more from the patient's baseline blood pressure. Different authors set different cutoffs as to what constitutes a hypotensive patient. Although in the past a systolic pressure of less than 90 mm Hg was thought hypotensive, this value has recently been suggested as being too low. For example, the

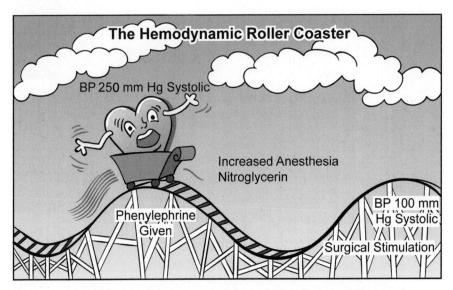

Figure 2–1. Anesthesia manipulations can often stress the heart and the patient. Although many healthy patients can tolerate these swings in blood pressure, the cardiac surgery patient may be unable to do so without developing myocardial ischemia and ventricular dysfunction. (Reproduced with permission from Wasnick JD: *Handbook of Cardiac Anesthesia and Perioperative Care*. Boston, MA: Butterworth Heinemann; 1998.)

new cutoff value for hypotension has been reset to 110 mm Hg systolic in trauma patients.[2] A mean arterial blood pressure less than 65 mm Hg has been associated with adverse outcomes perioperatively and should be corrected. However, at times during cardiac procedures surgeons may request relative hypotension to facilitate aortic cannulation or to control bleeding. At other times physical manipulation of the heart by the surgeons will transiently reduce blood pressure. Close communication between the surgeon and anesthesiologist is critical for effective hemodynamic management.

Each practitioner must determine for each individual patient what systemic pressures, high and low, warrant treatment. In the adult cardiac surgery patient, it is likely that any patient with a systolic blood pressure much less than 90 mm Hg would be considered in need of hemodynamic intervention of some kind depending upon the etiology of the hypotensive episode. Hypertension is also aggressively treated in the cardiac surgery patient. This chapter will examine how to approach the hypotensive cardiac patient and to apply appropriate therapy. Some of the causes of perioperative hypotension are presented in Table 2–1.

An understanding of hemodynamics, can help discern the numerous possible etiologies responsible for hypotension. Blood pressure (BP) gradients drive the delivery of blood throughout the circulation. BP is similar to Ohm's law that regulates the flow of current through a circuit:

Table 2–1. Differential Diagnosis of Perioperative Hypotension

Hypovolemia
Myocardial ischemia and infarction
Systolic ventricular failure
Pneumothorax
Pericardial tamponade
Arrhythmias
Dynamic left ventricular outflow obstruction
Pulmonary embolism
Right ventricular failure
Reduced sympathetic tone
Anaphylaxis
Sepsis

$$V = I \times R$$

where:

V = potential

I = current intensity (electron flow)

R = resistance (electrical)

The potential (V) in the circuit drives the current (I) through the resistance (R). Lowering the resistance increases current flow.

The basic formula for blood pressure is quite similar:

$$BP = CO \times SVR$$

where:

BP = blood pressure

CO = cardiac output (blood flow)

SVR = systemic vascular resistance

Thus, blood pressure has only two fundamental determinants: cardiac output and systemic vascular resistance. Consequently, when patients become hypotensive, they can do so only because of reductions in cardiac output, systemic vascular resistance, or both.

Indeed, all the disease states listed in Table 2–1 reduce blood pressure by having an impact on the patient's cardiac output or systemic resistance.

Cardiac Output

Cardiac output (CO) is the product of the stroke volume (SV) and the heart rate (HR). The normal cardiac output of 4 to 6 liters per minute (L/min) must be interpreted in relation to a patient's body surface area. An elderly, small woman with a small body surface area (BSA) will require less cardiac output to meet her metabolic needs than will a larger individual. The cardiac index (CI) {CO/BSA} ranges from

2.2 to 4.2 L/min/m^2. Ultimately when considering CO and CI, practitioners are really interested in making sure that an adequate amount of oxygen is being delivered to the tissues to maintain tissue viability. In general, a CI less than 2.2 L/min/m^2 is concerning as it may lead to anaerobic metabolism and metabolic acidosis. However, there are many factors that determine if a particular CI is adequate for an individual patient's metabolic needs. These include patient temperature, hemoglobin concentration, and oxygen saturation.

Stroke Volume (SV)

The SV reflects the output of the heart during an individual beat.

$$CO = SV \times HR$$
$$SV = CO/HR$$

Normal values = 50 to 100 mL/beat

There are a number of determinants that affect the SV. These include:

1. Volume: Patients must have an adequate preload to generate a normal SV. Hypovolemia due to various causes is one of the most obvious causes of reduced SV. Hypovolemic patients are often hypotensive and tachycardic with a reduced SV. SV can also be reduced when venous return to the heart is diminished such as from institution of positive pressure ventilation, pericardial tamponade, or pneumothorax.

2. Afterload: Recall, BP = CO × SVR. The SVR and the SV are inversely related; as the resistance against which the heart must pump increases, the SV will decrease, whereas when the SVR is reduced, the SV increases. Conditions, which reduce SVR, include those that produce vasodilatory states [e.g., sepsis, systemic inflammatory response syndrome (SIRS), and spinal shock]. Conditions, which increase SVR, are numerous but in general center upon an increase in sympathetic outflow (e.g., hypertension, heart failure, and hypothermia).

3. Myocardial contractility: Myocardial ischemia, myocardial infarction, valvular heart diseases, and cardiomyopathies can all affect the ability of the heart both to relax and to contract. Impaired contractility reduces stroke volume.

As mentioned SV represents the amount of blood ejected from the heart during a beat.

So, SV = left ventricular end-diastolic volume – left ventricular end-systolic volume.

The stroke volume can be depicted graphically through the pressure-volume loop (Figure 2–2).

Systemic Vascular Resistance

SVR is estimated as follows:

SVR = [Mean arterial pressure (MAP) – Central venous pressure (CVP)]/CO × 80

The normal calculated SVR is approximately 800 to 1200 dyne second/cm.^{5}

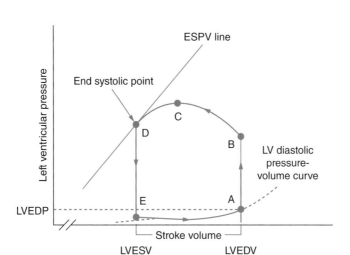

Figure 2–2. The pressure-volume loop depicts graphically the hemodynamic changes in the left ventricle during a heartbeat and the ejection of one stroke volume (SV). Segment A-B occurs at the beginning of systole after the mitral valve closes. (A) The left ventricular end-diastolic pressure is noted on the graph at the end of diastolic filling. Pressure in the ventricle gradually builds until point B is reached when the aortic valve opens (B) and blood is ejected from the ventricle. The aortic valve closes when ejection is complete at end systole. The line at point D identifies end systole. Moving the slope of this line to the reader's right represents a shift to a less contractile state. Moving the slope to the left reflects a more highly contractile ventricle. Segment D-E represents iso-volumetric relaxation. Once pressure in the ventricle is reduced, the mitral valve again opens (point E) and diastolic filling resumes in preparation for the heart's next systole. Left ventricular end-diastolic pressure (LVEDP), left ventricular end-diastolic volume (LVEDV), end-systolic pressure-volume (ESPV). (Reproduced with permission from Hoffman WJ, Wasnick JD: *Postoperative Critical Care of the Massachusetts General Hospital*, 2nd ed. Boston, MA: Wolters Kluwer; 1992.)

Hypotension and Hemodynamics

As discussed, hypotension can occur as a consequence of a reduction in cardiac output, systemic vascular resistance, or both. Still, the differential diagnosis of perioperative hypotension listed in Table 2–1 is rather large. It is important to understand the physiologic principles underlying hemodynamic instability to work through the differential and make the appropriate diagnosis of "*Why is my patient hypotensive?*"

When TTE is available, the FATE protocol can be used to immediately assess cardiac function and volume status. When not available, the CO can be determined to calculate the SV. Various methods and devices can be employed for the estimation of the CO.[3-5] These approaches include estimation of CO based on pulse contour analysis of arterial pressure tracings from the arterial line (Vigileo/ FloTrac, PiCCO, and Pulse CO). Many of these pulse contour analysis systems require calibration of their measurements with some other form of CO measure to be accurate.

Traditionally, the Swan-Ganz pulmonary artery (PA) catheter was used to estimate CO. However, there are a number of reports, which question the risk/benefit of pulmonary artery (PA) catheter placement.[6-9] Sandham et al.[6] reported no benefit in PA-guided therapy in American Society of Anesthesiology (ASA) physical status class 3 or 4 patients scheduled for elective or urgent surgery as compared with patients not monitored with a PA catheter. Harvey et al. showed no benefit in overall outcome in critically ill patients managed with a PA catheter compared to a less invasive CO measurement devices.[7] Moreover, studies have questioned the need to specifically measure CO in the cardiac surgery patient.[8,9] Cowie concludes that there is no clear evidence of benefit nor harm in cardiac, intensive care, or perioperative patients from PA catheter use.[10] As will be discussed later in this chapter, transthoracic echocardiography and transesophageal echocardiography have reduced the need to place specific monitors for CO determination since echocardiography can itself be used to measure hemodynamic parameters.[11]

Although the use of CO measurements to guide therapy according to specific protocols in critically ill patients may be controversial and the methods by which these measurements are obtained are ever changing, the use of hemodynamic monitoring remains ever present in perioperative management even if the PA catheter's heyday is long since over.

If the SV is elevated in the setting of hypotension, it is likely that the patient is vasodilated. Conversely, if the SV is reduced and the patient is hypotensive, then there are two fundamental possible etiologies to consider.

1. Abnormal pump function secondary to cardiomyopathy, ischemia, arrhythmia, valvular heart disease, and so forth.
2. Decreased preload secondary to hypovolemia, tension pneumothorax, or cardiac tamponade.

To distinguish between these two etiologies additional information from perioperative monitors is necessary.

Invasive Monitors

The cardiac surgical patient requires invasive arterial blood pressure monitoring as well as central venous access. As mentioned previously, the routine use of the PA catheter in heart surgery patients is controversial but remains widely employed perioperatively especially in the United States.

ARTERIAL MONITORING

There are perhaps as many varying techniques of arterial line placement as there are practitioners. Although approaches to arterial lines can be discussed and demonstrated, there is no substitution for trial and error as trainees develop their own approaches to line placement. Table 2–2 lists sites for arterial cannulation. The Allen test has been suggested as an approach to screen out the possibility of hand ischemia should ulnar arterial blood flow be inadequate in the setting of radial artery cannulation. During the Allen test both radial and ulnar arteries are occluded and the hand is observed after developing pallor. The ulnar artery compression is released and the time for the hand to return to normal color noted. Should color

Table 2–2. Arterial Cannulation Sites Helpful Hints

- Radial artery: Confirm radial artery not to be used for bypass grafts.
- Femoral artery: Confirm absence of distal vascular disease; useful if intra-aortic balloon pump is planned: confirm the site is not to be used for planned or backup cannulation.
- Axillary artery: A good alternative site if radials and femorals are unavailable.
- Brachial artery: Risks of reduced arterial flow to the arm must be considered if this site is employed.

---

fail to return to the hand after release of ulnar compression within 10 to 15 seconds, the test is positive and radial arterial cannulation avoided. This test is, however, controversial and is not universally employed.[12,13] Whatever site is chosen for line placement, there is always the risk of arterial bleeding, hematoma, embolization, and thrombosis. Sterile techniques should be employed and the pressure tubing used to connect the arterial line to the monitoring system purged of any air. The pressurized bag containing the normal saline flush solution should be at a pressure greater than arterial pressure to prevent back bleeding through the arterial line. It should be noted that the arterial pressure waveform changes depending upon the cannulation site. As arterial lines are placed in more distal arteries, there is a change in the waveform with a progressive loss of the dicrotic notch, a delay in transmission, and a higher measured systolic pressure. MAP and diastolic blood pressure (DAP) are less affected by line placement.

CENTRAL VENOUS ACCESS

Central access can be obtained through cannulation of the external jugular, internal jugular, subclavian, or femoral veins. Generally, the right internal jugular vein is cannulated due to ease of access and ease of flotation of the PA catheter should that be considered necessary (Figure 2–3).

Multiple complications may arise from obtaining central access. Infection is one of the most common complications and may lead to sepsis and multiple organ failure. The importance of using scrupulous sterile techniques must be emphasized, including the use of full body draping.[14,15] Other complications include inadvertent carotid artery catheterization, neck hematoma and airway compromise, pneumothorax, and air embolism.

Confirmation that the central venous circulation, and not an artery, has been identified for cannulation is *essential* prior to catheter placement. Numerous flawed confirmatory methods can and have been employed including:

- Color comparison between an arterial sample and one obtained from the proposed cannulation site. This *does not* reliably eliminate the possibility of arterial puncture.[16]
- Lack of pulsatility at the cannulation site *does not* reliably eliminate the possibility of arterial puncture.

Better methods include:

- Pressure measurements to determine venous waveform and pressure rather than arterial waveform and pressure at the cannulation site.

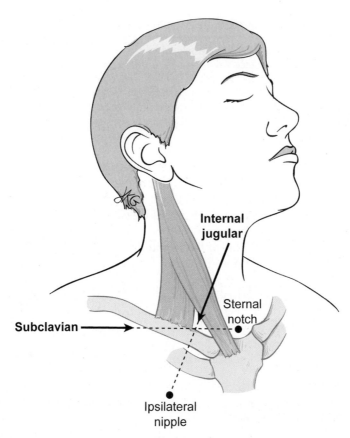

Figure 2–3. The subclavian and internal jugular veins are both used for central access perioperatively with the sternal notch and ipsilateral nipple in the direction of needle passage for each, respectively.

- Observation on TEE of guidewire placement in the right atrium (**Video 2–1**).
- Ultrasound-guided line placement (**Video 2–2**) with localization of the guide wire in the venous circulation.

 Lastly,

- Confirm radiographically the final position of the CVP catheter tip as soon as clinically possible. The catheter tip should lie in the superior vena cava.

 Ultrasound-guided placement has been shown to reduce complications of line placement.[17,18] Consequently, it is likely that ultrasound-guided placement will become ever more mandated in performing central venous access. However, ultrasound equipment is expensive and may not be universally available. Should arterial cannulation occur, surgical consultation is mandatory before removing the catheter.

Pulmonary Artery Catheterization

After having secured adequate central venous access, a PA (Swan-Ganz) catheter can be floated to assist in diagnosing the etiology of perioperative hypotension.[19-21]

Although other less invasive methods of determining CO, SVR, and SV are available, the PA catheter remains a routine component of hemodynamic monitoring for cardiac surgical patients in some hospitals.

Risks of PA catheterization include pulmonary artery rupture, rhythm disturbances, complete heart block, and knotting of the catheter. Figure 2–4 demonstrates the expected pressure patterns as the pulmonary catheter passes from the central venous circulation through the right atrium, the right ventricle, the pulmonary artery, and finally settles into the occlusive or wedge position. The PA catheter traditionally has aided patient management in multiple ways:

1. CO, SVR, and SV can be determined. CO measurements can be obtained using the thermodilution technique. The thermodilution technique determines cardiac output by using the temperature of the blood as an indicator. Cool or room temperature saline is injected into a proximal port of the PA catheter. At the end of the catheter there is a thermistor that can detect the change in temperature as fluid passes by. Temperature change is inversely proportional to cardiac output. The changes in temperature are then calculated by software incorporated, and a CO is estimated. Some PA catheters are equipped with fiber-optic capabilities, which enable them to determine mixed venous oxygen saturation. Mixed venous oxygen saturation (SvO_2) is normally 65% to 75%. Mixed venous oxygen partial pressure is normally 40 mm Hg. The SvO_2 may be measured in the blood gas lab by obtaining a blood sample from the distal PA port of the PA catheter. SvO_2 represents the venous hemoglobin saturation in the pulmonary artery after the mixing of venous blood from the superior vena cava, the inferior vena cava, and the coronary sinus. The following hemodynamic formula derived from the Fick equation defines the SvO_2:

$$SvO_2 = SaO_2 - VO_2/(CO \times 1.36 \times Hb)$$

where:

SaO_2 = arterial oxygen saturation

Hb = hemoglobin concentration

VO_2 = oxygen consumption

The Fick equation:

$$CO = VO_2/(C_aO_2 - C_vO_2)$$

where:

CO = cardiac output

VO_2 = oxygen consumption per minute

C_aO_2 = oxygen content of arterial blood [$S_aO_2 \times$ hemoglobin (g/dl) $\times$ 1.36 (mL O_2/g Hb)]

C_vO_2 = oxygen content of mixed venous blood [$S_vO_2 \times$ hemoglobin (g/dl) $\times$ 1.36 (mL O_2/g Hb)]

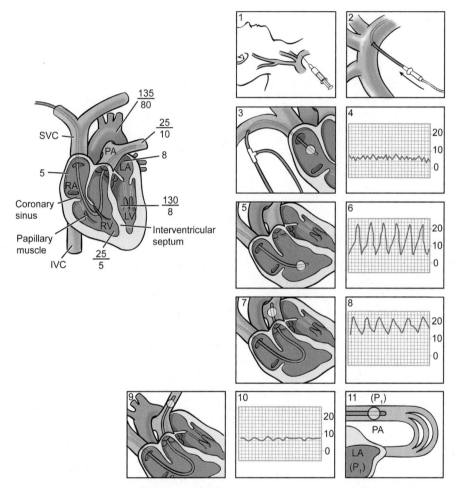

Figure 2–4. Although its utility is increasingly questioned, pulmonary artery catheters continue to be a part of perioperative management of the cardiac surgery patient. Following placement of a sheath introducer in the central circulation (panels 1, 2), the pulmonary artery catheter is "floated." Central line placement should always be completed using rigorous sterile technique; full body draping; and only after multiple, redundant confirmations of the correct localization of the venous circulation. Pressure guidance is used to ascertain the localization of the PA catheter in the venous circulation and the heart. Upon entry into the right atrium (panels 3 and 4), the central venous pressure tracing is noted. Passing through the tricuspid valve (panels 5 and 6) right ventricular pressures are detected. At 35 to 50 cm depending upon patient size, the catheter will pass from the right ventricle through the pulmonic valve into the pulmonary artery (panels 7 and 8). This is noted by the measurement of diastolic pressure once the pulmonic valve is passed.

Lastly, when indicated, the balloon-tipped catheter will "wedge" or "occlude" a pulmonary artery branch (panels 9, 10, 11). When this occurs, the pulmonary artery pressure equilibrates with that of the left atrium, which, barring any mitral valve pathology, should be a reflection of left ventricular end-diastolic pressure. (Reproduced with permission from Soni N: *Practical Proceduresin Anaesthesia and Intensive Care.* Boston, MA: Butterworth Heinemann; 1994.)

SvO_2 is reduced in settings of increased extraction of oxygen by the tissues or decreased oxygen delivery to the tissues. This occurs when there is reduced CO, anemia, or decreased arterial oxygen saturation. SvO_2 is increased when there is decreased utilization of oxygen by the tissues such as is the case in cyanide poisoning and hypothermia or in the presence of a left-to-right shunt.

2. Secondly, the PA catheter measures the pressure in the various chambers of the heart. The right atrial pressure (RAP) also known as the central venous pressure (CVP) estimates right ventricular filling. Elevated RAP greater than 20 mm Hg can be associated with right ventricular dysfunction.[22-30] Additionally, trends in RAP are often used to determine the adequacy of volume replacement. Although static indicators of volume load such as RAP have been traditionally employed, dynamic parameters such as stroke volume variation, pulse pressure variation, and systolic pressure variation have more recently been used to estimate volume status.

The PiCCO system employs a transpulmonary thermodilution technique, using a femoral arterial catheter, to detect changes in temperature following saline injection into the superior vena cava through a central line. Whereas pulmonary artery thermodilution estimates CO by the change in temperature at the thermistor located at the tip of the PA catheter, the PiCCO system employs thermodilution but does not require pulmonary artery catheterization. A specialized femoral arterial catheter equipped with a thermistor detects changes in temperature following saline injection into the superior vena cava via a central line (Figures 2–5 and 2–6).

The PiCCO system continually estimates the stroke volume from the arterial waveform, using the arterial catheter, following an initial calibration process using thermodilution, which calibrates the parameters. The algorithm is then capable of computing each single stroke volume.

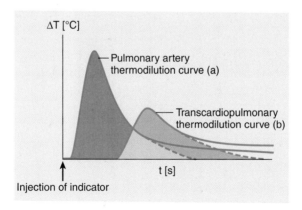

Figure 2–5. Comparison of thermodilution curves after injection of cold saline into the superior vena cava. The peak temperature change arrives earlier when measured in the pulmonary artery (a) than if measured in the femoral artery (b). Thereafter, both curves soon reapproximate baseline. [Reproduced with permission from Reuter D, Huang C, Edrich T, et al. Cardiac output monitoring using indicator dilution techniques: Basics, limits and perspectives. *Anesth Analg.* 2010 Mar 1;110(3):799-811.]

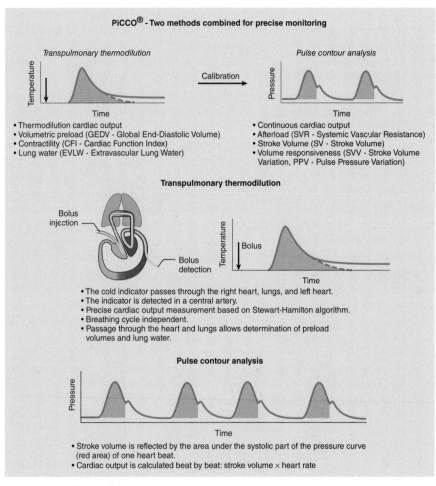

Figure 2–6. Two methods combined for precise monitoring. (Reproduced with permission from Philips Electronics.)

When using the PA catheter to estimate preload, central venous and pulmonary capillary wedge pressures (PCWP) are used as surrogates for the volume loads presented to the right and left heart, respectively. Pressure and volume are related to one another by ventricular compliance.

Compliance is defined by the formula:

$$C = \Delta V / \Delta P$$

where:

C = compliance

ΔV = change in volume

ΔP = change in pressure

In highly compliant systems, large volume changes are accommodated with minimal changes in pressure. In noncompliant systems, minimal changes in volume produce dramatic pressure changes. Compliance is encountered in many organ systems including the heart, lungs, and brain. For example, when the lungs are noncompliant, a positive pressure tidal volume breath will generate a greater inspiratory pressure than in a patient with normal lung compliance. In cardiac patients, the compliant heart accommodates volume with minimal increases in left ventricular end-diastolic pressure (LVEDP). The LVEDP is the pressure in the left ventricle at the end of diastolic filling. Compliant left ventricles fill with lower pressures (e.g., 5-10 mm Hg). On the other hand, a noncompliant left ventricle accommodates the left ventricular end-diastolic volume (LVEDV) with increased LVEDP. Figure 2–7 demonstrates compliance curves of normal, highly compliant, and noncompliant left ventricles.

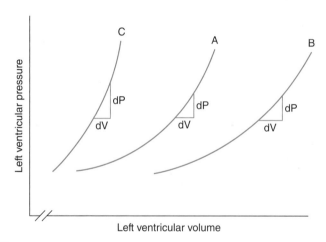

Figure 2–7. Pressure and volume are related in the ventricle through the compliance relationship depicted here. Normal compliance curve (A) relates changes in left ventricular volume to changes in left ventricular pressure. Moving along the normal curve, increases in left ventricular volume are initially tolerated with minimal changes in pressure. However, as end-diastolic volume increases, the left ventricular end-diastolic pressure rises. The less compliant curve (C) reflects a left ventricle as might be seen in a patient with a chronic pressure overload of the left ventricle such as in aortic stenosis or chronic hypertension. Here, left ventricular end-diastolic pressure rises rapidly with changing volume conditions. Consequently, such patients are at risk for the development of pulmonary edema with minimal increases in left ventricular end-diastolic volume. Conversely, the highly compliant curve (B) reflects a heart, which accommodates large changes in volume with minimal changes in pressure. Such conditions might be seen in patients with chronic, compensated aortic or mitral regurgitation, whereby the left ventricle is volume overloaded. In time, compensatory mechanisms fail and the ventricle becomes progressively noncompliant. (Reproduced with permission from Hoffman WJ, Wasnick JD: *Postoperative Critical Care of the Massachusetts General Hospital,* 2nd ed. Boston, MA: Wolters Kluwer; 1992.)

The PA catheter can indirectly determine the LVEDP. In the absence of mitral stenosis, the LVEDP should be reflected in the left atrial pressure (LAP), which in turn is estimated by the PCWP. So why is this useful? Utilizing estimates of both the SV and the LVEDP permits discernment of the cause of perioperative hypotension.

Recall that should the SV be reduced there are two main considerations, altered pump function or decreased preload.

The SV is obtained by dividing the CO by the heart rate (CO/HR). The PA catheter provides estimates of both the CVP and PCWP. The PCWP is an indirect measure of the LVEDP. Moreover, the LVEDP reflects the volume load of the heart depending on ventricular compliance. If the heart is noncompliant—such as in elderly patients—minimal changes in volume will produce somewhat exaggerated increases in LVEDP. Consequently, the LVEDP (estimated by PCWP) may not fully reflect the LVEDV.

Should a hypotensive patient have a low SV, the next approach using the PA catheter to determine the cause of hemodynamic instability is to estimate the LVEDP. If the patient is hypotensive with a low SV and a reduced LVEDP, then the patient is most likely hypovolemic except when the CVP is increased. Should the LVEDP be low and the CVP elevated, decreased left ventricular filling should be considered secondary to right heart failure, tension pneumothorax, or pericardial tamponade.

If the patient is hypotensive with a low SV and an elevated PCWP, then impaired left ventricular function should be suspected in the differential diagnosis.

Of course, PA catheter data should not be employed in isolation. Information obtained from other monitors must be used. The electrocardiogram is reviewed for signs of ischemia and arrhythmia. Medical history and physical examination should be reviewed regarding the possibility of tamponade, volume loss, cardiomyopathy, or pneumothorax.

Although the PA catheter and the approach outlined above was used for decades in cardiac surgery operating rooms and intensive care units to guide hemodynamic management, evidence supporting its ongoing routine use is lacking. Moreover, the availability of echocardiography, as this chapter will demonstrate, permits rapid diagnosis of hypotension. Cardiogenic, hypovolemic, and distributive (vasodilatory) shock states can be rapidly identified using established guidelines such as the FATE protocol (see Introduction to Perioperative Echocardiography).

Hypertension and Hemodynamics

Like hypotension, hypertension contributes to morbidity and mortality in the cardiac surgery patient. Patients routinely scheduled for cardiac surgery are treated with diuretics, beta-blockers, and angiotensin converting enzyme inhibitors to control long-standing hypertension. Antihypertensive medications are generally continued perioperatively.

Acute episodes of perioperative hypertension are usually secondary to increases in sympathetic tone associated with inadequate anesthesia, anxiety, and the natural response to surgical stress. Intraoperative management of hypertension is often treated with increasing anesthetic depth. Nitroprusside, nitroglycerin, clevidipine, nicardipine, and beta-blockers are used as needed. Recall that blood pressure is the product of cardiac output and systemic vascular resistance. Hypotension is treated either by increasing SVR and/or CO. To augment SVR, vasopressors are administered. Volume and/or inotropic agents increase CO. Interventions to lower BP likewise decrease SVR and CO.

THE PUMPING HEART: HOW DOES THE PUMP CONTRACT AND RELAX?

Ultimately, the function of the heart is to deliver oxygenated blood to the tissues. If the heart fails to do this, patients develop cardiogenic shock and metabolic acidosis. In the perioperative period, anesthetists can do much to either improve or hinder heart pump function. Hemodynamic fundamentals can assist the anesthesiologist in determining the adequacy of cardiac performance and in designing appropriate therapy to assist the failing heart.

Unfortunately, many patients today present to surgery and anesthesia with reduced ventricular function.[31-33] Chronic hypertension, myocardial ischemia, valvular heart disease, and cardiomyopathies often result in hearts that neither forcefully contract nor effectively relax and, therefore, manifest systolic and diastolic dysfunction, respectively.[34-36]

Systolic Function

Systolic ventricular dysfunction occurs when the left ventricle fails to contract resulting in a reduced SV. Patients attempt to compensate for this reduction in ejection fraction (EF, nl = 50% to 60%) by increasing sympathetic tone. An examination of hemodynamic principles is useful for understanding this compensatory mechanism.

Recall,

$$BP = CO \times SVR$$
$$SV = CO/HR$$
$$SV = LVEDV - LVESV$$
$$EF = SV/LVEDV \times 100\%$$

Therefore, the EF represents the percentage of blood volume ejected with each SV from the total volume filling the heart at the end diastole. Normal EF is 50% or more. Patients with varying degrees of systolic dysfunction have reduced EF. Indeed, anesthesiologists may be called to anesthetize patients with EF less than 20%. And yet, these patients with poor systolic function can nonetheless compensate for their dysfunction.

The body compensates for reduction in SV by attempting to augment vascular tone and heart rate through increased catecholamine release. Additionally, the renin-angiotensin-aldosterone system is activated to increase the volume load presented to the heart. Angiotensin is a vasoconstrictor, and aldosterone inhibits sodium urinary excretion leading to fluid retention.

By increasing sympathetic tone and heart rate, the low EF patient manages to maintain BP and organ perfusion in the setting of reduced SV. Although compensated at baseline, these patients may acutely and precipitously decompensate during delivery of general anesthesia. Anesthetic agents often decrease sympathetic outflow. Because sympathetic tone is critical to low EF patients to maintain blood pressure, these patients often suffer hemodynamic collapse during anesthetic induction. Anesthetic management of heart failure patients will be discussed in detail in Chapter 5.

The renin-angiotensin-aldosterone response to systolic failure increases the volume presented to the heart. This increase in preload is helpful secondary to the Frank-Starling relationship (Figure 2–8).

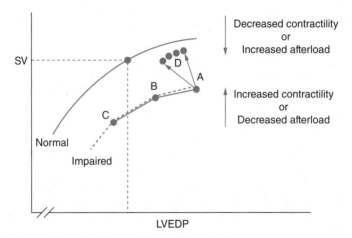

Figure 2–8. The Frank-Starling curves depicted here relate the loading conditions of the left ventricle [preload—as measured by left ventricular end-diastolic pressure (LVEDP)] and stroke volume. Stroke volume (SV) is the amount of blood ejected into the aorta by the heart with each beat.

Changes in afterload (vascular resistance), preload (volume delivered to the ventricle to eject), and contractility can all interact to change the stroke volume. Point A represents a patient with systolic heart failure. The LVEDP of this impaired patient is high, and the SV is low compared to that expected in the normal patient. Reducing the patient's preload moves the patient from point A to points B and C. The SV is relatively unchanged at point B; however, the LVEDP is reduced. This can occur secondary to the use of diuretic therapy. The lower LVEDP may reduce symptoms of fluid overload and congestion. However, advancing to point C, SV is further reduced bringing into question the adequacy of tissue oxygen delivery.

Increasing contractility and decreasing afterload through the use of inodilators such as milrinone will move the patient's Starling curve to points D, reflecting an increased SV and a lower LVEDP and thereby relieving both symptoms of congestive heart failure and improving tissue oxygen delivery. Note for the same LVEDP, the SV is lower in the patient with impaired ventricular function. (Reproduced with permission from Hoffman WJ, Wasnick JD: *Postoperative Critical Care of the Massachusetts General Hospital*, 2nd ed. Boston, MA: Wolters Kluwer; 1992.)

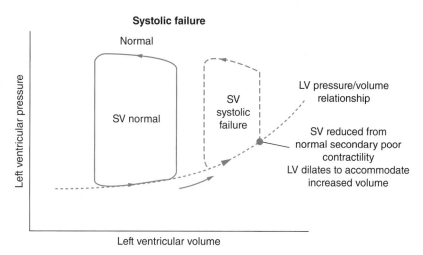

Figure 2–9. The pressure-volume loop of a patient with systolic failure. The heart dilates to accommodate increased volume to maintain the SV with minimal increase in LV pressure.

The Starling curve demonstrates that as the LVEDV increases, the SV increases up to a point. Consequently, to augment the SV, the body responds by increasing the size of the heart. Hence, many failing hearts are dilated and enlarged. As such, even if contracting very poorly during systole, the low EF heart is capable of generating an SV sufficient to meet the patient's metabolic needs at least under rest conditions (Figure 2–9). The effects of the compensatory responses to systolic failure are also responsible for many of the signs and symptoms often seen in the heart failure patient, which ultimately lead to a "downward spiral" of progressive myocardial dysfunction (Figure 2–10).

Diastolic Function

Diastolic ventricular dysfunction can present independently or associated with systolic ventricular dysfunction. Isolated diastolic dysfunction is often seen in hypertensive patients with a hypertrophied left ventricle. Once again, an understanding of hemodynamic basics can explain the development of this condition.
Recall,

$$BP = CO \times SVR$$
$$CO = SV \times HR$$

SV is determined by:

1. Preload or the volume presented to the left ventricle
2. Myocardial contractility
3. Afterload or the resistance against which the heart must pump

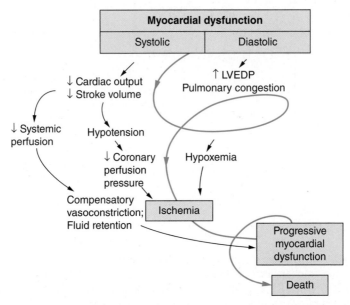

Figure 2-10. The "downward spiral" in cardiogenic shock. Stroke volume and cardiac output fall with left ventricle (LV) dysfunction, producing hypotension and tachycardia that reduce coronary blood flow. Increasing ventricular diastolic pressure reduces coronary blood flow, and increased wall stress elevates myocardial oxygen requirements. All of these factors combine to worsen ischemia. The falling cardiac output also compromises systemic perfusion. Compensatory mechanisms include sympathetic stimulation and fluid retention to increase preload. These mechanisms can actually worsen cardiogenic shock by increasing myocardial oxygen demand and afterload. Thus, a vicious circle can be established. LVEDP, left ventricular end-diastolic pressure. [Reproduced with permission from Hollenberg SM, Kavinsky CJ, Parrillo JE: Cardiogenic shock, *Ann Intern Med.* 1999 Jul 6;131(1):47-59.]

Increases in afterload maintain SVR but reduce CO and SV. In response to afterload increases, the heart compensates by hypertrophy. However, as discussed earlier, compensatory mechanisms present their own particular problems. In the case of the thickened myocardium, these problems include diastolic dysfunction and increased risk of ischemia.

The heart requires energy not only in systole but also in early diastole during relaxation to move calcium from the myocardial cell back to the cell's sarcoplasmic reticulum. The relaxed ventricle then fills with low pressures easily during diastole. The patient with diastolic dysfunction relaxes poorly resulting in an elevated LVEDP (Figure 2–11). The elevated LVEDP is transmitted to the pulmonary vasculature ultimately leading to pulmonary congestion and right ventricular failure. Diastolic dysfunction in the cardiac surgery patient will be discussed in Chapter 5.

Coronary Arteries Circulation

The blood supply to the heart is provided by the right and left coronary arteries (Figure 2–12).

Diastolic failure

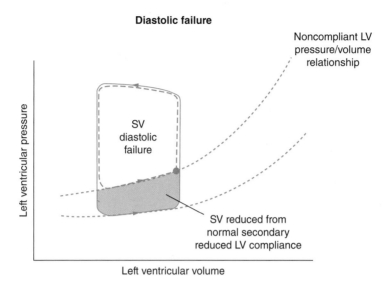

Figure 2–11. In patients with diastolic dysfunction, the SV is reduced due to impaired ventricular filling. LV pressure is higher for the same LV volume as compared to a normally compliant ventricle.

Coronary perfusion pressure (CPP) determines blood flow to the myocardium.

CPP = Diastolic blood pressure – Left (Right) ventricular end-diastolic pressure

Perfusion of the left ventricle occurs predominantly in diastole, while perfusion of the normal right ventricle, which operates at lower intracavitary pressures,

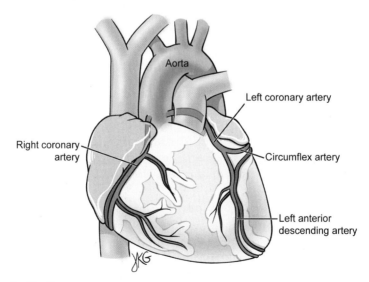

Figure 2–12. The coronary arteries.

occurs throughout the cardiac cycle. CPP is reduced when diastolic blood pressure is decreased (e.g., when a patient has wide-open aortic regurgitation and thus a low diastolic pressure) or when left or right ventricle EDP is increased (e.g., patients with noncompliant ventricles and diastolic dysfunction).

Tachycardia reduces diastolic time and as such puts the heart at risk for ischemia. Lastly, the oxygen content of the blood determines oxygen delivery to the heart as well as the other tissues. Anemia, decreased oxygen saturation, and hemoglobinopathies can all reduce the delivery of oxygen to the tissues and the heart.

Myocardial oxygen demand is increased by tachycardia, increased myocardial contractility, and increased myocardial wall tension.

Myocardial wall tension is expressed in the law of LaPlace.

LaPlace law:

$$\text{Myocardial wall tension} = \frac{(\text{Ventricular radius} \times \text{Ventricular pressure})}{2(\text{Ventricular wall thickness})}$$

Increased myocardial wall tension increases myocardial oxygen demand, and thickening of the ventricular wall reduces the wall tension. Consequently, in situations of increased afterload, the heart hypertrophies to decrease myocardial wall tension. Ultimately, this compensatory hypertrophy results in increased myocardial mass progressing to worsening heart failure and cardiac myocyte death. Brain natriuretic protein (BNP) is produced in response to myocyte distention associated with the failing heart and is a useful biomarker in heart failure patients as it reflects the heart's deleterious compensatory remodeling.

The Mechanism of Myocardial Contraction

Myocardial contraction is initiated by spontaneous depolarization of the conduction tissues. The generated action potentials are propagated throughout the heart. When the myocardial sarcolemma depolarizes, intracellular calcium concentration increases due to extracellular calcium entering the cell and due to release of calcium from the sarcoplasmic reticulum. Contraction is initiated when calcium binds to troponin C and results in a conformational change, which ultimately leads to cross bridging of actin with myosin. At the end of contraction, calcium is actively pumped back out of the cell and into the sarcoplasmic reticulum and relaxation begins.

Rhythm and conduction will be discussed in detail in Chapter 3.

Contraction results in thickening of the myocardium, inward movement of the endocardium, and twisting and torqueing of the heart (Video 2–3).

Right Heart Function

Right heart function is essential to overall cardiac performance.[37] When blood returns from the superior vena cava (SVC) and the inferior vena cava (IVC), it enters the right atrium. Right ventricular contraction then delivers the venous blood into the pulmonary circulation for gas exchange and further to the left heart for ejection into the systemic circulation (Video 2–4). The left heart must generate the systemic blood pressure, but the right heart and pulmonary circulation are low-pressure systems. The normal pulmonary arterial systolic pressures are often less than 20 mm Hg. When pulmonary artery pressures are elevated as seen in left heart failure, pulmonary disease, or protamine reaction, the right heart (a low-pressure system) can be overwhelmed. In such circumstances the right heart becomes distended and functions poorly (Video 2–5). Because the right heart and the left heart pump blood in series, right heart failure will ultimately lead to decreased CO and decreased organ perfusion.

Right heart failure is associated with increased CVP and often results in peripheral edema and hepatic engorgement.

PHARMACOLOGY AND HEMODYNAMICS: AN INTRODUCTION

There are many drugs and mechanical devices that can be employed to improve hemodynamic performance. Mechanical assistance of the failing heart is discussed in Chapter 11.

The pharmacologic armamentarium employed to manipulate hemodynamics must take into account the etiology of hemodynamic instability.

Hypertension

Generally in the perioperative period, hypertensive episodes are secondary to increased sympathetic outflow subsequent to inadequate anesthesia, surgical stress, or preexisting hypertension. Should a patient be found to be hypertensive, therapy can be directed at either reducing cardiac output or reducing sympathetic tone. There are many pharmacological agents available that will achieve these effects.

Drugs that reduce heart rate and myocardial contractility will have primary effects upon the CO. Such agents include the beta-blockers (esmolol, propranolol, metoprolol) and certain calcium antagonists. Other agents are primary vasodilators (nitroglycerin, nitroprusside, hydralazine, fenoldopam, nicardipine, clevidipine) (see Table 2–3). Many times intraoperatively, patients require supplemental anesthetic agents (e.g., fentanyl, inhalational agents, propofol, or midazolam). During recovery in the ICU, patients frequently become hypertensive as anesthetic effects wane or pain control is inadequate. Infusions of propofol, fenoldopam, dexmedetomidine, and calcium channel antagonists are frequently employed postoperatively. Nitric oxide and prostaglandin analogs (e.g., iloprost) are useful in treating pulmonary hypertension.

The specifics of anesthetic management of the cardiac surgery patient will be discussed in Chapter 4.

Hypotension

The pharmacologic management of perioperative hypotension in the cardiac surgical patient is of urgent concern. In the cardiac surgery patient, hypotension often leads to myocardial ischemia, which produces ventricular dysfunction followed by even more severe hypotension—ending in hemodynamic collapse and circulatory arrest.

Table 2–3. Vasodilators

Drug	Dosage
Clevidipine	1-16 mg/h
Fenoldopam	0.03-0.6 mcg/kg/min
Nicardipine	2.5-10 mg/h
Nitric oxide	10-60 ppm (inhaled)
Nitroglycerin	0.5-10 mcg/kg/min
Nitroprusside	0.5-10 mcg/kg/min
Prostaglandin E_1	0.01-0.2 mcg/kg/min

Reproduced with permission from Butterworth JF, Mackey DC, Wasnick JD: *Morgan & Mikhail's Clinical Anesthesiology*, 6th ed. New York, NY: McGraw-Hill Education; 2018.

Once again,

$$BP = CO \times SVR$$

Consequently, pharmacologic therapies are directed at the underlying fundamental cause of hypotension.

Should the patient be hypotensive because of reductions in SVR, vasoconstrictors are administered. The common practice of administering small doses of phenylephrine to treat peri-induction hypotension is one such example of the use of a vasconstricting drug to augment blood pressure following anesthesia induction. The indirect acting agent, ephedrine, similarly produces vasoconstriction through its release of endogenous norepinephrine. Infusions of phenylephrine or norepinephrine are frequently employed to augment vascular tone. Likewise, vasopressin as a 1 unit (U) intravenous bolus or by infusion (up to 0.08-0.1 U/min) can be administered to restore vascular tone.

Reductions in CO are somewhat more complicated. Should the CO be reduced because of hypovolemia, then volume administration is the appropriate response. If the CO is reduced secondary to an arrhythmia (e.g., atrial fibrillation with loss of atrial contraction or a ventricular arrhythmia), then correction of the rhythm disturbance would be immediately indicated. Similarly, if CO were to be reduced because of compression of the heart by pericardial tamponade or tension pneumothorax, then appropriate treatment of those conditions is warranted. In patients with systolic left ventricular failure, inotropes can be used to improve myocardial contractility.

A reduced SV can be restored by increasing ventricular volume, increasing myocardial contractility, or reducing the afterload.

Although administration of additional volume might increase SV in the patient with impaired left ventricle (LV) function, this may carry the cost of an increased LVEDP and pulmonary congestion depending where the LV is functioning along the Starling curve. Increased LVEDP will be reflected in increased PCWP and most likely increased pulmonary artery diastolic (PAD) pressure. Increased pressure in the pulmonary vasculature can lead to pulmonary edema and hypoxemia. The compensatory activation of the renin angiotensin aldosterone system in LV failure patients can contribute to dyspnea and acute congestive heart failure (CHF) perioperatively. Conversely, many cardiac surgery patients are hypovolemic preoperatively secondary to aggressive diuretic therapy and thus require volume administration to treat hypotension at the time of anesthetic induction. As will be seen in the upcoming section of this chapter, echocardiography answers many questions regarding both the patient's ventricular function and their volume status.

There are various inotropic agents that can be employed to increase LV contractility. Epinephrine, dobutamine, and dopamine are examples of agents that interact with the beta-1 sympathetic receptors on the heart to augment contractility by increasing Ca^{2+} in the myocyte.

The use of these agents is not without potential complications. The routine use of inotropes may contribute to increased patient morbidity and mortality.[38,39]

Catecholamine-like drugs such as epinephrine and dopamine can produce arrhythmias, tachycardias, and vasoconstriction. In addition to its inotropic effect, dobutamine can also produce vasodilation. This effect is often desirable because vasodilatation reduces the work against which the failing heart must pump. However, lower BP can potentially reduce the CPP.

Recall,

$$CPP = DBP - LVEDP$$

Fortunately, vasodilatation coupled with augmented SV could reduce mean LVEDP as well, therefore maintaining CPP.

Inodilators, such as milrinone, are frequently employed to both increase SV and decrease SVR. Milrinone is a phosphodiesterase inhibitor, which augments myocardial contractility.[40] Like catecholamines, milrinone can lead to hypotension and arrhythmia. Often it is necessary to support the blood pressure with a vasopressor to provide enough blood pressure for tissue perfusion (Figure 2–13).

Recently, a new class of inotropes, the calcium ion sensitizers (e.g., levosimendan 0.05 to 0.2 mcg/kg/min) has emerged. Rather than increasing intracellular calcium ion concentration, they sensitize troponin C to the intracellular calcium present resulting in enhanced myocardial contractility. The investigative drug, omecamtiv mecarbil, works as a cardiac myosin activator and increases the efficiency of cardiac muscle contraction.

Strategies in the inotropic treatment of the patient with systolic and diastolic heart failure will be discussed in greater detail in Chapter 5. Commonly employed vasopressors and inotropes are summarized in Table 2–4.

Right Heart Failure

The right heart and the left heart pump in series. Consequently, right heart failure can compromise left heart performance producing cardiogenic shock, reduced organ perfusion, and acidosis.[35]

Signs of right heart failure include peripheral edema and hepatic enlargement. Hepatic dysfunction may result in coagulopathy. Much as an elevated PCWP might indicate a noncompliant, distended, failing left heart, an increased CVP may herald a failing right heart.

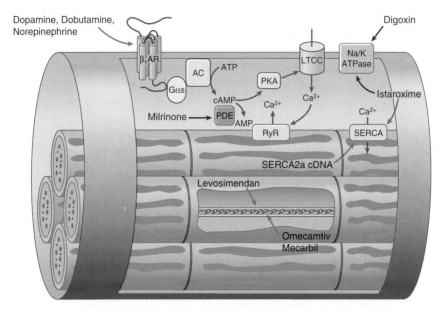

Figure 2–13. Diagram of intracellular signaling cascades within cardiomyocytes altered by inotropes. Dopamine, dobutamine, and norepinephrine activate the β1-adrenergic receptor, which activates the G protein Gαs, which in turn, activates adenylyl cyclase. Adenylyl cyclase converts ATP to cAMP when activated. cAMP can activate PKA, which then phosphorylates the L-type calcium channel, among other targets. cAMP is converted to AMP by PDE. Milrinone inhibits PDE-3 thereby increasing the effective concentration of cAMP. Calcium influx through the L-type calcium channel induces activation of ryanodine receptors, leading to calcium-induced calcium release. Free intracellular calcium interacts with troponin C, which changes the binding properties of tropomyosin and allows the interaction between actin and myosin. Levosimendan potentiates the interaction between troponin and calcium. It may also have PDE-3 inhibitor activity as well. Omecamtiv mecarbil increases the rate of ATP turnover and slows the rate of ADP release thereby increasing the number of myosin molecules bound to actin at any given time. SERCA is responsible for uptake of calcium into the sarcoplasmic reticulum while the Na/K ATPase participates in resetting the membrane potential of the cell. Istaroxime inhibits Na/K ATPase while also potentiating SERCA. Digoxin inhibits the Na/K ATPase. **Red arrows** denote agonists, whereas **black arrows** signify antagonists. AC = adenylyl cyclase; ADP = adenosine diphosphate; ATP = adenosine triphosphate; B1AR = β1-adrenergic receptor; cAMP = cyclic adenosine monophosphate; LTCC = L-type calcium channel; PDE = phosphodiesterase; PKA = protein kinase A; RyR = ryanodine receptor; SERCA = sarco/endoplasmic reticulum Ca^{2+}-ATPase. [Reproduced with permission from Francis GS, Bartos JA, Adatya S: Inotropes, *J Am Coll Cardiol.* 2014 May 27;63(20): 2069-2078.]

Often the right and left hearts do not fail in isolation but concurrently. A failed left heart results in an increased LVEDP. Elevated pulmonary artery pressures follow, leading to right ventricle (RV) dilatation and dysfunction. Severe tricuspid regurgitation can be seen in the setting of a dilated right ventricle.

Table 2–4. Vasopressors and Inotropic Agents*

	Bolus	Infusion	Adrenergic activity α	β	Indirect	Phosphodiesterase inhibition
Epinephrine	2-10 mcg	0.01-0.03 mcg/kg/min	+	+++	0	0
		0.04-0.1 mcg/kg/min	++	+++	0	0
		>0.1 mcg/kg/min	+++	+++	0	0
Norepinephrine		0.01-0.1 mcg/kg/min	+++	++	0	0
Isoproterenol	1-4 mcg	0.01-0.1 mcg/kg/min	0	+++	0	0
Dobutamine		2-20 mcg/kg/min	+	++	0	0
Dopamine		2-10 mcg/kg/min	+	++	+	0
		10-20 mcg/kg/min	++	++	+	0
Ephedrine	5-25 mg		+	++	+	0
Phenylephrine	50-200 mcg	10-50 mcg/min	+++	0	0	0
Inamrinone	0.5-1.5 mg/kg	5-10 mcg/kg/min	0	0	0	+++
Milrinone	50 mcg/kg	0.375-0.75 mcg/kg/min	0	0	0	+++
Vasopressin	1-2 units	2-8 units/h	0	0	0	0

*+, mild activity; ++, moderate activity; +++, marked activity.

Reproduced with permission from Butterworth JF, Mackey DC, Wasnick JD: *Morgan & Mikhail's Clinical Anesthesiology*, 6th ed. New York, NY: McGraw-Hill Education; 2018.

There are no specific drug therapies for RV failure. Efforts are generally directed at reducing pulmonary arterial pressures and increasing right ventricular contractility. Milrinone is frequently employed to treat RV failure perioperatively because of its inodilating properties.

Inhaled nitric oxide (NO) is a pulmonary vasodilator, which directly reduces PAP. The advantage of NO is that its effects are limited to the pulmonary circulation preserving systemic blood pressure.

RV failure and the treatment of pulmonary hypertension will be discussed in greater detail in Chapter 8.

TEE AND HEMODYNAMIC INSTABILITY: HOW TEE ADVANCES THE DIAGNOSIS OF HYPOTENSION?

Both transthoracic echocardiography (TTE) and transesophageal echocardiography (TEE) can be employed in the perioperative period to aid in the diagnosis of hemodynamic instability.[41,42]

The advantage of hemodynamically focused echocardiography is that it is not necessary to obtain calculated parameters to diagnosis the etiology of hypotension. Rather, the answer to *"Why is the patient hypotensive?"* is one or more of the following: volume depletion, vasodilation, pump failure, or external compression of the heart (e.g., pericardial tamponade, tension pneumothorax). Echocardiography identifies the sources of hemodynamic instability using imagery rather than pressure estimates and SV thermodilution calculations.

The introduction provided a review of the basic views and images, which can be obtained using transesophageal echocardiography. Usually the transgastric midpapillary short-axis view is useful to quickly assess the function of the heart. A normally contracting and adequately volume loaded ventricle is obvious to physicians with very little echocardiography experience.

In hypovolemic patients, the transgastric midpapillary short-axis view will show a hyperdynamic LV with the ventricular cavity obliterated with each heart beat due to very low LVEDV as well as an equally empty right ventricle (**Video Intro–14**). The hypovolemic patient is also likely to have a reduced SV, PCWP, and CVP. Reduced SVR (e.g., in patients with SIRS) can also produce a TEE image where the LV cavity is significantly diminished during systole but perhaps not to the extent as found in the setting of profound hypovolemia. As always, echocardiography diagnoses should be informed by the patient's medical history, physical examination, and laboratory studies. All this information can help distinguish between possible etiologies.

TEE examination can easily reveal mechanical compression of the heart (e.g., pericardial tamponade) as a cause of inadequate volume loading of the left heart and hypotension (**Video 2–6**).

TEE can likewise determine if the heart is not functioning adequately as a pump secondary to global LV dysfunction (**Video Intro–6**), RV dysfunction, or isolated areas of LV dysfunction secondary to myocardial ischemia (**Video 2–7**). In severe ventricular dysfunction, stasis of blood within the heart appears as a spontaneous echo contrast or "smoke" in the left atrium and occasionally in the LV (**Video 2–8**).

Such patients are likely to have a very limited ability to respond to the decrease in SVR, which occurs at the time of anesthetic induction.

RV failure can occur associated with LV failure or secondary to pulmonary arterial hypertension. In the transgastric mid-papillary view, the crescent moon that characterizes the image of the healthy RV becomes more spherical and the interventricular septum shifts toward the LV.

TEE also can detect areas of the heart that are dysfunctional. During myocardial infarction (MI), coronary artery thrombosis occludes blood flow to regions of the myocardium in the vessel's distribution. When that occurs, the myocardium becomes dysfunctional by failing to thicken and move inward with each systole (Video 2–9). Additionally, by identifying the area of the myocardium that is dysfunctional, it is possible to determine which of the coronary arteries is likely affected (Video 2–10).

Thus, by simple visual inspection it is possible to make rapid assessments of the causes of perioperative hemodynamic instability. Of course, echocardiography can also quantify LV function.

Estimates of ventricular function include measures of fractional shortening (Figure 2–14) and fractional area change (Video 2–11). Fractional area change measurements assess the function of the ventricle by examining changes not along a single line as in fractional shortening but by changes in the area of the ventricular cavity during systole and diastole.

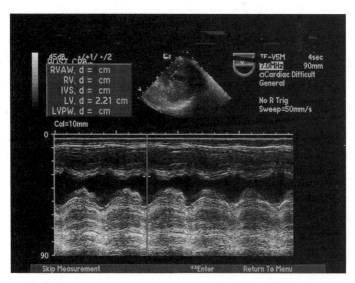

Figure 2–14A. M-mode echocardiography is used to estimate the left ventricular diastolic and systolic dimensions. M mode provides a one-dimensional image of the heart along the beam line. The diastolic dimension is measured here. The end-systolic and end-diastolic intracavitary diameters can be measured, and the fractional shortening can be calculated. Fractional shortening is a rough estimate of left ventricular myocardial performance in the absence of wall motion abnormalities.

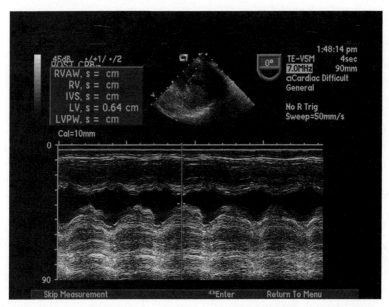

Figure 2–14B. Now, the measure is obtained when the ventricle contracts in systole to determine fractional shortening.

Fractional shortening = (LV end-diastolic diameter

− LV end-systolic diameter)/LV end-diastolic diameter × 100

Normal values = 25% to 45%

Fractional area change (FAC) = (LV end-diastolic area

− LV end-systolic area)/LV end-diastolic area × 100

Normal values range between 55% and 65%.

The modified Simpson rule "method of discs" attempts to estimate the LV volume in systole and diastole (Video 2–12). Using incorporated software, the LV volume can be estimated by considering the LV cavity as a series of stacked discs. The LV cavity is traced at the end of systole (fully contracted) and at the end of diastole (fully filled). The machine then generates a stack of discs. Much as a pile of pennies stacked on end would create a cylinder, the machine generates a series of discs of different size. The machine calculates the volume of the stack of discs using their area and thickness, which are known both during diastole and systole. Three-dimensional echocardiography can also be employed to assess ventricular function (Video 2–13). In truth, experienced echocardiographers in the operating room often use visual impressions rather than formally calculating the EF in this way.

Echocardiography can also be used to assess SV, CO, and intracavitary pressures as described in detail in the chapter "Introduction to Perioperative Echocardiography."

The SV can be calculated using echocardiography by knowing the area through which blood travels and the distance traveled during an individual heartbeat.

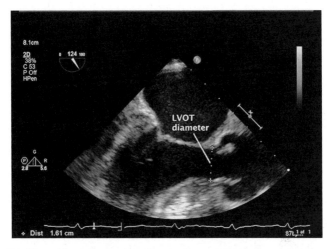

Figure 2–15. The mid-esophageal aortic valve long-axis view is used to determine the diameter of the left ventricular outflow tract (LVOT), which is 1.61 cm.

The left ventricular outflow tract provides a good location to make these determinations with TEE (Figure 2–15).

$$SV = Area_{LVOT} \times TVI_{LVOT}$$

By approximating the shape of the LVOT with a cylinder, the area of the LVOT can be calculated by measuring the LVOT diameter. By integrating the flow velocities of the blood passing through the LVOT, the distance that the blood travels is obtained [the time velocity integral (TVI)]:

$$LVOT\ area = \pi \times (d/2)^2$$

Therefore,

$$SV\ (cm^3\ or\ mL) = (0.785\ d^2) \times TVI$$

Now, CO can be calculated using the formula:

$$SV \times HR = CO$$

The left atrial pressure (LAP) can also be calculated by echocardiography. The Bernoulli equation was previously introduced.

$$Pressure\ gradient\ between\ two\ cardiac\ chambers = 4V^2$$

where V is the maximal blood flow velocity measured by Doppler from the high-pressure chamber to the low-pressure chamber.

To calculate the LAP using this method, the patient must have mitral regurgitation. When the LV contracts during systole if MR is present, some of the blood will be ejected not out the aorta but back through the closed mitral valve. Being ejected through the closed mitral valve the blood will likely move at a high velocity from the high-pressure LV to the lower-pressure LA. By using continuous wave Doppler the peak velocity of this regurgitant jet can be measured. Once the velocity is known, Bernoulli's equation can be employed to determine the LAP based on the pressure gradient between LV and LA during systole.

Because this flow of blood happens during systole, the pressure in the LV during systole is the same (assuming no aortic stenosis or obstruction to ventricular outflow) as the systolic arterial blood pressure obtained from other monitors.

So,

$$\text{Pressure gradient} = 4V^2$$

Also,

$$\text{LV systolic pressure} - \text{LA pressure} = 4V^2$$
$$(-)\text{LA pressure} = 4V^2 - \text{LV systolic pressure}$$

where, V is the maximal flow velocity of the mitral regurgitant jet.

Hence,

$$\text{LA pressure} = \text{LV systolic pressure} - 4V^2$$

Pressure estimates such as these are routinely done in the echocardiography laboratory; however, in the operating room such estimates are less frequently performed. Echocardiography is a very useful tool to determine why a patient might be hemodynamically unstable. Increasingly echocardiography is available not only in the operating room but in ICU settings. Consequently, the PA catheter is ever less likely to be employed in cardiac surgery patients to assist in perioperative hemodynamic management.

AVOIDING HEMODYNAMIC COLLAPSE: A CASE ILLUSTRATION

A 53-year-old man presents for exploratory laparotomy secondary to ischemic bowel. His vital signs are BP 70/40 mm Hg, HR 110 bpm, respiratory rate (RR) 29 breaths per minute, 102°F. A preoperative ECG demonstrates a left bundle branch block (LBBB). He denies other medical problems except for occasional episodes of chest tightness when he climbs stairs and he has three-pillow orthopnea. He has had no prior medical evaluations.

Obviously this patient presents a number of immediate concerns and possible etiologies to his hypotension. He may be hypovolemic secondary to volume loss from the perforated bowel, or he might be septic from peritonitis. On the other hand, his LBBB and intermittent chest pain could also suggest that his hypotension is cardiogenic in nature.

So basically, the patient presents with possible hypovolemic shock, cardiogenic shock, and/or vasodilatory (distributive) shock—and he is about to undergo general anesthesia.

Questions to Consider

1. What monitors will be of assistance in managing this case? What monitors are essential? What monitors are optional? What are the risks and potential complications?
2. How should the induction of this patient be managed?
3. Why is he hypotensive and how should his hypotension be treated?

Frankly, none of these questions are easy and as with so many things in anesthesiology there are no absolute answers.

Possible Answers

This is a critically ill patient at very high risk of experiencing severe hemodynamic compromise at the time of induction. Arterial pressure monitoring would appear indicated along with central access to provide for volume and/or vasoactive substance administration. The LBBB potentially complicates placement of a PA catheter. As the PA catheter passes through the right heart, it could produce a transient right bundle branch block leading to complete heart block. The LBBB also complicates the ECG diagnosis of myocardial ischemia, and thus TEE would be useful assuming there are no contraindications to its placement. (See Introduction to Perioperative Echocardiography.)

Assuming that arterial and central lines have been placed, the anesthesiologist will benefit from more information regarding the etiology of his hypotension and on how best to proceed with induction. Pulse contour analysis of the arterial waveform could be used to estimate CO. Likewise, measurements of stroke volume variation (SVV) in patients receiving positive pressure ventilation provide an estimate of volume responsiveness. SVV greater than 10% to 15% indicate that the patient will likely benefit from volume administration. However, many studies related to volume responsiveness in patients receiving positive pressure ventilation were performed before the routine use of perioperative protective ventilation strategies (tidal volume < 6 mg/kg). The CVP may be helpful but does not reflect LV performance. In this patient the RAP is 8 mm Hg and intravenous fluid is given. As the patient's BP increases to 95/60 mm Hg, general anesthesia is induced with etomidate and succinylcholine. After a successful intubation and application of positive pressure ventilation, the BP decreases to 60/40 mm Hg. Phenylephrine and additional fluid are administered with minimal response. A TEE probe is placed. What is demonstrated by this echo image (Video 2–14)? As can be seen, the patient appears to have a hyperdynamic heart. Indeed, the papillary muscles come together nearly obliterating the ventricular cavity during systole. In this setting, it appears that the patient may be hypovolemic and septic; therefore, vasoconstrictors and additional volume are given.

How would management have changed if Video 2–15 was observed at the time of probe placement? A grossly dysfunctional left ventricle is seen. Therapy with inotropic agents such as epinephrine to improve ventricular function would be indicated. Mechanical support might also be indicated to assist ventricular function.

Assuming the patient did not have an LBBB and a PA catheter was placed, what would be the SV and PCWP if the patient was in (a) primarily hypovolemic shock,

(b) primarily vasodilated shock, or in (c) cardiogenic shock? If the patient is hypovolemic, expect the patient to have a reduced SV with low PCWP. If the patient is vasodilated, the SV could be elevated with a midrange to low PCWP. On the other hand, if the patient is in cardiogenic shock, expect a reduced SV and high PCWP. Of course, the patient could be hypovolemic, septic, and in heart failure. In that setting, the picture becomes somewhat cloudy. Nonetheless, hemodynamic measures obtained from PiCCO or PA catheters along with echo images can be used concurrently to guide perioperative therapy. Whether there is definitive scientific evidence that any of these monitoring devices actually affect overall outcome remains uncertain. Essentially, when addressing hemodynamic instability, diagnostic tools are employed to guide therapy realizing that occasionally multiple etiologies might be at work making the patient hypotensive, thus requiring the use of a combination of therapies for treatment. Using all these diagnostic approaches, you can answer the question, "Why is the patient hypotensive?"

REFERENCES

1. Bijker J, van Klei W, Kappen T, et al. Incidence of intraoperative hypotension as a function of the chosen definition: literature definitions applied to a retrospective cohort using automated data collection. *Anesthesiology*. 2007;107(2):213-220.

2. Eastridge B, Salinas J, McManus J, et al. Hypotension begins at 110 mm Hg: redefining "hypotension" with data. *J Trauma*. 2007;63(2):291-299.

3. Gueret G, Rossignol B, Kiss E, et al. Cardiac output measurements in off-pump coronary surgery: comparison between NICO and the Swan-Ganz catheter. *Eur J Anaesthesiol*. 2006;23:848-854.

4. Missant C, Rex S, Wouters P. Accuracy of cardiac output measurements with pulse contour analysis (Pulse CO) and Doppler echocardiography during off pump coronary artery bypass grafting. *Eur J Anaesthesiol*. 2008;25:243-248.

5. Manecke G, Auger W. Cardiac output determination from the arterial pressure wave: clinical testing of a novel algorithm that does not require calibration. *J Cardiothorac Vasc Anesth*. 2007;21(1):3-7.

6. Sandham J, Hull R, Brant R, et al. A randomized controlled trial of the uses of pulmonary artery catheters in high-risk surgical patients. *NEJM*. 2003;348(1):5-14.

7. Harvey S, Welch C, Harrison D, et al. Post hoc insights from PAC-MAN—the UK pulmonary artery catheter trial. *Crit Care Med*. 2008;36(6):1714-1721.

8. Resano F, Kapetanakis E, Hill P, et al. Clinical outcomes of low risk patients undergoing beating heart surgery with or without pulmonary artery catheterization. *J Cardiothorac Vasc Anesth*. 2006;20(3):300-306.

9. Djaiani G, Karski J, Yudin M, et al. Clinical outcomes in patients undergoing elective coronary artery bypass graft surgery with and without utilization of pulmonary artery catheter generated data. *J Cardiothorac Vasc Anesth*. 2006;20(3):307-310.

10. Cowie B. Does the pulmonary artery catheter still have a role in the perioperative period? *Anaesth Intensive Care*. 2011;39:345-355.

11. Darmon P, Hillel Z, Mogtader A, et al. Cardiac output by transesophageal echocardiography using continuous Doppler across the aortic valve. *Anesthesiology*. 1994;80(4):796-805.

12. Kohonen M, Teerenhovi O, Terho T, et al. Is the Allen test reliable enough? *Eur J Cardiothorac Surg*. 2007;37:902-905.

13. Jarvis M, Jarvis C, Jones P, et al. Reliability of Allen's test in selection of patients for radial artery harvest. *Ann Thorac Surg*. 2000;70:1362-1365.

14. Krein S, Hofer T, Kowalski C, et al. Use of central venous catheter related bloodstream prevention practices by US Hospitals. *Mayo Clin Proc*. 2007;82(6):672-678.

15. Pawar M, Mehta Y, Kapoor P, et al. Central venous catheter related blood stream infections: incidence, risk factors, outcome and associated pathogens. *J Cardiothorac Vasc Anesth*. 2004;18(3):304-308.

16. American Society of Anesthesiologists Task Force on Central Venous Access. Practice guidelines for central venous access. *Anesthesiology*. 2012;116(3):539-573.

17. Riopelle J, Ruiz D, Hunt J, et al. Circumferential adjustment of ultrasound probe position to determine the optimal approach to the internal jugular vein: a noninvasive geometric study in adults. *Anesth Analg.* 2005;100:512-519.

18. Calvert N, Hind D, McWilliams R, et al. Ultrasound for central venous cannulation: economic evaluation of cost effectiveness. *Anaesthesia.* 2004;59:1116-1120.

19. Ramsay J. Pro: is the pulmonary artery catheter dead? *J Cardiothorac Vasc Anesth.* 2007;21(1):144-146.

20. Murphy G, Vender J. Con: is the pulmonary artery catheter dead? *J Cardiothorac Vasc Anesth.* 2007;21(1):147-149.

21. Bossert T, Gummert J, Bittner H, et al. Swan Ganz catheter-induced severe complications in cardiac surgery: right ventricular perforation, knotting and rupture of a pulmonary artery. *J Card Surg.* 2006;21:292-295.

22. Muller L, Louart G, Bengler C, et al. The intrathoracic blood volume index as an indicator of fluid responsiveness in critically ill patients with acute circulatory failure: a comparison with central venous pressure. *Anesth Analg.* 2008;107(2):607-613.

23. Buettner M, Schummer W, Huettemann E, et al. Influence of systolic pressure variation guided intraoperative fluid management on organ function and oxygen transport. *Br J Anaesth.* 2008;101(2):194-199.

24. Goepfert M, Reuter D, Akyol D, et al. Goal directed fluid management reduces vasopressor and catecholamine use in cardiac surgery patients. *Intensive Care Med.* 2007;33:96-103.

25. Della Rocca G, Costa M, Pietropaoli P. How to measure and interpret volumetric measures of preload. *Curr Opin Crit Care.* 2007;13(3):297-302.

26. Uchino S, Bellomo R, Morimatsu H, et al. Pulmonary artery catheter versus pulse contour analysis: a prospective epidemiological study. *Critical Care.* 2006;10(6):R174.

27. Hofer C, Ganter M, Zollinger A. What technique should I use to measure cardiac output? *Curr Opin Crit Care.* 2007;13(3):308-317.

28. Michard F. Volume management using dynamic parameters. *Chest.* 2005;128:1902-1903.

29. Michard F, Descorps-Declere A. The times are a-changin: Should we bury the yellow catheter? *Crit Care Med.* 2007;35(5):1427-1428.

30. Auler J, Galas F, Hajjar L. Online monitoring of pulse pressure variation to guide fluid therapy after cardiac surgery. *Anesth Analg.* 2008;106(4):1201-1206.

31. Talmor D. Risk stratification in the changing field of cardiac surgery. *Crit Care Med.* 2004;32(9):1970-1971.

32. Guyton R. Coronary artery bypass is superior to drug eluting stents in multivessel coronary artery disease. *Ann Thorac Surg.* 2006; 81:1949-1957.

33. Hannan E, Racz M, Walford G, et al. Long-term outcomes of coronary artery bypass grafting versus stent implantation. *NEJM.* 2005;352:2174-2183.

34. Bursi F, Weston S, Redfield M, et al. Systolic and diastolic heart failure in the community. *JAMA.* 2006;296(18):2209-2216.

35. Ammar K, Makwana R, Redfield M, et al. Unrecognized myocardial infarction: the association with cardiopulmonary symptoms and mortality is mediated via echocardiographic abnormalities of global dysfunction instead of regional dysfunctional: the Olmstead County heart function study. *Am Heart J.* 2006;151(4):799-805.

36. Groban L, Butterworth J. Perioperative management of chronic heart failure. *Anesth Analg.* 2006;103(3):557-575.

37. Woods J, Monteiro P, Rhodes A. Right ventricular dysfunction. *Curr Opin Crit Care.* 2007;13(5):532-540.

38. Fellahi J, Parienti J, Hanouz J, et al. Perioperative use of dobutamine in cardiac surgery and adverse cardiac outcome: propensity adjusted analyses. *Anesthesiology.* 2008;108(6):979-987.

39. Elkayam U, Tasissa G, Binanay C, et al. Use and impact of inotropes and vasodilator therapy in hospitalized patients with severe heart failure. *Am Heart J.* 2007;153(1):98-104.

40. Stevenson L. Clinical use of inotropic therapy for heart failure: looking backward or forward? Part 1: Inotropic infusions during hospitalization. *Circulation.* 2003;108:367-372.

41. Subramaniam B, Talmor D. Echocardiography for management of hypotension in the intensive care unit. *Crit Care Med.* 2007;35(8):S401-S407.

42. Poelaert J, Schupfer G. Hemodynamic monitoring utilizing transesophageal echocardiography. *Chest.* 2005;127:379-390.

Perioperative Rhythm Abnormalities

TOPICS

Alterations in heart rhythm and rate can have sweeping and at times ultimately fatal hemodynamic consequences perioperatively. Thus, the rapid interpretation of abnormal rhythms and their correction is critical in cardiac anesthesia practice.

THE ELECTROCARDIOGRAM

The electrocardiogram (ECG) remains one of the main monitors used by anesthesiologists. It is primarily employed in anesthesia practice to detect heart rate and rhythm changes and perioperative myocardial ischemia. The ECG detects electrical currents generated by the electrical activity of the heart. ECG leads are placed in different positions and provide various perspectives (depending upon where the lead is placed) of the electrical activity of the heart as electrical vectors point toward or away from the examining leads. Examining the ECG in multiple leads provides the anesthesiologist the ability to discern if perceived changes in the ECG pattern are widespread (found in multiple leads) or are perhaps less significant (motion artifact). At the end of diastole, atrial depolarization generates the "P" wave and is followed by atrial contraction. Following atrial contraction, the ventricle is loaded awaiting systole. Systole commences at the QRS beginning with isovolumetric contraction following a 120- to 200-ms conduction delay at the AV node. Subsequently, intracavitary pressure builds, the atrioventricular

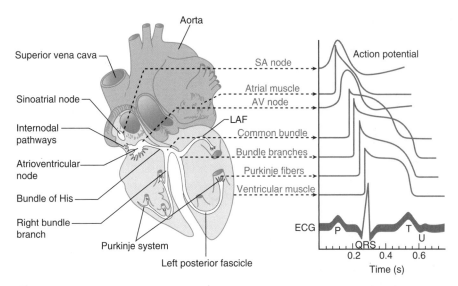

Figure 3–1. Conducting system of the heart. Left: Anatomic depiction of the human heart with additional focus on areas of the conduction system. Right: Typical transmembrane action potentials for the SA and AV nodes, other parts of the conduction system, and the atrial and ventricular muscles are shown along with the correlation to the extracellularly recorded electrical activity, that is, the electrocardiogram (ECG). The action potentials and ECG are plotted on the same time axis but with different zero points on the vertical scale for comparison. AV, atrioventricular; LAF, left anterior fascicle; SA, sinoatrial. (Data from Donahue JG, Choo PW, Manson JE, et al. The incidence of herpes zoster. *Arch Intern Med.* 155:1605–1609, 1995; Choo PW, Galil K, Donahue JG, et al. Risk factors for postherpetic neuralgia. *Arch Intern Med.* 1997;157:1217–1224.)

valves (e.g., mitral or tricuspid) close, and the arterioventricular valves (e.g., aortic, pulmonic) open resulting in ventricular ejection of the stroke volume (SV). The QRS represents the electrical activity generated by the depolarization of the left and the right ventricles. Depolarization proceeds from the AV node through the interventricular septum via the His-Purkinje fibers. The QRS segment lasts approximately 120 milliseconds. Repolarization of the ventricles produces the ST segment and the T wave. Electrolyte abnormalities (e.g., hypocalcemia) and drug effects (e.g., droperidol) can delay repolarization leading to a prolonged QT interval. This can result in potentially life-threatening ventricular arrhythmias (see Figures 3–1 and 3–2).

Pacemaker cells in the sinoatrial node spontaneously depolarize as their resting membrane potential becomes less negative through the gradual leakage of sodium ions. When the threshold is reached, calcium ions enter the cells and an action potential is generated. The action potential is then propagated throughout the heart generating the electrical activity that is reflected in the electrocardiogram. Repolarization then restores the baseline resting potential for the cycle to repeat.

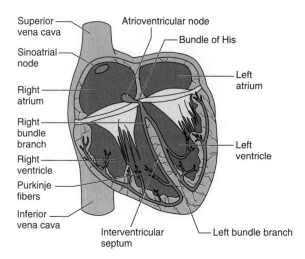

A.

B.

Figure 3–2A,B. The progression of cardiac conduction in the heart during a cardiac cycle. (Adapted with permission from Rushmer RF: *Cardiovascular Dynamics*, 2nd ed. Philadelphia, PA: Saunders; 1961.)

ECG ABNORMALITIES

Electrolyte disorders, heart structure abnormalities, and myocardial ischemia can cause aberrations in the patient's baseline ECG without producing an arrhythmia per se (Figure 3–3). Electrolyte abnormalities occur with some frequency periop-eratively. Hyperkalemia can present following cardioplegia administration dur-ing cardiopulmonary bypass (CPB), subsequent to iatrogenic administration of potassium, or associated with metabolic acidosis. As the potassium concentration increases, the T wave becomes progressively peaked. Hyperkalemia can ultimately produce broad, complex ventricular activity and asystole. Treatment is with immediate administration of calcium chloride. Glucose and regular insulin are given to lower the potassium concentration.

Hypokalemia lengthens the QT interval placing the patient at risk for *les torsades de pointes* type of ventricular fibrillation.

Hypocalcemia and hypomagnesemia likewise can prolong the QT interval placing the patient at risk for ventricular fibrillation (VF). Hypermagnesemia is associated with various conduction abnormalities and is seen from time to time in the obstetrical patient being treated for preeclampsia. Hypercalcemia can also cause T-wave abnormalities.

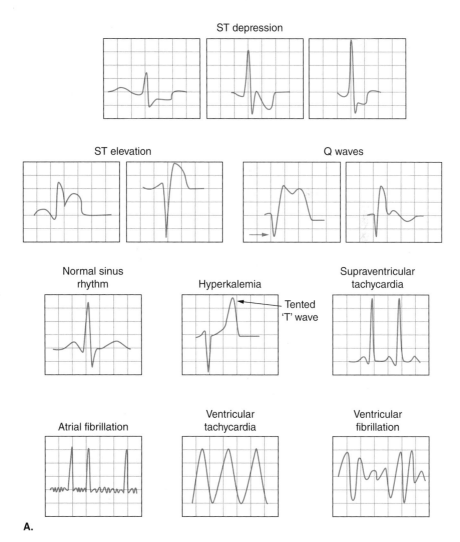

A.

Figure 3–3A. Common ECG findings during cardiac surgery.

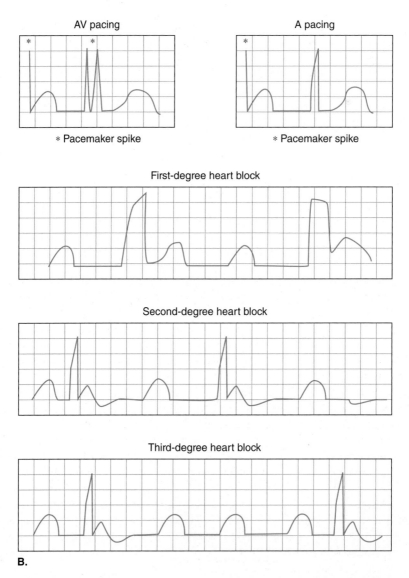

Figure 3–3B. AV sequential and atrial pacing are frequently employed during cardiac surgery as various degrees of heart block are often encountered perioperatively. Prolongation of the PR interval is seen in first-degree heart block here associated with the prolonged QRS complexes often seen during bundle branch blocks. In second-degree heart block the PR interval gradually lengthens until the impulse is no longer conducted to the ventricles. In third-degree block there is no association between atrial and ventricular beats. The atrial and the ventricular contraction are not coordinated.

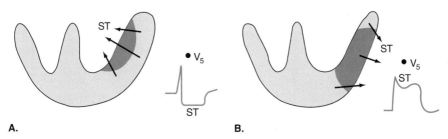

A. **B.**

Figure 3–4A,B Acute ischemia causes a current of injury. With predominant suben-docardial ischemia (A), the resultant ST vector will be directed toward the inner layer of the affected ventricle and the ventricular cavity. Overlying leads therefore will record ST depression. With ischemia involving the outer ventricular layer (B) (transmural or epicar-dial injury), the ST vector will be directed outward. Overlying leads will record ST eleva-tion. (Reproduced with permission from Jameson JL, Fauci AS, Kasper DL, et al: *Harrison's Principles of Internal Medicine*, 20th ed. New York, NY: McGraw-Hill Education; 2018.)

Ventricular hypertrophy, cardiomyopathies, and inherent conduction disorders can all alter the baseline ECG. Increased QRS amplitude in the left precordial leads (e.g., V5, V6) may indicate the presence of left ventricular hypertrophy associated with increased afterload and/or obstruction to left ventricular outflow tract (LVOT) ejection. Conversely, tall QRS waves in the right precordial leads (e.g., V1, V2) might indicate right ventricular hypertrophy secondary to pulmonary hypertension.

Right and left bundle branch blocks in addition to various prolongations in the QRS duration (> 0.12 seconds) are evidence of impaired cardiac conduction and often herald the presence of cardiac disease.

ST-segment elevations and depressions are associated with transmural and sub-endocardial ischemia, respectively. Pathologic (wide and deep) Q waves suggest myocardial infarction. TEE imagery demonstrating poorly contracting myocar-dium can be compared with ECG tracings to identify and to confirm the pres-ence of ischemic myocardium. Changes in the cardiac myocytes alter the electrical properties recorded by the ECG (Figure 3–4). By directing electrical vectors either away from (subendocardial ischemia) or toward (transmural ischemia) precordial ECG leads (e.g., V_5), characteristic changes such as ST depression or ST elevation patterns are respectively generated.

Access to the chest is limited during cardiac surgical procedures. Because ECG interpretation is critical throughout the procedure, it is very important that the leads be securely fixed to the patient to avoid having to replace them during the operation. ECG tracings should be clear at the start of the case to facilitate rhythm interpretation intra-operatively.

BRADYARRHYTHMIAS

Bradycardia and bradyarrhythmias routinely complicate the perioperative man-agement of the cardiac surgery patient. Hyperkalemia, myocardial ischemia, vagal effects, intrinsic cardiac disease, hypoxemia, and loss of sympathetic tone can all contribute to the development of varying degrees of heart block and/or sinus bradycardia at any time during heart surgery.

Sinus bradycardia (sinus rate < 60 bpm) frequently is associated with anesthesia induction, narcotic administration, a reflex response to systemic hypertension, and beta blockade. Sinus bradycardia is of little consequence assuming cardiac output is sufficiently preserved to maintain an acceptable blood pressure and tissue perfusion.

Recall,

Blood pressure = Cardiac output × Systemic vascular resistance

Cardiac output = Stroke volume × Heart rate

Therefore, if the heart rate falls—even if sinus rhythm is maintained—the patient may become hemodynamically unstable. Too slow a sinus rhythm provides other pacemaker cells in the heart the opportunity to emerge resulting in various other nodal or ventricular arrhythmias.

Treatment for sinus bradycardia must be determined on a case-by-case basis depending upon the patient's hemodynamic performance. Bradycardia in response to systemic hypertension is corrected by lowering the blood pressure. Sinus bradycardias resulting from anesthesia induction may need to be treated if they result in hypotension and low cardiac output. Atropine (IV) can be administered to correct the heart rate. The causes of sinus bradycardia should be sought and corrected. A slowing heart rate in the setting of hypoxemia is immediately worrisome and may indicate impending circulatory arrest. Ephedrine can be judiciously administered to the heart surgery patient experiencing hypotension and sinus bradycardia as a consequence of anesthesia induction. However, ephedrine's reliance upon release of native catecholamine reserves may make it a poor choice in the catecholamine-depleted patient. Likewise, various inotropic infusions [e.g., epinephrine (2 µg/min IV) infusion and upward, dobutamine (2-10 µg/kg/min) etc.] can be administered to increase the patient's heart rate. Of course, administration of catecholamines as well as atropine might lead to the development of accelerated nodal or ventricular rhythms. Temporary pacing can be used where available and when indicated to provide atrial, ventricular, or atrial-ventricular pacing as needed.

At times, patients will present with competing atrial pacemaker cells, each resulting in an atrial driven rhythm albeit at different rates and with differing "P"-wave morphologies. Nodal rhythms emanate from the AV node and result in inadequate filling of the left ventricle due to the absence of a coordinated atrial contraction. The contribution of the atrial contraction to effectively load the left ventricle at the end of diastole varies from patient to patient depending upon age and left ventricular compliance. The less compliant the left ventricle, the more dependent it becomes upon the contribution of the atrial contraction. When nodal rhythms emerge, hemodynamic consequences may be nil or great depending upon the individual patient and the patient's degree of diastolic dysfunction. Patients with a slow nodal rhythm may respond to administration of atropine and inotropic agents in a manner similar to the treatment of sinus bradycardia. On the other hand, some nodal rhythms develop into AV junctional tachycardia and require treatment as described below for supraventricular tachycardias.

Varying degrees of heart block are also quite common in the cardiac surgery patient. Impairment of the conduction system occurs frequently perioperatively secondary to ischemia; electrolyte disorders; and iatrogenic, surgically mediated injury to the heart's conduction system in the interventricular septum. First-degree heart block occurs when there is a prolongation in the AV interval. Second-degree heart block occurs when not all the atrial beats are conducted through the AV node to the ventricle. Mobitz type 1, or Wenckebach, block is associated with a gradual prolongation of the AV interval until a ventricular beat fails to occur. Often Mobitz type 1 block requires no direct therapy. Conversely, Mobitz type 2 block has a propensity to deteriorate to third-degree heart block. In this form of second-degree AV block, the atrial pacemaker beat is not always conducted through to the ventricle. Sporadically, atrial contractions can occur without a ventricular beat. In third-degree heart block, no atrial beats are conducted through to the ventricle. A slow ventricular pacemaker may emerge leading to the atria and ventricles contracting in a discordant fashion. The "P" waves can be seen marching through the ECG tracing without an associated QRS immediately thereafter. Hemodynamic instability often becomes manifest, and temporary pacing is required perioperatively.

Left and right bundle branch blocks are very common in heart surgery patients as they can portend the presence of intrinsic cardiac disease. In patients with a left bundle branch block, pulmonary artery catheterization can result in a mechanically induced concomitant right bundle branch block producing complete heart block and hemodynamic instability. A temporary pacing ability (e.g., external cutaneous pacing) should be available whenever right heart catheterization is planned in the left bundle branch block patient.

TEMPORARY PACEMAKER

The ability to provide temporary pacing is essential in cardiac anesthesia practice. Bradyarrhythmias as described earlier can present at any point in the patient's perioperative course. Many patients require some form of pacing to separate from CPB even if only for a few minutes until the heart is reperfused and/or the potassium concentration is reduced. Transient perioperative ischemia can also produce varying degrees of heart block necessitating some form of emergent pacing. Temporary pacing must be distinguished from permanent pacing. Permanent pacemakers are increasingly being implanted in patients for the treatment of heart failure.[1] Permanent biventricular pacing for cardiac resynchronization therapy (CRT) provides a more effective myocardial contraction in the heart failure patient by reducing the width of the QRS complex synchronizing septal and lateral ventricular wall contraction. Additionally, many permanent pacemakers contain the ability to sense an increase in respiratory rate and thus are able to increase the pacing rate in response to exercise. Finally, with an ever-increasing number of patients at risk for sudden cardiac death (SCD), these devices contain a defibrillation or anti-tachycardia function permitting electrical conversion of malignant rhythms [implantable cardioverter defibrillator (ICD)]. Permanent pacemaker/defibrillators are discussed in Chapter 15.

Temporary pacemakers in general are designated by a three-letter code relating to their function: The first letter identifies the chamber or chambers of the heart paced [A for atrium, V for ventricle, D for dual (both A and V) and O for none]. The second letter identifies which, if any, of the chambers are sensed. The third letter indicates the response of the device to a sensed beat (I for inhibited, D for both inhibition and triggering). Thus, a temporary VVI pacemaker would pace the ventricle, sense the ventricle, and be inhibited if a ventricle beat was detected. Likewise, a DDD temporary pacemaker would pace both the atrium and the ventricle, sense both chambers, and either be inhibited or deliver a beat depending upon what the device senses.

There are many different modes of temporary pacing available to anesthesiologists perioperatively. Transcutaneous pacing is usually available as a part of most modern cardioverter/defibrillator devices. Pacing/defibrillation patches are applied to the chest, and ventricular pacing is initiated by setting the pacing rate and the output from the device until the heart is captured and a beat generated. Transcutaneous pacing is ventricular pacing, and as such the atrial contribution to the cardiac output is lost. Often pacing patches are placed prophylactically in cardiac surgery patients to provide for a quick pacing capability should the rhythm be lost before the heart is exposed and epicardial pacing wires placed. In reoperative heart surgery patients, access to the heart may be difficult thus preventing rapid sternal opening and application of epicardial pacing wires. Placement of transcutaneous pacing pads perioperatively is especially suggested in these cases to provide for a temporary ventricular beat and emergent defibrillation.

Temporary esophageal pacing systems can be used to pace the atrium. They have limited application in the heart surgery patient because this atrial pacing modality (AOO) does not provide for ventricular capture. Moreover, a TEE probe frequently occupies the esophagus during cardiac surgical procedures.

Temporary epicardial pacing has been used in cardiac surgery since the 1960s.[2] Surgeons routinely place epicardial pacing wires to provide for both atrial and ventricular pacing. These wires are passed from the surgical field to the anesthesiologist and attached to a pulse generator. The anesthesiologist next chooses the pacemaker mode and settings. Generally, the DDD mode is chosen to provide for temporary pacing. To set the pacemaker, the anesthesiologist selects:

1. Heart rate: The rate can be set lower than the patient's own rate to provide an emergency backup pacing function or can be set at any rate desirable. Often rates of between 80 and 100 bpm are selected.

2. Output: The electrical output (up to 20 mA) of both the atrial and ventricular pacing components is set so to establish capture of the signal by the heart to generate a beat. The threshold for pacing, which is the minimal output required to generate an action potential in the myocardium, is checked after insertion and the output is set a few milliamps higher than the triggering threshold. Too high an output will lead to formation of fibrosis at the lead/myocardium interface.

3. Sensitivity: The sensitivity of the device is set to determine which signals will result in inhibition of the pacemaker function, for example, atrial sensitivity of 0.5 mV and ventricular sensitivity of 2.0 mV.

4. Pulse width duration: Generally, of short duration (1 millisecond).

5. AV interval: 150 to 200 milliseconds.

Pacemaker settings are adjusted to achieve the best possible hemodynamics. Usually this occurs when the atrial and ventricular contractions are timed to provide for sufficient loading of the left ventricle during diastole. As with all pacing functions, inappropriate delivery of a paced beat during repolarization of the heart can initiate VF. Consequently, asynchronous ventricular pacing modes (VOO, DOO) are best avoided. Recently, CRT through biventricular epicardial pacing perioperatively has been suggested to improve ventricular function when separating from CPB.[3] Biventricular pacing provides for a reduced width of the QRS resulting in better coordination of left ventricular contraction and improved hemodynamics.

From time to time, anesthesiologists may place either a temporary transvenous pacing catheter or a pulmonary artery catheter with pacing capabilities. A balloon-tipped pacing wire can be placed in the right heart following central venous access. The output of the pulse generator is adjusted until beat capture is achieved.

Various pulmonary artery catheter designs have either electrodes built into them or additional channels by which transvenous pacing wires can be placed. These leads are attached to a temporary pulse generator, and pacing can be initiated as appropriate. However, in the overwhelming majority of instances, the anesthesiologist will employ temporary epicardial pacing to wean from CPB or emergent transcutaneous pacing during resuscitative efforts. From time to time, patients with heart block will present for surgery with a temporary pacer wire previously placed by the cardiology staff. Placement of a pulmonary artery flotation catheter can readily dislodge both temporary transvenous pacemakers as well as recently placed permanent transvenous wires.

SUPRAVENTRICULAR TACHYCARDIAS

Both sinus tachycardias and various supraventricular arrhythmias are common in the perioperative cardiac surgery patient. Rapid heart rates can have profound hemodynamic consequences perioperatively resulting from inadequate ventricular filling secondary to the loss of atrioventricular synchrony and/or reduced diastolic filling time. The causes of perioperative sinus tachycardia include hyperthermia, hypovolemia, anemia, light anesthesia, vasoactive infusions, and sympathetic stimulation to name a few. Correction of the underlying initiating mechanism of sinus tachycardia will generally resolve the issue. Often in the cardiac surgery patient, the intense surgical stimulation of sternal opening can lead to both a hypertensive and tachycardic response necessitating administration of additional narcotics and increased concentrations of inhalational agents.

Supraventricular tachycardias (SVTs) also frequently occur perioperatively. Very fast sinus tachycardias can be difficult to distinguish from SVTs. SVTs, of course, lack the "P" wave that would be found in a sinus tachycardia. SVTs are

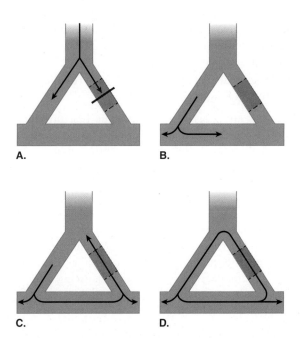

Figure 3–5. When areas in the myocardium differ in electrical conductivity or refractoriness, it is possible for a re-entrant loop to be established. A unidirectional block develops (A). It is conducted (B,C) back to the first pathway, which has repolarized permitting a re-entrant loop leading to a supraventricular tachycardia (D). (Reproduced with permission from Butterworth JF, Mackey DC, Wasnick JD: *Morgan & Mikhail's Clinical Anesthesiology*, 6th ed. New York, NY: McGraw-Hill Education; 2018.)

generally produced through re-entrant mechanisms. Re-entrant arrhythmias occur when conduction tissues in the heart (either within the AV node or through accessory conduction pathways) depolarize and repolarize at varying rates.[4] In this way a self-perpetuating loop of repolarization and depolarization within the AV node can occur resulting in the development of SVTs (Figure 3–5).

SVTs occur frequently during both cardiac and noncardiac surgery. SVTs producing ischemia or hemodynamic collapse are routinely treated in the cardiac surgery patient with synchronized cardioversion. Adenosine 6 to 12 mg IV can be given to slow AV node conduction potentially disrupting the re-entrant loop. Attention should be paid because adenosine can result in a third-degree atrioventricular block in heart transplant patients. Various beta-blockers and calcium antagonists can also be employed in patients with SVT with the exception of the SVTs as a manifestation of Wolff-Parkinson-White (WPW) syndrome. In patients with WPW, preexcitation syndrome amiodarone, adenosine, digoxin, and nondihydropyridine calcium antagonists are avoided as they can accelerate the ventricular rate response. Procainamide or ibutilide may be given to restore sinus rhythm in patients with a high ventricular response rate and who are hemodynamically stable. Cardioversion is indicated if the patient is hemodynamically unstable. Occasionally an SVT with an intraventricular conduction block can appear as wide QRS complex tachycardia similar in appearance to ventricular tachycardia (VT) and should be treated as VT until otherwise proven.[5]

Atrial fibrillation/flutter (AF) can likewise complicate the perioperative management of the cardiac surgery patient. AF is classified as paroxysmal, persistent, long-standing, or permanent. Paroxysmal AF is defined as at least two episodes of AF that terminate spontaneously within 7 days. Persistent AF occurs when the duration of AF is longer than 7 days or lasts for any duration but requires pharmacologic or electrical cardioversion. Long-standing AF has a duration of more than 1 year. In permanent AF, a decision has been made not to attempt restoration of sinus rhythm but rate control and anticoagulation will still be achieved. Many patients with impaired ventricular function and/or valvular disease present to cardiac surgery already in AF as a baseline. Such patients tend to have very dilated atria (Video 3–1) and must be screened for the presence of an intra-atrial clot if they have been in AF without having been anticoagulated (TEE Videos 3–2 and 3–3). The incidence of new postoperative atrial fibrillation (AF) ranges from 17% to 35% following cardiac surgery.[5] Prophylaxis against postoperative AF is usually undertaken perioperatively with beta-blockers in those patients without contraindications. Amiodarone (IV and PO) can be given in combination with beta-blockers to further reduce the new onset of AF, postoperatively. Sotalol can likewise be employed to reduce the incidence of perioperative AF.

Patients brought to surgery with long-standing AF associated with valvular heart disease (e.g., mitral stenosis) may undergo the Cox-Maze procedure at the time of surgery. The procedure consists of performing right and left atrial lesions and left atrial appendage exclusion to disrupt conduction pathways at the level of the atria. Amiodarone by infusion is also started (150 mg IV load followed by infusion 1 mg/min for 6 h and 0.5 mg/min for 18 h) followed by oral therapy.

AF can also appear unexpectedly during cardiac surgical procedures secondary to manipulation of the heart, the inflammatory response, and changing autonomic tone. The irregular ventricular response can become rapid (> 150 bpm) leading to hemodynamic collapse necessitating internal synchronized cardioversion. Surgeons can place internal paddles on the heart and effectively restore sinus rhythm with a relatively low energy of 10 to 20 J. External cardioversion often requires 50 to 200 J depending upon patient factors (e.g., size); however, newer biphasic devices require less energy delivery to be effective.

The American Heart Association/American College of Cardiology (AHA/ACC) have produced voluminous guidelines on the management of all aspects of atrial fibrillation.[6] These guidelines include suggestions for the management of postoperative atrial fibrillation. Class I (benefits far outweigh risks) guidelines suggest the use of beta-blockers to treat AF in cardiac surgery patients if not contraindicated. Moreover, they suggest use of a nondihydropyridine calcium antagonist if refractory to beta-blocker therapy. Additionally, amiodarone is suggested in cardiac surgery patients thought at risk for perioperative AF development (Class IIa benefit is greater than risk). Additionally, the guidelines suggest that it is reasonable to administer antiarrhythmic medications to maintain sinus rhythm in those patients

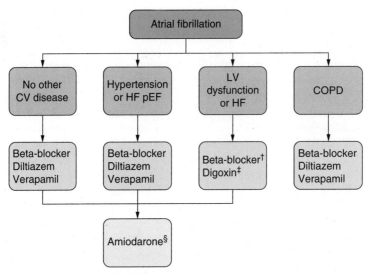

Figure 3–6. Approach to selecting drug therapy for ventricular rate control.*
*Drugs are listed alphabetically. †Beta blockers should be instituted following stabilization of patients with decompensated HF. The choice of beta blocker (eg, cardioselective) depends on the patient's clinical condition. ‡Digoxin is not usually first-line therapy. It may be combined with a beta blocker and/or a nondihydropyridine calcium channel blocker when ventricular rate control is insufficient and may be useful in patients with HF. §In part because of concern over its side-effect profile, use of amiodarone for chronic control of ventricular rate should be reserved for patients who do not respond to or are intolerant of beta blockers or nondihydropyridine calcium antagonists. COPD indicates chronic obstructive pulmonary disease; CV, cardiovascular; HF, heart failure; HFpEF, heart failure with preserved ejection fraction; and LV, left ventricular. [Reproduced with permission from January CT, Wann LS, Alpert JS, et al: 2014 AHA/ACC/HRS guideline for the management of patients with atrial fibrillation: a report of the American College of Cardiology/American Heart Association Task Force on Practice Guidelines and the Heart Rhythm Society, *J Am Coll Cardiol.* 2014 Dec 2;64(21):e1-76.]

with recurrent or refractory AF. Lastly, anticoagulation therapy and attempts at cardioversion should be applied as in nonsurgical patients assuming no contraindications exist. The AHA recommends the following approach for ventricular rate control of AF patients (Figure 3–6).

AHA class I and II recommendations for the management of post cardiac surgery atrial fibrillation are listed in Figure 3–7.

VENTRICULAR TACHYCARDIA AND FIBRILLATION

Perioperative VF represents an immediate threat to the patient's life and requires the simultaneous generation of a differential diagnosis, defibrillation, and therapy to prevent VF recurrence. Ventricular arrhythmias are associated with myocardial ischemia, heart failure, hypoxemia, various cardiomyopathies, electrolyte

Recommendations	COR
Postoperative cardiac and thoracic surgery	
A beta blocker is recommended to treat postoperative AF unless contraindicated	I
A nondihydropyridine calcium channel blocker is recommended when a beta blocker is inadequate to achieve rate control with postoperative AF	I
Preoperative amiodarone reduces AF with cardiac surgery and is reasonable as prophylactic therapy for patients at high risk of postoperative AF	IIa
It is reasonable to restore sinus rhythm pharmacologically with ibutilide or direct-current cardioversion with postoperative AF	IIa
It is reasonable to administer antiarrhythmic medications to maintain sinus rhythm with recurrent or refractory postoperative AF	IIa
It is reasonable to administer antithrombotic medications for postoperative AF	IIa
It is reasonable to manage new-onset postoperative AF with rate control and anticoagulation with cardioversion if AF does not revert spontaneously to sinus rhythm during follow-up	IIa
Prophylactic sotalol may be considered for patients with AF risk after cardiac surgery	IIb
Colchicine may be considered postoperatively to reduce AF after cardiac surgery	IIb

Figure 3–7. Summary of Recommendations for Specific Patient Groups and AF. COR = Class of Recommendation. [Data from January CT, Wann LS, Alpert JS, et al: 2014 AHA/ACC/ HRS guideline for the management of patients with atrial fibrillation: a report of the American College of Cardiology/American Heart Association Task Force on Practice Guidelines and the Heart Rhythm Society, *J Am Coll Cardiol.* 2014 Dec 2;64(21):e1-76.]

abnormalities, prolonged QT syndrome, inotrope administration, and mechanical manipulation of the heart. The AHA/ACC have developed extensive guidelines for the management of ventricular arrhythmias.[7] Both VF and pulseless ventricular tachycardia (VT) require immediate resuscitative efforts as systemic blood flow ceases during these arrhythmias. Defibrillation should be undertaken immediately for VF and cardioversion for VT. In the operative setting, the open sternum permits the delivery of defibrillation current through the use of internal paddles. Additionally, should the rhythm fail to be restored, open chest cardiac massage can be initiated. Also, immediate institution of CPB can be undertaken to preserve tissue perfusion while efforts are made to restore cardiac function. External pads should be applied especially to patients who undergo re-do sternotomy because timely access to the heart is compounded and delayed by presence of scar tissue from previous surgeries. If refractory VF is present and access to the heart is delayed, institution of CPB can proceed through femoral cannulation.

Any wide QRS complex tachycardia should be assumed to be VT even if a pulse is present. When VT provides an acceptable blood pressure, pharmacological therapy (e.g., procainamide, amiodarone) can be employed. Most likely in the perioperative period the surgeon will attempt cardioversion should such a rhythm occur. Intravenous lidocaine may be useful in patients where ischemia is a causative factor in the etiology of the rhythm aberrancy. VT associated with a prolonged QT interval produces *les torsades de pointes.* The sine wave appearing ECG with polymorphic VT indicates the presence of torsades. Correction of any electrolyte abnormalities and discontinuation of any drugs that promote QT-interval prolongation is mandatory.

Other causes of perioperative VF include air embolism in the coronary vessels or bypass grafts, myocardial ischemia, heart failure, migration of the pulmonary artery catheter into the RV or RV outflow track, and pacemaker misfires (R on T phenomenon). VF can occur at any time perioperatively. Correction of metabolic derangements prior to separation from CPB is useful in reducing the occurrence of VF perioperatively. During periods of patient transfer it is critically important that the patient is monitored at all times and defibrillators are available to treat compromising dysrhythmias. The loss of an arterial pressure trace concurrent with the disappearance of the ECG and a falling end-tidal carbon dioxide measurement should immediately suggest the possibility of a lethal arrhythmia. Should VF be refractory to defibrillation, CPR can be initiated and maintained until the patient can be placed on CPB. Administration of epinephrine may be needed to successfully defibrillate the patient. Often only surgical repair of the patient's underlying cardiac pathology and emergent institution of CPB will permit patient survival.

Common antiarrhythmic drugs are classified according to their effects through the Vaughan-Williams classification (Table 3–1).

These agents have various effects on the cardiac cycle (Table 3–2).

Table 3–1. Vaughan-Williams Classification of Antiarrhythmic Drugs

Class	Action	Example drugs
I	Sodium channel blockade	
Ia	Block sodium channel in open state with an intermediate recovery from block; also, inhibit I_{Kr} at relatively lower concentrations; moderate phase 0 depression and conduction slowing, prolonging of action potential duration	Quinidine, procainamide, disopyramide
Ib	Block sodium channel in inactivated state with a fast time constant of recovery from block; minimal effect on phase 0 upstroke; no change or slight shortening of action potential duration	Lidocaine, mexiletine
Ic	Block sodium channel in open state with slow recovery from block; marked phase 0 depression and conduction slowing; small or no effect on repolarization	Flecainide, propafenone
II	β-Adrenergic receptor blockade	Propranolol, metoprolol, atenolol, esmolol, acebutolol, pindolol, nadolol, carvedilol, labetalol, and bisoprolol
III	Potassium channel blockade and/or inward current enhancer	d,l-Sotalol, dofetilide, amiodarone, bretylium, ibutilide, dronedarone
IV	Calcium channel blockade	Verapamil, diltiazem

Reproduced with permission from Fuster V, Harrington RA, Narula N, et al: *Hurst's The Heart*, 14th ed. New York, NY: McGraw-Hill Education; 2017.

Table 3–2. Clinical Pharmacological Properties of Antiarrhythmic Drugs

Drug	Effect on SA nodal rate	Effect on AV nodal refractory period	PR interval	QRS duration	QT interval	Usefulness in arrhythmias		Half-life
						Supraventricular	Ventricular	
Adenosine	Little	↑↑↑	↑↑↑	0	0	++++	?	< 10 s
Amiodarone	↓↓[1]	↑↑	↑↑	↓	↑↑↑	+++	+++	(Weeks)
Bretylium	↑↓[2]	↑↓[2]	0	0	0	0	+	4 h
Diltiazem	↓↓	↑↑	↑	0	0	+++	–	4-8 h
Disopyramide	↑↓[1,3]	↑↓[3]	↑↓[3]	↑↑	↑↑	+	+++	6-8 h
Dofetilide	↓?	0	0	0	↑↑	++	None	7 h
Esmolol	↓↓	↑	↑↑	0	0	+	+	10 min
Flecainide	None	↑	↑↑	↑↑↑	0	+[4]	++++	20 h
Ibutilide	↓(?)	0	0	0	↑↑	++	?	6 h
Lidocaine	None[1]	None	0	0	0	None[5]	+++	1-2 h
Metopolol	↓↓	↑↑	↑↑	0	0	+	+	8 h
Mexiletine	None[1]	None	0	0	0	None[6]	+++	12 h
Moricizine	None	None	↑	↑↑	0	None	+++	2-6 h[6]
Procainamide	↓[1]	↑↓[3]	↑↓[3]	↑↑	↑↑	+	+++	3-4 h
Propafenone	0	↑	↑↓[3]	↑↑↑	0	+	+++	5-7 h
Quinidine	↑↓[1,3]	↑↓[3]	↑↓[3]	↑↑	↑↑	+	+++	6 h
Sotalol	↓↓	↑↑	↑↑	0	↑↑↑	+++	+++	7 h
Tocainide	None[1]	None	0	0	0	None[5]	+++	12 h
Verapamil	↓↓	↑↑	↑↑	0	0	+++	–	7 h

[1]May suppress diseased sinus nodes.
[2]Initial stimulation by release of endogenous norepinephrine followed by depression.
[3]Anticholinergic effect and direct depressant action.
[4]Particularly in Wolff-Parkinson–White syndrome.
[5]May be effective in atrial arrhythmias caused by digitalis.
[6]Half-life of active metabolites is much longer.
Reproduced with permission from Butterworth JF, Mackey DC, Wasnick JD: *Morgan & Mikhail's Clinical Anesthesiology*, 6th ed. New York, NY: McGraw-Hill Education; 2018.

TEE AND THE ECG

ECG is a vital part of any TEE examination and should be placed whenever any echo examination is planned. The ECG is correlated with TEE imagery to determine when the patient is in diastole and when in systole. It is important to remember that mechanical events in the heart slightly lag behind the appearance of their corresponding electrical signals on the ECG.

Patients with AF frequently have dilated atria, which are readily apparent on TEE. Poor flow associated with a poorly contractile atrium can be seen as spontaneous echo contrast "smoke" swirling in the left atrium. Pulse wave Doppler can be used to determine the velocity of flow in the left atrial appendage (LAA). The left atrial appendage appears as a beak-like structure on TEE examination. Reduced velocity in the LAA less than 45 cm/s increases the risk of a clot developing in the LAA (Figure 3–8 and Video 3–4).

Patients presenting for cardioversion who have not been placed on anticoagulation for more than 24 hours require TEE prior to cardioversion to minimize the risk of embolization of atrial thrombus following the restoration of sinus rhythm.

Although beyond the scope of basic TEE, tissue Doppler and speckle tracking techniques can be employed to determine the varying velocities of different segments of the myocardium during each cardiac beat. Tissue Doppler examines the velocities of the myocardium by filtering out the velocities of the red blood cells. Therefore, the various velocities and timing of different ventricular segments during systole can be compared. Speckle tracking uses ultrasound image speckles and tracks their velocity and movement during the cardiac cycle to determine strain, the length deformation of the myocardium. When patients develop heart failure, the effectiveness of their conduction system in the ventricle becomes impaired. The septal wall often contracts before the lateral wall making overall contraction of

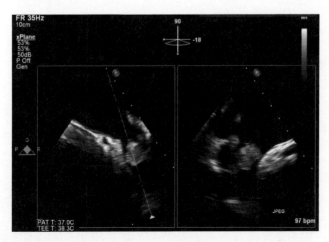

Figure 3–8. A clot is seen in the left atrial appendage.

the ventricle less effective. Cardiac resynchronization therapy attempts to restore efficiency of the ventricular contraction by concomitant pacing of the left and right ventricle with two separate ventricular pacing leads. Tissue Doppler and speckle tracking may assist in selecting patients who would benefit from CRT; however, these techniques are subject to ongoing study.

CASE SCENARIO

A 65-year-old patient presents for elective cardioversion for atrial fibrillation.

What constitutes the anesthesia preoperative examination?

Although elective cardioversion is a brief procedure, a full anesthesia history should be obtained. Particular attention should focus on the presence of valvular heart disease, systolic and diastolic heart failure, and the patient's anticoagulation status.

When should a TEE examination be completed prior to cardioversion?

In any patient with AF for more than 24-hour duration without initiation of anticoagulation, a TEE examination should be performed immediately prior to cardioversion.

Assuming relatively preserved cardiac function, what anesthetic approach should be used for the TEE and cardioversion?

Provided there are no contraindications, deep sedation with propofol can be employed along with topicalization of the oropharynx. Patients should be sufficiently awake to aid in the TEE examination by swallowing the probe following topicalization.

Looking at **Video 3–3**, should the cardioversion be performed?

The left atrial appendage demonstrates the absence of a clot. The cardioversion may be performed.

REFERENCES

1. Trohman R, Kim M, Pinski S. Cardiac pacing: the state of the art. Lancet. 2004;364:1701-1719.
2. Hasan S, Lewis C. A new method of temporary epicardial atrioventricular pacing utilizing bipolar pacing leads. *Ann Thorac Surg.* 2005;79:1384-1387.
3. Berberian G, Quinn T, Kanter J, et al. Optimized biventricular pacing in atrioventricular block after cardiac surgery. *Ann Thorac Surg.* 2005;80:870-875.
4. Delacretaz E. Supraventricular tachycardia. *NEJM.* 2006;354(10):1039-1051.
5. DiDomenico R, Massad M. Pharmacologic strategies for prevention of atrial fibrillation after open heart surgery. *Ann Thorac Surg.* 2005;79:738-740.
6. January CT, Wann LS, Alpert JS, et al. 2014 AHA/ACC/HRS guideline for the management of patients with atrial fibrillation: a report of the American College of Cardiology/American Heart Association Task Force on Practice Guidelines and the Heart Rhythm Society. *J Am Coll Cardiol* 2014;64:e1-76.
7. Zipes D, Camm A, Borggrefe M, et al. ACC/AHA/ESC 2006 Guidelines for management of patients with ventricular arrhythmias and the prevention of sudden cardiac death—executive summary. *Circulation.* 2006;114:1088-1132.

Routine Cardiac Surgery and Anesthesia*

4

TOPICS

In decades past, the otherwise healthy patient for coronary bypass surgery was the "ideal" patient for cardiac surgery/anesthesia teams. Such patients often presented with one- or two-vessel coronary artery disease in need of surgical revascularization. Perhaps the patient had suffered a myocardial infarction but, overwhelmingly, ventricular function tended to be preserved. Free from both systolic and diastolic ventricular dysfunction, such patients tolerated anesthesia induction, maintenance, and emergence easily. Often these patients were relatively young, in their forties, fifties, and sixties and lacked other organ system diseases. Time on cardiopulmonary bypass tended to be short because the patients often required only one or two vessel revascularizations.

Today, patients presenting for coronary artery surgery are anything but "routine." Frequently they will have already undergone numerous percutaneous coronary interventions (PCIs) prior to being referred for surgery. Many patients will have had a history of recurrent small myocardial infarctions, anginal episodes, and catheterizations. Over time, myocardial

---

Warning: There is no such thing as routine cardiac anesthesia.

damage accrues, leaving some patients with systolic and diastolic ventricular dysfunction. Other patients are referred for coronary bypass surgery because they have complex coronary artery lesions not readily amenable to PCI (e.g., patients with high SYNTAX scores—see Chapter 1) or they have concurrent valvular heart disease.

Although few of today's patients for coronary revascularization are "easy" to manage, review of the anesthesia management for this particular surgical procedure provides an overview of the anesthesia maneuvers necessary in the management of almost all adult cardiac surgeries. In other words, the skills and techniques applied in managing the "routine" coronary artery bypass graft (CABG) surgery also apply when managing anesthesia for more complex procedures.

IMMEDIATE PREOPERATIVE ASSESSMENT AND ANTIBIOTIC PROPHYLAXIS

Increasingly, patients are admitted to the hospital for elective CABG on the day of surgery. In that instance, the anesthesiologist may have very few moments to meet and to assess the patient for cardiac surgery. Most institutions operating a same-day admission cardiac surgery program will have arranged for the patient to be evaluated in a preoperative anesthesia clinic well before the day of surgery. If that is the case, the anesthesiologist reviews the evaluative work completed in the outpatient clinic. Still, it is critically important that the anesthesiologist completes an immediate assessment prior to preparing the patient for surgery.

Patients should be questioned regarding any change in their overall health since their preoperative evaluation. They are asked if they are currently experiencing any dyspnea or anginal pain. Patients should be monitored at this time with electrocardiogram, pulse oximeter, and automatic blood pressure cuff. Supplemental oxygen should be provided.

Most patients will have continued their medications, including beta-blockers, on the morning of surgery as instructed. Angiotensin converting enzyme inhibitors can lead to perioperative hypotension, and many patients will have been instructed to discontinue these medications. However, there may be outcome benefits in continuing ACE therapy perioperatively. Anesthesiologists should be aware of potential perioperative hypotension in patients continuing ACE inhibitors and angiotensin receptor blockers (ARBs) up to the day of surgery. A complete review of the patient's current anti-hypertensive regimen is warranted preoperatively, and consensus as to therapeutic approaches achieved between surgeon, cardiologist and anesthesiologist. Diabetes regimens must also be adjusted perioperatively. Both hyper- and hypoglycemia can occur in diabetic cardiac surgery patients. Close monitoring of glycemia is critical throughout the entire perioperative period.

A brief neurological examination will establish an immediate preoperative baseline. The eyes should be examined to note pupillary responses and pupillary size. The patient's lungs are auscultated to detect the presence of any wheezes or rales indicative of heart failure.

Patients reporting anxiety and assuming they are free of conditions likely to lead to imminent cardiac collapse (e.g., tight stenotic valvular disease, severely impaired ventricular function) can be medicated in the holding area with intravenous midazolam 0.5 to 2 mg. Resuscitative equipment should be available and the anesthesiologist immediately at hand. Inpatients are occasionally given oral lorazepam as a preoperative medication. Although the authors tend to avoid all premedication except for that given intravenously under immediate anesthesiology supervision, individual institutions are likely to have their own accepted protocols for preoperative sedation.

Prior to administering any sedative or anxiolytic, correctly identify the patient according to hospital policies and make sure all consents are in proper order.

Antibiotic prophylaxis is administered within 1 hour of surgery incision time. This is a frequent anesthesiology quality assurance indicator and must be dutifully performed and charted. In patients free of methicillin-resistant *Staphylococcus aureus,* a first-generation cephalosporin is indicated.[1] Later-generation cephalosporins have better gram-negative and less gram-positive coverage. Because gram-positive *S. aureus* is most frequently implicated in cardiac surgical infections, the earlier cephalosporins, such as cefazolin or cefuroxime, are best for antibiotic prophylaxis. If the patient has a presumed, known, or anticipated colonization with methicillin-resistant *S. aureus,* use of both a cephalosporin (cefazolin) and a glycopeptide (vancomycin) has been suggested to expand prophylaxis.[1] If a patient has a beta-lactam allergy, vancomycin is employed for antibiotic prophylaxis. However, since vancomycin provides no gram-negative coverage, administration of an aminoglycoside for one to two doses is suggested.[1] Mupirocin topical antibiotic eliminates nasal colonies of all types of *S. aureus.* Because the nose is considered a depository for bacteria that lead to infection following cardiac surgery, treatment with mupirocin is recommended to commence on the day before surgery and continue from 2 to 5 days following.[1]

When indicated cefazolin 2 g (patient weight > 60 kg) should be administered within 1 hour of surgical incision. Assuming normal renal function, a repeat dose of 1 g should be given every 4 hours while the chest is open.

Vancomycin (15 mg/kg) is administered as a slow IV infusion for more than 1-hour duration. When a beta-lactam antibiotic is contraindicated secondary to allergy, gentamicin is also given within 1 hour of surgery along with vancomycin.

MONITORING AND VASCULAR ACCESS

Chapter 2 discussed in detail the placement of invasive monitors and their use in managing perioperative hemodynamic instability.

Depending upon institutional protocols, both the types of monitors employed and the location where such monitors are placed varies. All patients should be provided with a large-bore intravenous catheter. Inpatients often arrive to the holding area with either a #22- or #20-gauge catheter in place. There is often temptation to use such small catheters for anesthesia induction. Although it may be acceptable to do so, if veins of sufficient size are available, placement of a large-bore catheter will facilitate rapid fluid and medication delivery should that be needed and central access not yet established following induction.

Central venous access with or without the use of a pulmonary arterial (PA) flotation catheter can be accomplished either before or after the induction of general anesthesia. In the author's practice, central access is completed following anesthesia induction. In other institutions, central access is done with the patient sedated. The utility of PA catheters perioperatively was discussed in detail in Chapter 2. Placement of a PA catheter remains the individual choice of the physicians involved. Once again, institutional norms are likely to determine whether all, some, or no patients are monitored using a PA catheter.

Arterial line monitoring is of course essential and is customarily placed prior to anesthetic induction. The anesthesiologist should confirm that the radial arteries are not to be harvested for bypass graft conduits. Additionally, the anesthesiologist should consider femoral artery cannulation if needed. Compared with the aortic pressure pulse waves, peripheral pulse waves are narrower with higher systolic pressures and lower diastolic pressures. The mean blood pressures obtained from either a central arterial pressure tracing or from a peripheral arterial line are usually quite similar.

Both transesophageal echocardiography (TEE) and epiaortic ultrasound are routinely used in all patients when not contraindicated. The intraoperative use of TEE dramatically reduces the utility of the PA catheter in managing patients intraoperatively. Nonetheless, the PA catheter is often employed in the ICU setting to aid in the management of postoperative hemodynamic instability. Bispectral index (BIS), although controversial, may be useful as cardiac surgery patients have a high incidence of awareness. Cerebral near infrared spectroscopy is also employed to estimate the adequacy of brain tissue oxygen delivery. Near infrared spectroscopy (NIRS) detects reflected light from cerebral tissue. Cerebral oximetry largely reflects the absorption of light by venous hemoglobin. Saturations reduced 20% from baseline or less than 40% overall may indicate inadequate brain tissue oxygenation. Decreased brain oxygen delivery can be secondary to many factors including increased cerebral vascular resistance (e.g., secondary to reduced $PaCO_2$), low hemoglobin, reduced cardiac output, and increased cerebral metabolic rate.

Immediate preoperative laboratory values should be obtained including blood gas, activated clotting time, thromboelastography, electrolytes, blood glucose concentration, and ionized calcium. Additionally, tests of kidney and hepatic function should be reviewed.

ANESTHETIC INDUCTION AND MAINTENANCE

Induction of patients undergoing cardiac surgery should be performed with the perfusionist and a member of the surgical team capable of performing sternotomy in the operating room, in case the need for emergent institution of cardiopulmonary bypass (CPB) arises secondary to intractable hemodynamic instability.

All patients are preoxygenated. Choice of induction agents varies according to the individual practitioner and the particular anesthesia-related issues at play.

There is no magic formula that can be universally applied that will ensure hemo-dynamic stability during anesthetic induction. Every possible combination of nar-cotics, inhalational agents, and intravenous anesthetics can be employed in the management of the cardiac surgical patient.

Determining which combination of agents to employ is of course the task of the attending anesthesiologist. In making this choice the following must be considered:

1. How will the induction affect the balance between myocardial oxygen supply and myocardial oxygen demand?
2. Does the patient have ventricular dysfunction to the degree that the patient will not be able to tolerate a decrease in venous return, myocardial depression, or vasodilatation at the time of induction?
3. What other anesthetic considerations might influence the choice of agents?

Imbalance between myocardial oxygen supply and myocardial oxygen demand can readily lead to postinduction ischemia. Inadequate anesthesia and analgesia contribute to the development of tachycardia and hypertension leading to increased myocardial wall tension, greater myocardial oxygen demand, and decreased myo-cardial oxygen delivery. Consequently, historically many anesthesiologists have used large doses of synthetic narcotics (e.g., fentanyl 50-100 µg/kg) to blunt the hypertensive and tachycardic response to stimulation. Various amounts of intrave-nous midazolam (2-10 mg) along with non-depolarizing muscle relaxants are also employed in the anesthetic induction.

Currently, most anesthesiologists use a lower narcotic dose and manage peri-induction hypertension and tachycardia with inhalational anesthetics (e.g., sevo-flurane) and short-acting beta-blockers (e.g., esmolol), assuming the patient has a relatively normal ventricular function. Propofol and/or ketamine are routinely included in induction regimens for the cardiac surgery patient. Should hypoten-sion develop at the time of induction, it should be treated with phenylephrine, vasopressin or other vasopressors, volume administration, and the stimulation of direct laryngoscopy and intubation.

Ultimately, the anesthesiologist will attempt to prevent peri-induction myocar-dial ischemia by being both proactive and reactive. Proactive management implies that the anesthesiologist is prepared for and aware of the hemodynamic changes likely to occur with induction of any cardiac patient. In this way, the anesthesi-ologist prevents hemodynamic instability. Predicting the hemodynamic course of the patient is a hallmark of a skilled cardiac anesthesiologist. Concurrently, the anesthesiologist is immediately reactive, prepared to respond to changes during the induction through constant surveillance of the many hemodynamic monitors employed.

Should myocardial ischemia occur following induction, it can produce new wall motion abnormalities on TEE (Videos 4–1 and 4–2), ST-segment elevation or depression on ECG, and/or an increase in PA pressure. The anesthesiologist will respond accordingly by treating the triggering event thought to provoke ischemia. Inotropes (e.g., epinephrine, milrinone) could be administered by infusion to improve ventricular function. The surgery and perfusion teams should be alerted that the patient has become acutely ischemic in the event that emergency institution of CPB becomes necessary. Fortunately, most inductions are conducted in such a manner that the balance of myocardial oxygen supply and demand is maintained. Nonetheless, acute coronary syndrome secondary to coronary artery thrombosis unrelated to transient imbalances in myocardial oxygen supply/demand can also become manifest perioperatively leading to large ST-segment elevations.

More than ever, patients with both diastolic and systolic dysfunction present for cardiac surgery and the cardiac anesthesiologist must often induce patients at risk for both myocardial ischemia and perioperative hemodynamic collapse.[2] Patients with systolic dysfunction maintain their stroke volume (SV) through several compensatory mechanisms: expansion of the circulating blood volume, increased sympathetic tone, and ventricular dilatation. Although the heart may contract poorly (Video 4–3), the adaptive responses mentioned above may maintain an adequate cardiac output for vital organ perfusion. Anesthetic induction reduces sympathetic tone, lowers blood pressure, and decreases venous return. Positive pressure ventilation similarly reduces venous return to the heart. Therefore, following induction, the cardiac output can decrease profoundly as the anesthesiologist perturbs the patient's compensatory mechanisms. Coronary perfusion pressure may decrease, and the patient may develop myocardial ischemia leading to further hypotension and circulatory collapse.

At times, concern for severe hemodynamic instability may prompt the placement of an intra-aortic balloon pump prior to induction (see Chapter 11). Other patients may present supported by a percutaneous left ventricular assist device (Chapter 11).

Anesthesiologists planning the induction of the cardiac surgery patient must consider the routine anesthetic concerns found in all patients. With all anesthetics the fundamentals of ABC (airway, breathing, and circulation) apply. Patients with airway problems undergoing cardiac surgery require special consideration. The American Society of Anesthesiologists' algorithm for the management of difficult airways[3] is applicable to both cardiac surgery and noncardiac surgery populations. Awake intubation when needed should be undertaken in the cardiac surgery patient with the understanding that careful hemodynamic monitoring is necessary to prevent stress-induced tachycardias and myocardial ischemia. While the airway is being secured, one member of the anesthesia team should be constantly focused upon the patient's hemodynamics to respond to any intubation-related perturbations. Nasal intubations should be avoided if possible, as many patients are treated with various anticoagulation regimens and all will be systemically heparinized if CPB is planned.

Maintenance of anesthesia consists of a combination of narcotics, non-depolarizing muscle relaxants, inhalational agents, and, possibly, propofol. Anesthetic agents are titrated to optimize blood pressure and heart rate and to respond to the needs of the surgery team. Systolic blood pressure is generally reduced to less than 100 mm Hg at the time of aortic cannulation. During surgery, the heart is often lifted, compressed, or manipulated leading to transient periods of hypotension. Communication with the surgical team during times of heart manipulation and careful anesthetic titration will allow the patient to better tolerate hemodynamically these interventions. Reductions in mean arterial pressure less than 65 mm Hg or 20% from patient baseline are not advised and may lead to perioperative kidney injury or other adverse outcomes.

For many years it was thought that there were no specific benefits of one anesthetic regimen over another as long as the patient's hemodynamics were maintained. However, inhalational agents may provide a cardioprotective effect independent of their use in maintaining the balance between myocardial oxygen supply and demand.[4-8] Anesthetic preconditioning, similar to ischemic preconditioning, has been suggested as a mechanism by which the use of volatile anesthetics may permit the heart to better tolerate ischemic injury during surgery.

When myocardial ischemia occurs, the muscle cells die if the blood flow is not restored. However, even after blood flow is restored, the myocyte may yet be impaired or die through reperfusion injury. Ischemic preconditioning is the process through which repeated short episodes of ischemia protect the myocardium against a subsequent ischemic insult. The mechanisms by which the cell adapts are multifactorial and well beyond the scope of this text. However, preservation of cellular mitochondrial function through the activation of the mitochondrial K-ATP channel may be central to the preconditioning effect.[8] Anesthetic preconditioning is thought to offer a pharmacological equivalent to ischemic preconditioning ultimately preserving cellular mitochondrial function during periods of ischemic stress. Various clinical studies have attempted to demonstrate improved myocardial preservation or reduced biomarkers of perioperative myocardial injury; however, the overall impact of the use of inhalational agents on clinical outcomes such as mortality and morbidity remains unclear.[7] Nonetheless, the inclusion of inhalational anesthetics in the management of patients at risk for myocardial ischemia may have a protective benefit.

Patient positioning is checked to make sure that the arms are padded and that the face is free of any pressure.

Prior to surgical incision a *time-out* is performed so that all healthcare staff in the room re-identify the patient and the surgical procedure. The surgeon completes the sternotomy while assistants harvest saphenous vein graft conduits or the radial arteries. During sternotomy, the anesthesia team deflates the lungs to reduce the potential for the sternal saw to create lung injury. The surgeon next dissects free from the sternum the left internal mammary artery (LIMA). This graft is usually anastomosed to the left anterior descending artery and has been shown to benefit the coronary artery disease patient greatly, having a significantly lower rate of stenosis compared with vein grafts. The right internal mammary artery (RIMA) may also be harvested and used as a free conduit.

INSTITUTION OF CARDIOPULMONARY BYPASS

After dissecting of the arterial and vein conduits, the surgeon next prepares for the initiation of CPB [assuming surgery is not performed off-pump (see Chapter 13)]. The anesthesiologist administers 300 to 400 U/kg of heparin into a central line. The patient's activated clotting time (ACT) is measured, and an arterial blood gas is obtained. The surgeon will next examine the ascending aorta to identify a location for placement of the aortic perfusion cannula. Epiaortic ultrasound is often used to identify areas free of atherosclerotic plaque buildup. The aortic perfusion cannula is placed. At this time the anesthesiologist will lower the patient's blood pressure to less than 100 mm Hg systolic. This can be done gradually through the use of increased inhalational agents, intravenous anesthetics, or antihypertensive agents (e.g., nitroglycerin). Next the surgeon will place the venous cannula. A snare suture is placed in the right atrial appendage. Often, manipulation of the heart leads to various atrial and/or ventricular dysrhythmias. In general, these abnormal rhythms stop when the heart is no longer being manipulated. However, occasionally a patient will become unstable with rapid atrial or ventricular fibrillation. Should this occur, the patient can be placed on CPB emergently assuming the ACT is greater than 400 to 480 seconds or the patient can be cardioverted. Using internal paddles, the surgeon can cardiovert or defibrillate the patient. At times, pressor support is necessary to maintain blood pressure following heparin administration. In the event of hypotension, the anesthesiologist can also request that the perfusionist administer volume through the aortic perfusion cannula. This should be discussed with the surgeon who will confirm that all line clamps have been removed and that the cannula is correctly positioned in the aorta and free of air bubbles. Following placement of various cardioplegia cannulas, the surgeon will initiate CPB by releasing the clamps on the venous cannula. At this time the venous return is directed toward the venous reservoir on bypass machine. Pulmonary artery blood flow decreases as noted by the fall in PA pressures. The heart deflates in the chest. When the perfusionist notes that they are at "full flow," and the heart is no longer ejecting blood in the pulmonary and systemic circulation, ventilation to the patient can be discontinued; however, low tidal volume ventilation during CPB has been advocated by some to prevent atelectasis and reduce lung ischemia reperfusion injury since only the bronchial circulation continues to supply the deflated lungs during CPB. However, the long-term impact of ventilation strategies during CPB is not as of yet established.[9] At "full flow," venous return from the patient is directed to the bypass machine and not to the right heart and pulmonary artery; therefore, the lungs no longer oxygenate the venous blood. The patient's face is checked for swelling to rule out inadequate drainage from the superior vena cava. The surgeon next places the aortic cross clamp, thus isolating the coronary arteries from systemic aortic blood flow. Potassium-rich cardioplegia solution is next administered arresting the heart so that the surgical repair may proceed. Cardiopulmonary bypass management is discussed in detail in Chapter 17.

SEPARATION FROM CPB

After completion of coronary revascularization (and/or other surgical interventions), the patient must be separated from the bypass machine. The process of separation begins when the surgeon removes the aortic cross clamp. Blood from the aorta now flows through the coronary arteries and the venous bypass grafts. The patient is gradually rewarmed until core temperature is greater than 36°C and peripheral temperature is at least 35.5°C. During this time, the heart will begin to beat as the cardiac rhythm is restored either by epicardial pacing or the return of the heart's intrinsic rhythm. After the aortic cross clamp is removed, the flow of arterial blood into the heart washes out the cardioplegia solution, the cardiac rhythm is restored, and the heart contracts. Arterial blood gases are checked to confirm that the heart's metabolic environment is sufficiently normalized such that it can be expected to function in a normal manner. The frequency of blood samples obtained for analysis during CPB and the laboratory values measured vary from institution to institution. Most frequently they include:

- Potassium concentration: Hyperkalemia is usually secondary to cardioplegia solution. Spontaneous diuresis frequently results in a potassium concentration less than 6 mEq/L. Should the potassium concentration be elevated, restoration of an effective cardiac rhythm is unlikely. Administration of 10 units of regular insulin along with 1 ampule of dextrose 50% will temporarily shift potassium intracellularly. Correction of any metabolic acidosis will also lower serum potassium concentration. Administration of furosemide will promote diuresis reducing potassium as well. Kidney failure patients at times need urgent dialysis following heart surgery as they lack the ability to eliminate potassium through the kidneys.
- Glucose concentration: Blood glucose concentration is maintained perioperatively through the use of regular insulin infusions. Excessively tight blood glucose control is avoided to prevent possible hypoglycemia. Individual institutions have their own protocols for perioperative glucose management during cardiac surgery. (See Chapter 5.)
- Sodium concentration: Hyponatremia and hypernatremia are not routinely encountered during cardiac surgery. Balanced crystalloid solutions are preferred to normal saline infusions because saline may generate a hyperchloremic metabolic acidosis.
- Ionized calcium concentration: Calcium chloride 300 to 1000 mg IV can be administered to correct symptomatic hypocalcemia. Because of calcium's role in cellular injury, routine use of calcium chloride at separation from CPB is not recommended in the absence of hypocalcemia.
- pH: Assuming an uneventful bypass run, the patient should not have accumulated any metabolic acids. However, should metabolic acidosis occur, the differential diagnosis would include gut ischemia (e.g., secondary to gut hypoperfusion), kidney failure with acid buildup, and diabetic ketoacidosis. Lactate acidosis secondary to systemic hypoperfusion might also occur; however, during the bypass run venous oxygen saturation is usually closely monitored by the perfusionist to ensure adequate tissue oxygen delivery.
- Hematocrit: There is much controversy in the literature regarding the triggers for the perioperative transfusion of packed red blood cells during heart surgery. Red blood cell transfusion must be determined on an individual patient basis following discussion between the anesthesiologist, the surgeon, and the perfusionist. Generally, hematocrits lower than 18% are treated with red blood cell transfusion. Hemoconcentration during CPB permits the perfusionist to reduce the patient's plasma volume, thereby augmenting the hematocrit. Blood component therapy in the cardiac surgery patient is discussed in detail in Chapter 16.

Before the patient can be separated from CPB, the heart must return to its normal activity—rhythmically contracting and relaxing to effectively pump blood to the tissues. Following removal of the cross clamp and the washout of cardioplegia solution, the heart often returns to a normal sinus rhythm. However, at times upon removal of the aortic cross clamp the heart may fibrillate and thus must be defibrillated. Lidocaine, magnesium, and amiodarone may be given to facilitate defibrillation. Still other patients develop varying degrees of heart block (Chapter 3) requiring pacing. Surgeons routinely place epicardial pacing wires so that the institution of dual-chamber (DDD) pacing may facilitate CPB separation. A heart rate of 80 to 100 bpm is usually needed for an adequate cardiac output at separation from bypass.

The lungs are next inflated, and ventilation commenced. Inflation of the lungs is watchfully done so as to not overinflate and overdistend the lungs, which could potentially compromise the LIMA to left anterior descending artery bypass graft. Both the anesthesiologist and surgeon observe the lungs rising in the chest. Should the pleura have been opened perioperatively, the surgeon evacuates any blood that might have collected in the thoracic cavity.

With the patient ventilated, the rhythm restored, and the myocardial metabolic environment normalized, it is possible to begin the process of separation from the bypass machine.

Recall, the basics of hemodynamics:

Blood pressure = Cardiac output × Systemic vascular resistance

At the point of separation from CPB, the anesthesiologist must determine how to influence the patient's vascular tone and cardiac output to create the conditions to wean from CPB. The anesthesiologist is able to influence a number of parameters when weaning a patient from bypass. Vascular tone can be increased or decreased using vasoconstrictors (norepinephrine, vasopressin) or vasodilators (nitroglycerin, inhalational anesthetics). The patient's preload can be adjusted by giving additional volume. Lastly, the heart's contractility can be augmented using inotropes such as milrinone, epinephrine, and levosimendan. How each of these parameters is manipulated is individualized depending upon the patient.

Using TEE and/or the PA catheter the anesthesiologist acquires additional necessary information to separate the patient from the bypass machine.

The surgeon will gradually reduce the flow into the venous cannula; thereafter, the heart, which previously had no volume, begins to fill. Many surgeons will have the pump flow reduced to about 2 L/min of flow. In doing so, the patient is delivered 2 L of cardiac output from the pump with additional cardiac output produced by their own beating heart. With the pump flow reduced to 2 L/min, the anesthesiologist and the surgeon assess how likely the patient is to be able to maintain a suitable blood pressure with the newly repaired heart doing all the work of pumping the blood.

In the majority of patients, the heart is clearly seen beating in the chest. Although the anesthesiologist can usually see only the right heart beating, a vigorous contractile heart is a good first indicator that the patient will be weaned easily from bypass support.

Next, the anesthesiologist uses TEE to examine the heart's function and integrity. A highly contractile heart is clear. Likewise, a heart, which is poorly contractile, is also rather obvious even to new echocardiographers.

If the patient has a strongly contractile heart and a mean blood pressure of greater than 70 mm Hg, pump flow is further reduced from 2 L/min and the patient is weaned from bypass support. On the other hand, if the heart is strongly contracting and the mean blood pressure is less than 50 mm Hg, that patient is likely vasodilated. A number of patients following CPB develop vasoplegia.[10,11] Vasodilatation following CPB is thought to be secondary to the inflammatory response associated with surgery and CPB. Even though these patients have a very contractile heart, they are so vasodilated that they cannot maintain a suitable blood pressure. These patients are treated with vasoconstrictors.

Vasopressin 1 to 6 U/h by infusion can be titrated to effect. Norepinephrine can likewise be used. Methylene blue has also been suggested in cases of refractory vasoplegia syndrome. Methylene blue is an inhibitor of guanylate cyclase–mediated vasodilatation. With restoration of vascular tone, the patient is successfully weaned from bypass support.

A patient with left, right, or biventricular failure requires improved contractility to separate from the bypass machine. Whereas the heart with normal systolic function beats energetically in the chest, the poorly functioning heart will distend as it is filled upon separation from CPB. As the surgeon retards flow to the bypass machine, the failing heart will increasingly distend. As it is volume loaded, its poor compliance leads to increases in left ventricular end-diastolic pressure and pulmonary arterial pressures. On TEE the heart looks distended and contracts poorly. Mean blood pressure quickly falls along with mixed venous oxygen saturation. In such instances the heart has failed to separate from bypass and bypass machine flow must be restored.

The failed heart is managed with inotropic agents. Dobutamine, milrinone, levosimendan, and epinephrine can all be employed. Often multiple agents are administered to simultaneously increase contractility and vascular tone. Mechanical assistance (e.g., intraaortic balloon pump, ventricular assist devices) can be employed as well, should pharmacological means fail to separate the patient from CPB. (See Chapter 11.)

Once the patient is separated from the bypass machine, additional amounts of volume can be transfused judiciously as needed depending upon the loading conditions required. TEE can assess the adequacy of volume loading along with PA pressure measurements. An underloaded ventricle appears on TEE as the ventricular cavity is obliterated with each beat at end systole. Assuming relatively normal compliance, falling PA pressures and central venous pressures indicate the need for additional volume administration. Cardiac output determinations can likewise be obtained to help guide inotropic, vasoconstrictor, and volume therapies. A low stroke volume (SV) in the setting of high PA pressures and poor contractility on TEE suggests that the patient would benefit from inotropic therapy. An increased SV in the setting of low blood pressure suggests a vasodilated patient in need of vasoconstrictors. Lastly, the hypotensive patient with a low SV, low PA pressures, and good contractility on TEE might benefit from volume administration.

Of course many patients are hypovolemic, vasodilated, and hypokinetic concurrently and as such separation from bypass requires the anesthesia team to rapidly adjust their responses depending upon the patient's progress.

When the patient is considered stable and after the adequacy of any valve repair or replacement has been evaluated by TEE, heparin anticoagulation is reversed through the administration of protamine. Protamine is slowly administered in a 1 mg:100 U ratio with heparin or less, depending on the last dosing of heparin and last ACT on CPB. When heparin concentration assays are used perioperatively, they will determine the protamine dose to be given. Protamine interacts with heparin eliminating its antithrombin effect.

Protamine is slowly administered as it can be associated with a number of adverse reactions. Rapid administration results in histamine release and can lead to decreased vascular tone and hypotension. Fulminant anaphylaxis can also occur, resulting in circulatory collapse, edema, and bronchoconstriction. Pulmonary hypertension and right ventricular failure are also associated with protamine administration. Unlike allergic or histamine-mediated responses to protamine, circulatory collapse in this setting is due to increased pulmonary vascular resistance (PVR) thought secondary to production of thromboxane in response to heparin protamine complexes and accompanying right ventricular failure. Should pulmonary hypertension occur, protamine delivery should be suspended and inotropes should be employed to support the right heart. Full heparinization and reinstitution of CPB may be required. Subsequent protamine administration may result in similar episodes of hemodynamic instability. Should heparin not be reversed, ongoing bleeding can be expected until the heparin is metabolized. Blood product administration is likely. However, most patients tolerate protamine administration uneventfully when administered gradually.

Protamine has the potential for immediate patient death if given inadvertently while on cardiopulmonary bypass.

Clotting of the bypass circuit can occur if anticoagulation is reversed in a patient while on CPB. Should this error occur, results are catastrophic. Protamine should be kept separate from all other drugs employed during cardiac anesthesia and administered only after discussion between the attending cardiac surgeon and the attending anesthesiologist.

Following protamine, the activated clotting time is normalized. Nonetheless, many patients require ongoing blood product administration. Coagulopathy, hemodilution, and platelet dysfunction all contribute to bleeding. Coagulation tests are obtained, and blood products are administered as needed. Often therapy is empiric as laboratory results are too slow to successfully guide blood product delivery and many operating rooms lack the capacity of point-of-care testing for coagulation (see Chapter 16 for discussion of point-of-care coagulation management). Hypothermia should be avoided following separation from CPB as it leads to vasoconstriction, low cardiac output, and coagulopathy.

STERNAL CLOSURE AND PATIENT TRANSPORT

With the mediastinum sufficiently "dry," sternal wires are placed and the chest closed. During sternal closure the TEE should be examined both before and after closure. Patients can become hypotensive following chest closure particularly if the right heart is dysfunctional and distended. Compression of the heart by the sternum can lead to inadequate loading and hypotension. At times a clot can accrue around the heart leading to tamponade in the operating room. Reopening the sternum and evacuating any clot will relieve tamponade and restore hemodynamic stability. In certain patients the heart can be so dysfunctional and edematous that sternal closure is not possible. In such instances the sternum is left open, covered with a membrane, and the patient transported to the ICU for ongoing management until chest closure is feasible.

With full monitoring in place and both emergency drugs and emergency airway equipment ready, the stable patient is transported to the ICU.

COMMONLY USED VASOACTIVE DRUGS IN THE CARDIAC SURGERY PATIENT

Inotropic agents are used to improve myocardial contractility.[12] These agents work by increasing intracellular calcium or by affecting the interaction between the myofibrillar proteins. The catecholamines, dobutamine (2-10 µg/kg/min), epinephrine (0.01-0.15 µ/kg/min), and the phosphodiesterase inhibitor milrinone (50 µg/kg load, 0.375-0.75 µg/kg/min) increase the intracellular concentration of calcium ion as a last step of their mechanism of action leading to increased contractility. Unfortunately, the use of these drugs may result in an increased incidence of arrhythmias, worsened diastolic function, and increased myocardial oxygen demand. Also, they have been associated with increased mortality in patients being medically treated for heart failure. Nonetheless, these agents remain an important part of the anesthetic armamentarium as they do transiently improve ventricular function. In the perioperative period, transient support is often necessary to separate from CPB. Perioperative administration of inotropic agents should never be done routinely according to a mandatory protocol but only in response to specific needs for such support.[13]

Levosimendan (0.05-0.2 µg/kg/min) renders the myofibrillar proteins more sensitive to the intracellular calcium already present in the cell, therefore prolonging the cross-bridging time in systole. It avoids the calcium ion overload associated with the catecholamines and PDE inhibitors. Levosimendan produces vasodilation through its effects upon K^+ channels causing smooth muscle membrane hyperpolarization.[14] Levosimendan has also been reported to open the mitochondrial K-ATP channels, which are thought to provide a pharmacological preconditioning to ischemic injury.[15] Levosimendan exerts mild lusitropic effects improving diastolic relaxation. The intraoperative use of levosimendan may be complicated by its potential to produce vasodilatation leading to the need for vasoconstrictor support of the blood pressure. Additionally, recent studies have questioned the utility of levosimendan to improve outcome endpoints (e.g., 30-day mortality) in patients with left ventricular dysfunction undergoing cardiac surgery.[16,17]

Vasoplegia syndrome following CPB is treated with the administration of vasoconstrictors. Norepinephrine stimulates primarily alpha-receptors producing vasoconstriction. It is titrated to effect starting at 0.02 µg/kg/min. Vasopressin (1-6 U/h) is also employed to restore vascular tone following separation from CPB. Vasopressin acts to increase intracellular calcium through the V_1 receptor in the vascular smooth muscle.[18] Vasopressin and norepinephrine may act synergistically to restore tone in vasoplegic patients such as those treated preoperatively with angiotensin converting enzyme inhibitors.

CASE ILLUSTRATION

A 72-year-old man is scheduled for coronary revascularization.

What preoperative information is required to manage the patient?

The usual preanesthetic examination is completed. The anatomy of the coronary arteries is reviewed on the catheterization film and reported. The patient's ejection fraction is noted along with the presence of any other cardiac condition such as valvular disease or diastolic dysfunction. The patient's medical regimen is reviewed. Discontinuation of any medications preoperatively such as antiplatelet agents, anticoagulants, or antihypertensives is made *only* after consulting with the patient's cardiologist and surgeon.

The patient is found to have more than 60% stenosis of the left main coronary artery. His EF is preserved; he has had some dyspnea on exertion. How should induction proceed?

Following placement of invasive monitors, the patient is induced with the use of midazolam, fentanyl, muscle relaxants, and propofol. Following induction the blood pressure drops to 60 mm Hg systolic and the ST segments in leads V4 to V6 are noted to rise.

How should the anesthesia team respond?

The ECG shows signs of ischemia in the setting of hypotension upon induction. A vasoconstrictor such as phenylephrine is administered with restoration of the BP to 120 mm Hg. However, the ECG continues to show signs of ischemia. PA pressures are noted to have increased to 75/40 mm Hg.

The TEE reveals anterior wall hypokinesis and the presence of acute mitral regurgitation. The PA and systemic pressures equalize at 60/40 mm Hg. The surgeon proceeds to emergently open the chest. What other maneuvers might assist this patient?

It appears that the patient is having acute ischemia and does not respond to restoration of blood pressure with a vasoconstrictor. An intra-aortic balloon pump can be placed. In the setting of acute ischemia, emergency institution of CPB is warranted. The anesthesiologist administers a full (300-400 U/kg) dose of heparin. Following heparinization, the patient is placed on emergent CPB and the bypass grafts completed.

During an attempt at weaning from CPB, the pump flow is reduced to 1 L/min. The mean arterial blood pressure is 40 mm Hg. The PA pressures are 60/40 mm Hg. What does the TEE video clip show (**Video 4–4**)?

The patient has a clearly dysfunctional heart. Inotropic therapy with epinephrine is started. Vasopressin is used to restore vascular tone. Mean blood pressure increases to 70 mm Hg, and PA pressures decline to 40/20 mm Hg. TEE reveals improved ventricular function.

Protamine is slowly given to reverse heparin anticoagulation in a 1 mg:100 U ratio with heparin. However, following the delivery of two-thirds of the protamine dose, PA pressures are noted to increase to 75/60 mm Hg with a systemic pressure of 90/60 mm Hg. TEE now shows a dysfunctional right heart in the setting of a protamine reaction. What should the anesthesiologist do?

Protamine is immediately discontinued. A complete heparin dose for the reinstitution of CPB is also prepared. Inotropic and vasoconstrictor medications are adjusted. The patient improves. Additional protamine is not given, and the sternum is closed.

SUMMARY

Routine management of the cardiac surgery patient is anything but routine. Anesthesia teams must constantly respond to the hemodynamic challenges presented not only by the patient's primary cardiac disease but also by the surgical manipulations of the heart and the hemodynamic consequences of CPB. Anesthesiologists integrate information obtained from visualization of the beating heart, echocardiography, and invasive monitors to determine the best approaches to maintain hemodynamic stability. In subsequent chapters, various pathological conditions are introduced and their specific implications for anesthetic management discussed. However, all cases utilizing CPB basically involve the same four stages of management: induction and prebypass, bypass, separation from bypass, and sternal closure and transport.

REFERENCES

1. Engelman R, Shahian D, Shemin D, et al. The Society of Thoracic Surgeons practice guideline series: antibiotic prophylaxis in cardiac surgery, part II: antibiotic choice. *Ann Thorac Surg.* 2007;83:1569-1576.
2. Couture P, Denault A, Shi Y, et al. Effects of anesthetic induction in patients with diastolic dysfunction. *Can J Anesth.* 2009;56(5):357-365.
3. ASA taskforce on management of the difficult airway. Practice guidelines for management of the difficult airway. *Anesthesiology.* 2003;98:1269-1277.
4. Landoni G, Gignami E, Oliviero F, et al. Halogenated anaesthetics and cardiac protection in cardiac and non-cardiac anaesthesia. *Ann Card Anesth.* 2009;12(1):4-9.
5. Tritapepe L, Landoni G, Guarracino F, et al. Cardiac protection by volatile anaesthetics: a multicentre randomized controlled study in patients undergoing coronary artery bypass grafting with cardiopulmonary bypass. *EJA.* 2007;24:323-331.
6. DeHert SG. Anesthetic preconditioning: how important is it in today's cardiac anesthesia? *J Cardiothorac Vasc Anesth.* 2006;20:473-476.
7. DeHert SG, Van der Linden P, Cromheecke S, et al. Choice of primary anesthetic regimen can influence intensive care unit length of stay after coronary surgery with cardiopulmonary bypass. *Anesthesiology.* 2004;101:9-20.
8. DeHert SG. Cardioprotection with volatile anesthetics: clinical relevance. *Curr Opin. Anaesth.* 2004; 17(1):57-62.
9. Schreiber J, Lance M, de Korte M, et al. The effect of different lung protective strategies in patients during cardiopulmonary bypass: a meta-analysis and semiquantitative review of randomized trials. *J Cardiothorac Vasc Anesth.* 2012 Jun; 26(3):448-454.
10. Mekontso-Dessap A, Houel R, Soustelle C, et al. Risk factors for post-cardiopulmonary bypass vasoplegia in patients with preserved left ventricular function. *Ann Thorac Surg.* 2001;71:1428-1432.
11. Leyh R, Kofidis T, Struber M, et al. Methylene blue: the drug of choice for catecholamine-refractory vasoplegia after cardiopulmonary bypass? *J Thorac Cardiovasc Surg.* 2003;125:1426-1431.

12. Hannon J, Housmans P. Inotropic therapy. In: Housmans P, Nuttall G (eds). *Advances in Cardiovascular Pharmacology.* Baltimore, MD: Lippincott Williams & Wilkins;2008:1-15.

13. Fellahi J, Parienti J, Hanouz J, et al. Perioperative use of dobutamine in cardiac surgery and adverse cardiac outcome: propensity adjusted analyses. *Anesthesiology.* 2008;108(6):979-987.

14. Pierrakos C, Velissaris D, Franchi F, et al. Levosimendan in critical illness: a literature review. *J Clin Med Res.* 2014;6(2):75-85.

15. Toller W, Archan S. Levosimendan. In: Housmans P, Nuttall G (eds). *Advances in Cardiovascular Pharmacology.* Baltimore, MD: Lippincott Williams & Wilkins, 2008:17-42.

16. Landoni G, Lomivorotov V, Alvaro G, et al. Levosimendan for hemodynamic support after cardiac surgery. *NEJM.* 2017;376:2021-2031.

17. Mehta R, Leimberger J, van Diepen, et al. Levosimendan in patients with left ventricular dysfunction undergoing cardiac surgery. *NEJM.* 2017;376:2032-2042.

18. Kan R, Berkowitz D. In: Housmans P, Nuttall G (eds). *Advances in Cardiovascular Pharmacology.* Baltimore, MD: Lippincott Williams & Wilkins. 2008:67-90.

The Complicated Patient for Cardiac Anesthesia and Surgery

The elective patient for cardiac anesthesia and surgery free of other disease processes is increasingly a *rara avis*. Prior to advances in percutaneous interventions, the routine cardiac surgery patient was an otherwise healthy middle-aged biological male in need of a one to two vessel coronary artery bypass—How times have changed. Today's cardiac surgery patient is likely to be quite elderly with multiple medical problems presenting for combined revascularization and valvular replacement surgery. Moreover, many patients will have had over the course of their lives other cardiac procedures including previous operations and/or percutaneous interventions. Further complicating matters, many of these patients suffer from both systolic and diastolic dysfunction.

THE PATIENT WITH IMPAIRED SYSTOLIC AND DIASTOLIC VENTRICULAR FUNCTION

Systolic Dysfunction

In past decades, patients presented for cardiac surgery in need of one to two vessel bypass grafts. Usually, their chief complaint was angina and they had no or minimal myocardial damage. Patients with ejection fractions (EFs) of greater than 60% were the rule and not the exception.

Such patients tended to tolerate the peri-induction period well and were readily separated from cardiopulmonary bypass (CPB) with little need for pharmacological or mechanical support. Ventricular function tended to be preserved throughout surgery and recovery, assuming acceptable myocardial preservation and surgical techniques.

Today's cardiac surgical patient is far more challenging. Patients are older with varying degrees of systolic and diastolic dysfunction frequently presenting in congestive heart failure.

Congestive heart failure affects more than 5 million Americans with coronary artery disease (CAD) as a primary etiology.[1] Cardiac surgical outcomes are worse in patients with previous episodes of congestive heart failure, chronic obstructive pulmonary disease, increased age, and peripheral vascular disease (Figure 5–1).

However, preserved right ventricular function in the setting of a severely compromised left ventricle (EF < 25%) may improve perioperative outcomes[2] (Figure 5–2). Impaired LV diastolic function produces an increase in left ventricular end-diastolic pressure (LVEDP) that is transmitted to the pulmonary circulation. A patient whose right ventricle functions well and tolerates any perioperative worsening in LV diastolic dysfunction has a potentially better surgical outcome than a patient with biventricular failure.

What is certain is that long-term survival in the heart failure (HF) population is low compared with patients with preserved function[3] (Figure 5–3). Operative mortality (< 30 day postoperative) in patients with EF < 30% undergoing surgical revascularization has been reported as high as 4.6% compared with 1.9% in patients with preserved ventricular function.[3] However, low EF patients treated with surgical revascularization have a better long-term survival than those treated medically.[3] Thus, although immediate short-term morbidity and mortality are high compared to patients with normal ventricular function, surgical revascularization may offer improved survival over the long-term when compared to low EF patients treated medically. Consequently, an ever-increasing number of patients with compromised systolic left ventricular function may become candidates for surgical revascularization.

Heart failure (HF) in cardiac surgical patients may be secondary to ischemia, valvular heart disease, infectious agents, or myriad cardiomyopathies.[4] Measurements of brain natriuretic peptide (BNP) are routinely used to identify the heart failure patient. A BNP concentration of > 500 pg/mL is indicative of heart failure. BNP produces arterial and venous vasodilatation as well as diuresis. Recombinant BNP (nesiritide) has been employed to manage acute episodes of congestive heart failure. Unlike inotropes, it does not affect heart rate or myocardial contractility but rather unloads the failing heart through vascular smooth muscle cell relaxation.

In response to ventricular failure the body attempts to compensate for failing LV systolic function through the sympathetic and the renin-angiotensin-aldosterone systems. Consequently, the HF patient experiences salt retention, volume expansion, sympathetic stimulation, and vasoconstriction.[4] The heart dilates and remodels to maintain stroke volume (SV) in spite of decreased contractility. Augmented sympathetic tone preserves blood pressure. However, these compensatory mechanisms ultimately fail and contribute to many of the symptoms associated

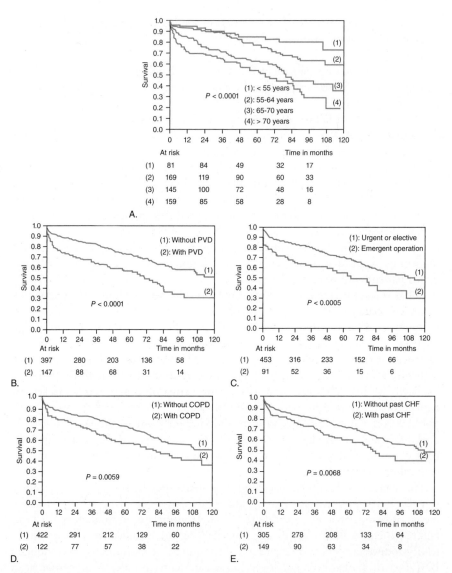

Figure 5–1. In a retrospective analysis of 525 patients with ejection fractions less than 25%, long-term outcomes were identified in these Kaplan-Meier survival curves. Increasing age (A), presence of peripheral vascular disease (B), emergent nature of surgery (C), presence of chronic obstructive pulmonary disease (D), and previous episodes of pulmonary congestion (E) all predict a poorer long-term outcome following coronary artery bypass surgery. [Reproduced with permission from DeRose JJ Jr, Toumpoulis IK, Balaram SK, et al: Preoperative prediction of long-term survival after coronary artery bypass grafting in patients with low left ventricular ejection fraction, *J Thorac Cardiovasc Surg.* 2005 Feb;129(2):314-21.]

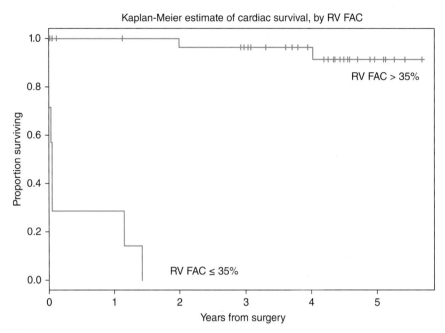

Figure 5–2. Survival of patients with poor left ventricular systolic function (EF < 25%) is influenced by right ventricular function as estimated by TEE measures of right ventricular fractional area contraction (RVFAC). Patients with normal right function (RVFAC 35%) had superior short- and long-term survival following coronary artery bypass surgery. [Reproduced with permission from Maslow AD, Regan MM, Panzica P, et al: Precardiopulmonary bypass right ventricular function is associated with poor outcome after coronary artery bypass grafting in patients with severe left ventricular systolic dysfunction, *Anesth Analg.* 2002 Dec;95(6):1507-1518.]

with HF including fluid overload, peripheral and pulmonary edema, tachycardia, and decreased organ perfusion. Ventricular remodeling of the failing heart is the result of multiple factors which produce a dilated, dysfunctional LV. The benefit from the use of angiotensin converting enzyme inhibitors (ACE-I) in HF patients is secondary to their vasodilatory properties and inhibition of ventricular remodeling. However, ACE-I can exacerbate hypotension upon anesthetic induction. Angiotensin receptor blockers (ARBs) are also employed as an alternative to ACE inhibitors with similar potential to lead to peri-induction hypotension. Aldosterone inhibitors when used may be associated with hyperkalemia. The American Heart Association provides extensive guidelines on the management of the heart failure patient with both preserved (HFpEF) and reduced ejection fraction (HFrEF) (Figure 5–4).

The patient with LV systolic dysfunction and reduced EF can present for surgery with acute exacerbation or with chronic compensated heart failure. The acute heart failure patient may appear with a greatly reduced EF following a recent myocardial infarction. Other patients will present for surgical revascularization with long-standing ischemic cardiomyopathy. Chronic HF patients usually have

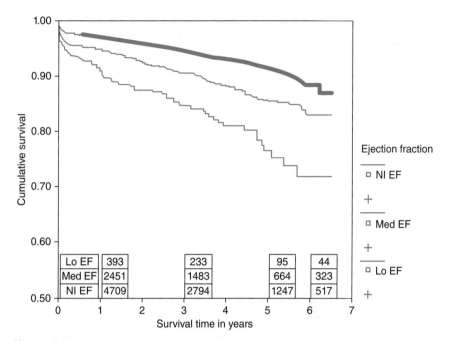

Figure 5–3. 7841 patients were studied between 1996 and 2001 who underwent coronary artery bypass surgery in Canada. Patients were divided into three groups: lo EF (EF < 30%), med EF (EF between 30% and 50%), and NI EF (EF > 50%). Patients with low ejection fractions had significantly reduced long-term survival following bypass surgery compared with those with preserved function. [Reproduced with permission from Appoo J, Norris C, Merali S, et al: Long-term outcome of isolated coronary artery bypass surgery in patients with severe left ventricular dysfunction, *Circulation.* 2004 Sep 14;110(11 Suppl 1):II13–II17.]

undergone numerous PCIs or perhaps previous cardiac surgery interventions. Pre-operative evaluation should focus on the review of catheterization and echocardiography reports. Knowledge of baseline left and right heart function is paramount. Pulmonary arterial pressures will often give clues as to the extent of LV dysfunction and provide insight into the pressure load against which the right heart must work to deliver the stroke volume (SV) to the LV. Often the patient with a reduced EF and/or with active myocardial ischemia will have had placed an intra-aortic balloon pump (IABP)[5] to increase coronary perfusion pressure and augment cardiac output during surgery.

The IABP is placed through the femoral artery into the descending thoracic aorta with the tip just below the takeoff of the left subclavian artery (Figure 5–5, Video 5–1). The IABP provides counter-pulsation to *assist* the heart in its pumping function. The IABP requires a working heart capable of producing a cardiac output to be effective—it is not to be confused with other mechanical supports for ventricular function that more or less assume the pumping duty of the ventricle. The IABP works opposite to the beating of the heart. When the heart contracts during systole, the IABP deflates assisting in drawing blood from the LV into the aorta.

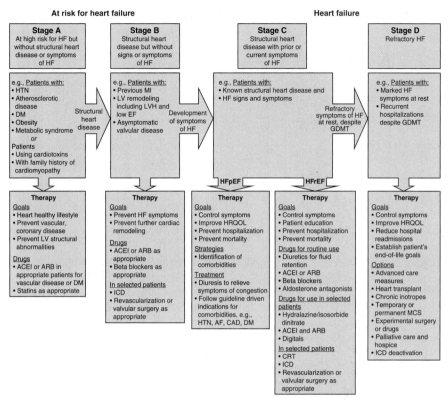

Figure 5–4. Stages in the development of HF and recommended therapy by stage. ACEI indicates angiotensin-converting enzyme inhibitor; AF, atrial fibrillation; ARB, angiotensin-receptor blocker; CAD, coronary artery disease; CRT, cardiac resynchronization therapy; DM, diabetes mellitus; EF, ejection fraction; GDMT, guideline-directed medical therapy; HF, heart failure; HFpEF, heart failure with preserved ejection fraction; HFrEF, heart failure with reduced ejection fraction; HRQOL, health-related quality of life; HTN, hypertension; ICD, implantable cardioverter-defibrillator; LV, left ventricular; LVH, left ventricular hypertrophy; MCS, mechanical circulatory support; and MI, myocardial infarction. [Reproduced with permission from Hunt SA, Abraham WT, Chin MH, et al: 2009 Focused update incorporated into the ACC/AHA 2005 Guidelines for the Diagnosis and Management of Heart Failure in Adults A Report of the American College of Cardiology Foundation/American Heart Association Task Force on Practice Guidelines Developed in Collaboration With the International Society for Heart and Lung Transplantation, *J Am Coll Cardiol.* 2009 Apr 14;53(15):e1-e90.]

When the heart relaxes during diastole and the aortic valve is closed, the IABP inflates increasing diastolic blood pressure and improving coronary perfusion pressure (CPP). Timing of IABP inflation and deflation is accomplished by a triggering mechanism, which can be synchronized to the heart's cycle using either the ECG, or through the arterial pressure wave. The patient with low EF and myocardial ischemia benefits from IABP placement because the increased diastolic pressure can

Systole: IABP deflated

Diastole: IABP inflated

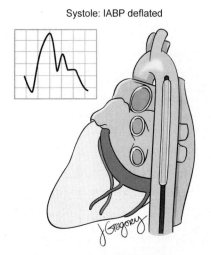
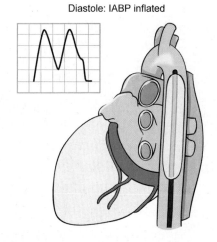

Figure 5–5. An intra-aortic balloon pump (IABP) is positioned distal to the subclavian artery in the descending thoracic aorta. The balloon inflates during diastole. The timing of IABP inflation is adjusted to maximally augment the diastolic pressure. The insets show a normal arterial pressure wave form with the IABP deflated during 1:1 ballooning. During diastole the balloon inflates producing the characteristic "M"-shaped arterial pressure waveform seen here.

improve coronary perfusion increasing myocardial oxygen supply. Additionally, by reducing afterload in systole, LV wall tension is decreased, reducing myocardial oxygen demand. IABP placement is contraindicated in patients with moderate to severe aortic insufficiency (inflation during diastole would increase regurgitant flow across the aortic valve), aortic aneurysms, aortic dissections, and in patients with severe peripheral vascular disease. In most cardiac surgery teams, the perfusionist manages the IABP. The IABP can be adjusted to provide various levels of assistance to the heart, triggered with every heartbeat or with every 1:2 or 1:4 beats. Likewise, the degree to which the balloon is inflated can be adjusted on the control panel. The IABP produces an easily recognizable arterial pressure waveform with increased diastolic pressure. Correct timing of balloon inflation and deflation is necessary to maximize the benefit of IABP placement to the patient. IABPs are not risk free and can produce vascular injury, thrombosis, and leg ischemia. More details on the IABP are found in Chapter 11.

Other patients suffering from cardiogenic shock secondary to reduced left ventricular function may be supported with percutaneous left ventricular assist devices (e.g., Impella). These percutaneous devices pump oxygenated blood from the left ventricle into the ascending aorta and deliver several liters of blood flow past the aortic valve into the systemic circulation (Figure 5–6) (see Chapter 11).

Patients with chronic low EF are also frequently treated with implantable cardioverter-defibrillators (ICDs) and cardiac resynchronization therapy (CRT) to both improve ventricular performance and mitigate the effects of any life-threatening dysrhythmias. The ICD is placed in the therapy-off mode during most

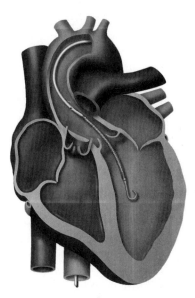

Figure 5-6. Impella 2.5® a percutaneous microaxial blood pump. (Reproduced with permission from Abiomed® 2019.)

surgical procedures including cardiac surgery so as not to trigger aberrantly during surgery. External defibrillation pads are placed when the ICD defibrillation function is turned off. These patients require continuous monitoring throughout the perioperative period until ICD function is restored and the device reprogrammed (see Chapter 15).

There are no anesthetic agents, which offer specific benefits in the induction and maintenance of patients with systolic left heart failure. Various combinations of anesthetic drugs can be used effectively with attention focused on how best to minimize hemodynamic instability in patients with limited cardiac reserve. Whatever agents are employed, all can or will impact the three determinants of stroke volume (SV): the volume delivered to the LV to eject (preload), the contractility of the LV, and the resistance against which the LV must work to deliver the SV into the systemic circulation (afterload). The patient with preserved cardiac function has the reserve to respond to a decrease in loading conditions (preload and afterload) that routinely accompany anesthesia induction. In the patient with CAD and preserved ventricular function, the main peri-induction task of the anesthesiologist is to avoid myocardial ischemia. Tachycardia and reduced CPP in the CAD patient can lead to myocardial ischemia as heralded by ST-segment changes and segmental wall motion abnormalities on TEE. However, if the anesthesiologist is able to maintain coronary perfusion and keep the balance between myocardial oxygen supply and demand favorable, the induction and maintenance of anesthesia can be readily achieved. In contrast, the systolic HF patient has limited ability to increase myocardial contractility in response to changed loading conditions. The loss of sympathetic tone, institution of positive pressure ventilation, and vasodilatation can lead to hemodynamic collapse. In a patient with chronic compensated heart failure, the enlarged heart contracts and ejects enough of a SV to generate a blood pressure and a cardiac output to meet the patient's metabolic needs.

Recall,

$$BP = CO \times SVR, \text{ where } CO = SV \times HR$$

However, when the loading conditions of the heart are reduced, and compensatory mechanisms are impaired, the blood pressure collapses with anesthetic induction. This reduction in blood pressure then decreases CPP leading to myocardial ischemia further worsening cardiac dysfunction. Anesthetic induction in the HF patient can lead to hemodynamic collapse resulting in ventricular fibrillation and the need for the immediate institution of CPB.

Therefore, induction of anesthesia in the HF patient can be stressful for patient and anesthesiologist alike. Plans should be made in advance for the institution of emergency CPB. Both the surgeon and the perfusionist should be closely at hand during anesthesia induction, and the bypass circuit should be primed. The placement of an IABP or temporary ventricular assist device prior to anesthetic induction can be useful in the patient with severe failure and/or myocardial ischemia.

Any anesthetic agent can be employed as long as its impact upon the loading conditions of the heart is managed. Large venous catheters should be in place to assist in volume delivery. Because IABPs carry their own risks including limb ischemia and embolization, they are not always placed in patients with borderline ventricular function. In such patients a femoral arterial catheter can be inserted before induction for systemic blood pressure monitoring. Should the patient deteriorate, that line can be rewired to permit IABP placement. Additionally, femoral arterial line monitoring provides a more central invasive blood pressure measurement than that obtained by a radial arterial catheter.

Following induction, management can be greatly informed by the use of TEE. TEE is employed to determine both the etiology of hypotension following induction. The patient with systolic dysfunction usually presents with a dilated and poorly contractile left ventricle. With anesthesia induction the patient's poorly contracting LV cannot increase stroke volume. Systemic blood pressure decreases along with systemic vascular resistance. Hemodynamic collapse can readily follow. Of course, peri-induction hypotension can also occur in the patient with well-preserved left ventricular function in the setting of hypovolemia and/or vasodilatation. With minimal TEE training, the anesthesiologist can quickly determine the contractile and/or the volume status of the heart in the transgastric mid-papillary short-axis view.

Should the patient become hemodynamically unstable, efforts are made to restore vascular tone and to improve contractility. Vasopressin 1 to 2 U bolus or as an infusion (up to 6 U/h) can be employed to increase vascular tone especially in those patients treated with an ACE-I. Inotropes are administered to improve myocardial contractility. TEE is used to guide volume loading of the heart and determine ventricular function as described in Chapter 2.

Diastolic Dysfunction

TEE is also used to diagnose diastolic dysfunction. Recall that many patients present with symptoms of heart failure with a relatively well-preserved EF. In patients with clinical heart failure, approximately 50% will nonetheless have preserved their ejection fraction (HFpEF).[6] Failure of the heart to relax in diastole leads to an increase in left ventricular end-diastolic pressure (LVEDP) that is transmitted to the pulmonary vasculature leading to symptoms of congestion and heart failure. Decreased activity of the sarcoplasmic endoreticulum calcium ATPase (SERCA) pump slows the removal of calcium from the myocyte cytoplasm hindering relaxation.[7] Echocardiography can be used to detect the presence of LV diastolic dysfunction through the use of pulsed wave (PW) Doppler. Recall that PW Doppler measures the velocity of flow at a specific point determined by the position of the sample gate. Placing the PW Doppler sample gate at the tips of the mitral valve during left ventricular filling will result in a characteristic transmitral diastolic flow pattern seen using transthoracic echocardiography (TTE) (Figure 5–7). For patients in sinus rhythm there are two peaks in the velocity of blood flow entering the LV during diastole. One peak occurs during early filling after the opening of the mitral valve (MV) (E wave), and the other peak occurs during atrial contraction (A wave) seen using transesophageal echocardiography (TEE) (Figure 5–8). The E and A waves are above or below the baseline depending upon whether diastolic flow is directed respectively toward or away from the examining echo probe. Consequently, the waveform deflections above and below the baseline are different when seen using TTE versus TEE.

In subjects with normal diastolic function the ratio between E and A velocities varies from 0.8 to 2. The isovolumetric relaxation time (IVRT) is the very first phase of diastole and represents the time from the end of systolic outflow until the opening of the mitral valve. Normal IVRT is between 70 and 90 ms. The deceleration time (DT) of the E wave represents the time necessary for the pressure gradient between the left atrium (LA) and the LV to equalize, and it is a surrogate for LV compliance. The DT is normally between 150 and 300 ms. In patients with restrictive diastolic and very poor LV compliance, the DT is very short (< 150 ms) because there is rapid equalization of atrial and ventricular pressures because of poor ventricular compliance.

There are various grades of severity of diastolic dysfunction. In early stages of diastolic dysfunction, the primary abnormality is impaired relaxation. When LV relaxation is delayed, the initial pressure gradient across the MV at the beginning of diastole is lower than normal. The reduced transmitral pressure gradient results in a decline in the early filling with a greater proportion of filling seen during atrial contraction resulting in a decreased E velocity, increased A velocity, a lower E/A ratio, and a prolonged IVRT and DT (Figure 5–9). This filling pattern represents grade I diastolic dysfunction or impaired relaxation. The impaired relaxation filling pattern can also be seen in the elderly due to less vigorous relaxation of the LV. Thus, loss of the atrial contraction during periods of atrial fibrillation in older patients can significantly reduce the SV and lead to hemodynamic collapse. In healthy, younger patients, the atrial contraction does not play as essential a role in diastolic filling. Consequently, loss of the "P" wave on the ECG and atrial contraction is better tolerated hemodynamically.

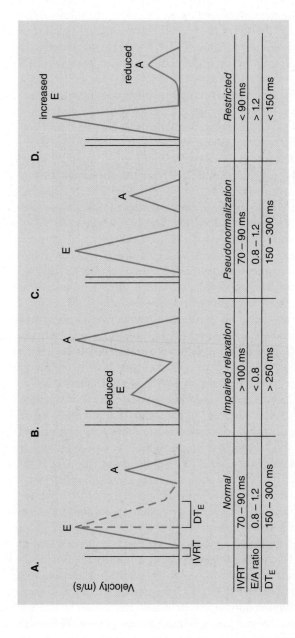

Figure 5–7. Doppler echocardiography of diastolic flow across the mitral valve. A–D (from left to right) represents increasing severity of diastolic dysfunction. A, peak atrial systolic flow; DTE, deceleration time of E; E, early diastolic flow; IVRT, isovolumic relaxation time. (Reproduced with permission from Butterworth JF, Mackey DC, Wasnick JD: *Morgan & Mikhail's Clinical Anesthesiology*, 6th ed. New York, NY: McGraw-Hill Education; 2018.)

	Normal	Impaired relaxation	Pseudonormalization	Restricted
IVRT	70 – 90 ms	> 100 ms	70 – 90 ms	< 90 ms
E/A ratio	0.8 – 1.2	< 0.8	0.8 – 1.2	> 1.2
DTE	150 – 300 ms	> 250 ms	150 – 300 ms	< 150 ms

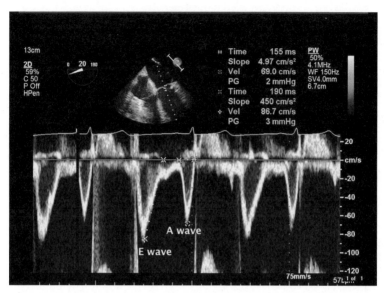

Figure 5–8. Normal mitral inflow pattern is seen here. The E wave is larger than the A wave. The A wave occurs during atrial contraction. The midesophageal four-chamber view at the top of the image shows the positioning of the PW Doppler gate to sample the flow velocities at that point.

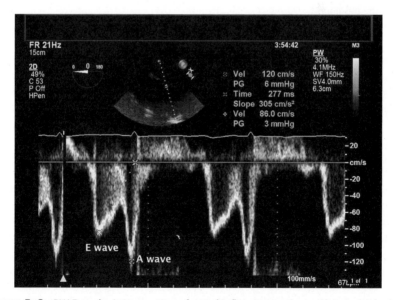

Figure 5–9. PW Doppler interrogation of mitral inflow in a patient with impaired relaxation. Note that in this instance the "A" wave is taller than the "E" wave. The velocity of flow into the left ventricle is provided by the scale at the right. A maximal "A" velocity of 120 cm/s is detected. The "E" velocity is 86 cm/s. The E/A ratio is less than 1.

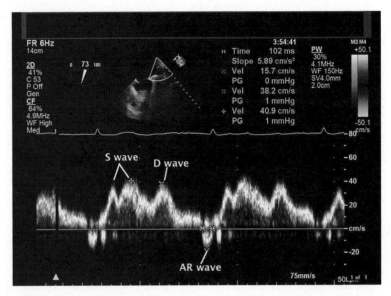

Figure 5-10. Pulse wave Doppler has now been placed in the left upper pulmonary vein. PWD flow from the pulmonary vein into the left atrium is above the baseline because flow is directed toward the transducer located in the esophagus. Note that in this normal tracing the maximal velocities of both the systolic and diastolic components are 40.9 cm/s and 38.2 cm/s, respectively. Flow is reversed during atrial contraction (AR) as indicated by the velocities of blood now moving away from the transducer (velocities below the baseline).

Over time, the progression of diastolic dysfunction results in an increase in the LA pressure. This increased pressure will restore the transmitral pressure gradient to its normal values resulting in a pseudonormalized transmitral pattern, which characterizes grade II diastolic dysfunction. In the pseudonormal pattern, the E to A ratio is essentially the same as one would find in a normal healthy patient. Thus, examining only the transmitral flow, PW Doppler flow patterns could indicate normal diastolic function when in fact relaxation is impaired. Fortunately, the pseudonormal pattern can be distinguished from the normal pattern by other uses of PW Doppler. The PW Doppler sample gate can be placed in one of the pulmonary veins at the opening in the LA (Figure 5-10 and Video 5-2). The spectral image of the velocities of blood flow from the pulmonary veins entering the LA shows three waveforms: two positive, above the baseline, the systolic waveform (S), and the diastolic waveform (D), and a negative waveform, below the baseline during atrial contraction (AR). In a healthy subject, the systolic peak velocity is equal or slightly larger than the diastolic peak velocity (Figure 5-11). In a patient with more advanced diastolic dysfunction (e.g., those with a pseudonormalized or restrictive mitral inflow pattern), the increased pressure in the LA will lead to a diminution of the systolic component of pulmonary vein flow as compared to the diastolic component (Figure 5-12).

Pulmonary Vein PW Doppler Flow Patterns

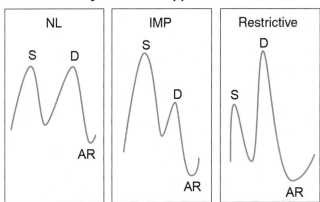

Figure 5–11. PV Doppler flow patterns can be used to assist in the classification of diastolic failure. In healthy adults (NL), the systolic (S), and diastolic (D) velocities of pulmonary vein flow are somewhat similar. However, when patients develop impaired relaxation (IMP), the systolic component of left atrial filling is augmented. As diastolic dysfunction progresses to a pseudonormal or restrictive pattern (restrictive), PV flow during diastole predominates. Additionally, AR velocity and duration increase.

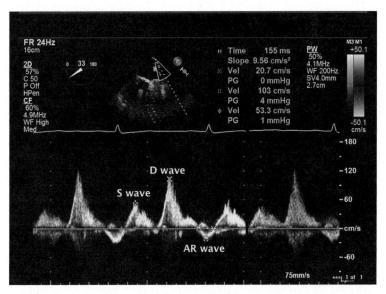

Figure 5–12. In this pulse wave Doppler interrogation of the pulmonary vein, the systolic component of flow is much reduced compared to that of the diastolic component reflecting increased left ventricular filling pressures.

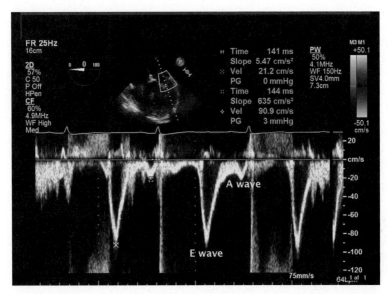

Figure 5–13. As diastolic dysfunction progresses, a restrictive pattern appears. Here, the maximal E velocity (90.9 cm/s) far exceeds that of the A wave (21.2 cm/s). The E/A ratio is greater than 2:1.

In patients with severe, restrictive diastolic dysfunction, the ventricle relaxes so poorly and is so stiff that there is a great buildup of pressure in the LA resulting in a high transmitral gradient at the beginning of diastole. When the MV opens, the blood rushes into the LV at great velocity leading to an increased E-wave velocity. However, due to the very noncompliant LV, the velocity of flow falls rather quickly resulting in a tall, narrow E wave greater than twice the size of the peak A velocity (Figure 5–13). The noncompliant LV is already full at the beginning of the atrial contraction, and the atrial contraction will contribute very little to the final LV volume. Therefore, the velocity and duration of the A wave will be very small. Both the IVRT and DT are of short duration.

Tissue Doppler provides another method to identify diastolic dysfunction. Although Doppler has thus far been used to determine the velocity and direction of blood flowing in the heart, that is not its only use. The myocardium itself moves during the cardiac cycle—albeit at velocities much lower than that of the blood. Tissue Doppler measures myocardial velocities and displays them either as a 2-D color map or as a spectral Doppler signal. Myocardial velocities are usually less than 15 cm/s. During systole as the heart contracts, the mitral annulus moves toward the apex of the heart and away from the TEE transducer (Figure 5–14). When the heart fills during diastole, the mitral annulus moves toward the probe and produces two positive Doppler signals, e′ during early filling and a′ during atrial contraction. The e′ and a′ waves correspond to the E and A diastolic transmitral filling waveforms. An e′ less than 8 cm/s is consistent with diastolic dysfunction (Figure 5–15). Like Doppler transmitral inflow patterns, tissue

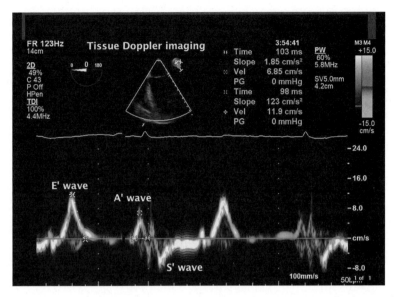

Figure 5-14. Tissue Doppler at the lateral mitral annulus. During diastole the annulus moves toward the TEE transducer. Thus, the E′ and A′ waves are above the baseline and correspond to diastolic inflow. During systole the mitral annulus moves away from the transducer producing the S′ wave of ventricular systole. Note that tissue velocities (8-15 cm/s) are much slower than those seen with blood (100 cm/s).

Doppler can be used to distinguish between normal and impaired diastolic function. Unlike, the E wave, the e′ wave remains diminished in patients with grade II (pseudonormal) diastolic dysfunction and is therefore helpful in distinguishing normal from pseudonormal diastolic dysfunction. Beyond using transmitral flow and mitral annulus velocities, the current guidelines issued by the American Society of Echocardiography and the European Association of Cardiovascular Imaging recommend taking into consideration other factors such as left atrial volume index (abnormal if more than 34 mL/m²) and the tricuspid regurgitation velocity (TR velocity > 2.8 m/s).[8]

The American Society of Echocardiography and the European Association of Cardiovascular Imaging provide extensive guidelines for the diagnosis of diastolic dysfunction. Figure 5–16 summarizes the use of both tissue Doppler and measurements of transmitral flow to diagnose diastolic dysfunction.

It is important to note that many heart surgery patients manifest both systolic and diastolic failure and their clinical symptoms and hemodynamic behavior often reflect both types of perioperative dysfunction. HFpEF patients tolerate volume challenges poorly and can readily develop pulmonary congestion secondary to diastolic heart failure perioperatively. Close attention to fluid management is critical so to not volume overload the patient with diastolic heart failure.

Hypotension, arrhythmias, and increased PA pressures are signs of decompensating heart failure. When the chest is open, the right heart can be easily seen from the anesthesiologist's position. If the RV is distended like a muscular balloon, it is a good indication that things are not going well. Increased central venous pressure (CVP) will also herald RV failure. However, it is TEE that provides an immediate assessment of right and left heart function. A distended right heart (Video 5–3) with a dilated right atrium indicates RV dysfunction. Tricuspid regurgitation can be seen in right ventricular failure, left heart disease with elevated PA pressures, or primary pulmonary hypertension. A noncontractile LV also cannot be mistaken when seen on TEE. Management of right heart dysfunction is discussed in Chapter 8.

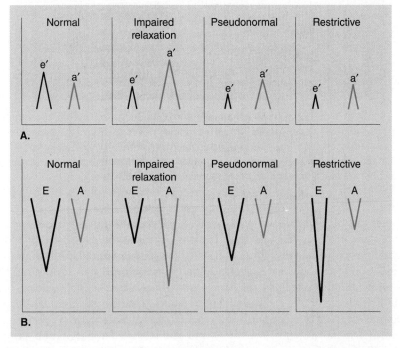

Figure 5–15. (A) Tissue Doppler at the lateral mitral annulus. During diastole the annulus moves toward the transesophageal examination transducer in the esophagus. Thus the e′ and a′ waves of diastolic filling are positive deflections above the baseline. (B) When transesophageal examination is used to measure transmitral diastolic inflow, the E and A waves of early and late filling are below the baseline because flow is moving away from the Doppler probe in the esophagus. Note that in the transthoracic Doppler measurements illustrated in Figure 5–7 the flow is above the baseline as the blood is moving in this case toward the transthoracic echo probe. Tissue Doppler can be used to distinguish normal from pseudonormal diastolic inflow pattern because the e′ wave remains depressed as diastolic dysfunction progresses. (C) Unlike mitral inflow velocity patterns where the E/A ratio changes, the E′ wave of mitral annular tissue Doppler remains reduced during pseudonormalized and restrictive diastolic dysfunction.

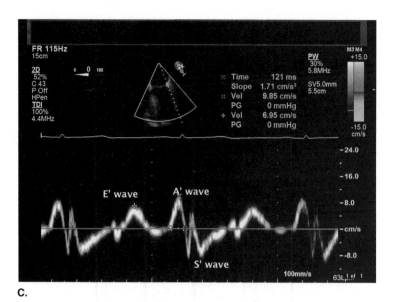

C.

Figure 5–15. *(Continued)*

If heart function is impaired, various inotropic agents are available that can be used to restore LV function. Catecholamines [e.g., dobutamine (2-15 μg/kg/min), epinephrine (0.03-0.15 μcg/kg/min), and phosphodiesterase inhibitors (e.g., milrinone 0.3-0.5 μg/kg/min) work by different mechanisms (beta-adrenergic receptor stimulation, phosphodiesterase inhibition) to increase c-AMP in the myocyte leading to increased intracellular calcium and increased contractility]. A newer agent, levosimendan is a myofilament calcium sensitizer, which enhances contractility by binding to troponin C and prolonging the cross-bridging time. It does not increase the intracellular calcium concentration.[9] Levosimendan has beneficial lusitropic effects and thus promotes diastolic relaxation. The use of inotropic agents without specific indications has been questioned.[10,11] Inotropes should not be started for routine separation from CPB but rather employed when needed to improve ventricular function.

Failure to separate from bypass support is indicated by the heart becoming increasingly distended on TEE, the PA pressures rising, the systemic BP falling, and the RV ballooning. When this occurs, CPB should be reinstituted immediately, the heart should be left to rest and reperfuse, and inotropic support should be adjusted. Often a vasoconstrictor such as norepinephrine (2-10 μg/min) or vasopressin (1-6 U/h) is necessary to support the blood pressure and counteract the vasodilatory properties of inodilators such as milrinone. Weaning the poor EF patient from CPB is a dynamic process with drug therapy titrated to the patient's changing condition. Dosage of drugs has little meaning in this sense, as the infusion rates of the various agents are continuously altered as the three determinants of SV are in constant flux. PA pressures, cardiac index determinations, visual

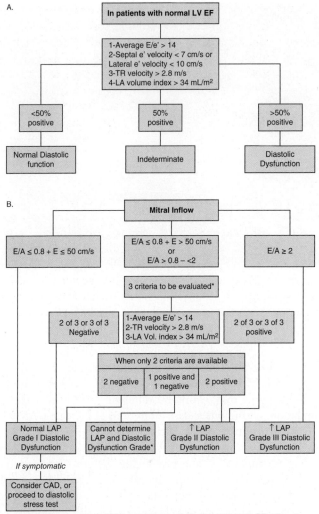

A.

In patients with normal LV EF

1-Average E/e' > 14
2-Septal e' velocity < 7 cm/s or
Lateral e' velocity < 10 cm/s
3-TR velocity > 2.8 m/s
4-LA volume index > 34 mL/m²

<50%
positive

50%
positive

>50%
positive

Normal Diastolic
function

Indeterminate

Diastolic
Dysfunction

B.

Mitral Inflow

E/A ≤ 0.8 + E ≤ 50 cm/s

E/A ≤ 0.8 + E > 50 cm/s
or
E/A > 0.8 – <2

E/A ≥ 2

3 criteria to be evaluated*

2 of 3 or 3 of 3
Negative

1-Average E/e' > 14
2-TR velocity > 2.8 m/s
3-LA Vol. index > 34 mL/m²

2 of 3 or 3 of 3
positive

When only 2 criteria are available

2 negative

1 positive and
1 negative

2 positive

Normal LAP
Grade I Diastolic
Dysfunction

Cannot determine
LAP and Diastolic
Dysfunction Grade*

↑ LAP
Grade II Diastolic
Dysfunction

↑ LAP
Grade III Diastolic
Dysfunction

If symptomatic

Consider CAD, or
proceed to diastolic
stress test

(* : LAP indeterminate if only 1 of 3 parameters available. Pulmonary vein S/D ratio < 1
applicable to conclude elevated LAP in patients with depressed LV EF)

Figure 5–16. (A) Algorithm for diagnosis of LV diastolic dysfunction in subjects with normal LVEF. (B) Algorithm for estimation of LV filling pressures and grading LV diastolic function in patients with depressed LVEFs and patients with myocardial disease and normal LVEF after consideration of clinical and other 2-D data. [Reproduced with permission from Nagueh SF, Smiseth OA, Appleton CP, et al: Recommendations for the Evaluation of Left Ventricular Diastolic Function by Echocardiography: An Update from the American Society of Echocardiography and the European Association of Cardiovascular Imaging, *J Am Soc Echocardiogr.* 2016 Apr;29(4):277-314.]

inspection of the heart, and most importantly TEE images are used in conjunction to determine the appropriate mix of volume, vasoconstrictors, and inotropes to employ to successfully wean the patient with poor ventricular function from CPB support. Patients with high PA pressures and RV dysfunction, in addition to treatment with inotropes such as milrinone, may benefit from the use of inhaled nitric oxide. Should weaning from CPB not be accomplished with combined inodilator and vasoconstrictor support, an IABP will at times be inserted. If all these interventions fail, temporary mechanical ventricular assistance devices can be used to salvage the patient (see Chapter 11).

THE REOPERATIVE PATIENT

Reoperative surgery is very common in the cardiac surgery population.[12,13,14] Patients with previous operations often need revascularization or valve repair or replacement. Reoperative patients are challenging for the anesthesiologist and surgeon in two ways. From a surgical standpoint, adhesions, which develop following primary surgery, can make surgical exposure difficult. Previous coronary artery bypass grafts can become entrapped in fibrotic tissue and can be inadvertently cut leading to bleeding and ischemia. The right ventricle can adhere to the sternum and be lacerated during sternotomy producing bleeding and hemodynamic collapse. Patients following chest radiation therapy and those with previous pericardial disease processes can also develop various adhesions, which can make sternotomy challenging.

When surgically indicated, a thoracotomy approach can be used to gain exposure to the heart for mitral or aortic valve replacement to avoid adhesions altogether. At times surgeons will change the cannulation strategy, establishing central cannulation through a peripheral approach, femoral vein for venous drainage and femoral or axillary artery for return of oxygenated blood from the CPB. Cannulation may be established before sternotomy for rapid institution of CPB if needed. External transcutaneous defibrillation pads should be placed on the patient to provide cardioversion/defibrillation in the event of an arrhythmia prior to the surgeon being able to adequately expose the heart to deliver a direct shock. With careful surgical management, reoperation in and of itself has not been shown to be a particular risk factor for operative mortality.

However, patients presenting for reoperative surgery are generally befallen with severe cardiac symptoms. Patients may be directed toward surgical treatment later, only after having failed medical management.[15] Consequently, patients often present in heart failure after various medical therapies have been exhausted. Catheter-based interventions increasingly provide an alternative to reoperative surgery in certain instances (e.g., valve-in-valve aortic valve placement) (see Chapter 6).

Considerations in the reoperative patient include:

- Risk of surgical laceration of the heart or previous bypass grafts upon sternotomy.
- Potential for increased post bypass bleeding.
- Poor ventricular function and other comorbidities in the reoperative patient population.

THE DIABETIC PATIENT AND PERIOPERATIVE GLUCOSE CONTROL

Patients with and without diabetes mellitus (DM) are at risk for perioperative hyperglycemia. Obviously, DM patients are well represented in the cardiac surgery population secondary to their propensity for vascular disease; however, any patient may experience hyperglycemia perioperatively. Perioperative glucose control in diabetic and nondiabetic patients alike has become the subject of interest as a pay for performance indicator of quality anesthetic management and, as such, is closely monitored by regulatory and hospital authorities. In spite of this interest, exactly what is an "acceptable" perioperative blood glucose remains elusive and the management strategies to achieve this "acceptable" standard are rather varied.

Perioperative hyperglycemia is not uncommon in the cardiac surgery patient. Hypothermia, the hormonal response to surgical stress, the effects of CPB all can contribute to the development of hyperglycemia secondary to increased gluconeogenesis or relative insulin resistance.[16] Some surgeons employ a glucose-containing cardioplegia solution, thereby delivering a glucose challenge to the patient during CPB. Poor blood glucose control has been associated with a worsened hospital outcome following cardiac surgery.[17]

Tight control of perioperative glucose concentration has been suggested by Van den Berghe et al. to reduce morbidity and death in critically ill patients.[18] Hyperglycemia is associated with poor wound healing, infection, and impaired immune function. Additionally, hyperglycemia has been associated with adverse effects on neurological outcomes and renal function.

Gandhi et al. randomly assigned patients undergoing on-pump cardiac surgery procedures to an insulin intensive therapy group to maintain blood sugars between 80 and 100 mg/dL and a conventional therapy group where insulin was given when blood sugar exceeded 200 mg/dL.[19] Interestingly, in spite of tighter intraoperative control of blood glucose concentrations, outcomes such as stroke and death were worse where glucose was intensively controlled, as opposed to traditionally controlled. In a study comparing liberal (121-180 mg/dL) and strict (90-120 mg/dL) glucose management protocols, long-term follow-up of CABG patients managed with either approach failed to demonstrate a survival benefit or improved life quality.[20]

Moreover, when tight intraoperative blood glucose control is undertaken, there remains the risk of inadvertent hypoglycemia.

There are many suggested protocols on how best to infuse insulin to achieve various "ideal" blood glucose concentration endpoints. A target in cardiac surgery patients of between 120 and 150 mg/dL has been offered as a compromise between the deleterious effects of perioperative hyperglycemia and unwanted, iatrogenic hypoglycemia. Various regular insulin infusion protocols are available, but most likely each institution has or should have a protocol for the perioperative insulin infusion targeted to set goals and with appropriate monitoring to detect effectiveness. Knowledge of the protocol used in each practitioner's institution is essential when undertaking management of the cardiac surgery patient. At all times the rate of infusion and the need for an initial insulin bolus must be individualized and regulated based upon information from hourly blood glucose concentration monitoring.

THE VASCULAR DISEASE PATIENT IN NEED OF CARDIAC SURGERY

Patients frequently present for cardiac surgery with other major vessels affected by vascular disease. Disease of the aorta, carotids, and femoral arteries can complicate cardiac surgery and anesthetic management. Vascular disease can lead to noncompliant vessels resulting in wide swings in blood pressure, which can further contribute to perioperative morbidity and mortality.

Occlusive vascular disease creates gradients between central aortic pressure and blood pressure measured from a peripheral arterial catheter. Such gradients can complicate patient management especially at the time of separation from CPB where a "root-radial" pressure gradient can be profound. Central aortic pressure can often be measured should a peripheral arterial waveform appear reduced and unexpectedly low.

Atherosclerosis in the aorta presents a high risk of embolic injury during cardiac surgery.[21] TEE and epiaortic echocardiography can be used to examine the aorta prior to surgical manipulation to reduce the incidence of embolic stroke.[22] The severity of atherosclerotic plaque in the aorta has been graded and associated with the incidence of stroke. Placement of the surgical cross clamp in an area of atheromatous aorta can produce devastating emboli or aortic tears and dissections (Video 5–4). The incidence of adverse embolic effects can be reduced when efforts are taken to avoid areas of aortic plaque.

Because the interposition of the trachea and main bronchi precludes TEE examination of much of the distal ascending aorta and proximal aortic arch, epiaortic ultrasound (EAU) examinations can be used to examine the aorta in detail allowing the surgical team to avoid areas of severe atherosclerosis.

Patients with vascular disease have a relatively noncompliant vasculature.[23] Noncompliant vessels increase pulse pressure. Pulse pressure is the difference between systolic and diastolic blood pressure. Increases in pulse pressure can augment afterload and decrease cerebral, renal, and coronary perfusion. Additionally, an increased pulse pressure creates shear stress on vessel walls leading to plaque rupture, thrombosis, and injury. Increased pulse pressure in cardiac patients has been associated with both kidney dysfunction and neurological injury.[24,25] Consequently, the patient with vascular disease requires tight blood pressure control perioperatively. In particular, the patient with poorly compliant vasculature may experience wide swings in pulse pressure as the anesthesiologist attempts to determine the appropriate loading conditions for the heart both before and after CPB.

The vascular patient may also manifest varying degrees of carotid artery disease. Patients with concomitant disease may be offered combined carotid endarterectomy and coronary bypass surgery.[26] Conversely, carotid endarterectomy may be performed prior to taking the patient for coronary revascularization in patients with stable angina. Ultimately, the patient's cardiologist and surgeons will determine an individualized management approach.

Obviously if carotid surgery is planned at the time of cardiac surgery, anesthesiologists should avoid any central line placement in the carotid surgical field. If the patient has tight unilateral carotid stenosis, central line placement in the contralateral internal jugular vein should be approached cautiously and under ultrasound guidance given the potential for carotid artery injury. If carotid repair is to precede cardiac surgery, neurophysiologic monitoring with EEG may be employed. The anesthesiologist should consult with the vascular surgeon to determine if any monitoring of neurophysiologic function is to be used during the carotid endarterectomy as the anesthetic may need to be tailored to avoid interference with monitoring. The patient for a combined procedure is prepared and draped for cardiac surgery concurrently with the carotid surgical procedure. In this manner, should the patient experience cardiovascular collapse, institution of CPB can and should be expeditiously undertaken.

Patients taken for cardiac surgery at times will require repair of femoral arterial aneurysms acquired during cardiac catheterization. Additionally, many cardiac surgery patients will have at one point or another undergone various vascular surgery procedures with possible aortic or lower extremity bypass grafts or stents having been placed. Knowledge of past vascular surgery procedures and anatomy is critical should femoral arterial monitoring be considered or if IABP placement is indicated so as to avoid potentially damaging previous stents and bypass grafts or contributing to lower extremity vascular injury.

THE KIDNEY FAILURE PATIENT AND CARDIAC SURGERY

Considering that many patients with DM and vascular disease are in need of cardiac surgery, it is not surprising that many patients also present with kidney failure. Patients with end-stage renal disease on dialysis therapy are relatively common in cardiac surgical operating rooms.[27] Other patients may have various degrees of kidney function impairment on presentation to cardiac catheterization and cardiac surgery and are at risk to develop worsening kidney injury postoperatively.

The renal failure patient may manifest perioperatively volume overload, volume depletion (if too much fluid has been removed during dialysis), hyperkalemia, acidemia, hypertension, and hemodynamic instability. Cardioplegia solutions administered during CPB contain potassium and can lead to postoperative potassium overload in the dialysis patient. Glucose and insulin can be administered to shift potassium intracellularly, and acidosis should be corrected to temporarily lower extracellular potassium concentrations. Should the patient demonstrate ECG effects of hyperkalemia, calcium chloride is given. Most renal failure patients tolerate mild hyperkalemia up to 6 mEq/L without difficulty. Dialysis or continuous renal replacement therapy will correct perioperative hyperkalemia and should be readily available postoperatively if needed to lower an increased potassium concentration and/or remove excessive volume.

Kidney failure patients are usually anemic and therefore may require blood transfusion during cardiac surgery. However, transfusion should be undertaken with the knowledge that blood transfusion may make tissue matching for any future renal transplant more difficult. Additionally, such patients are somewhat prone to perioperative bleeding due to impaired platelet function. DDAVP (arginine vasopressin) is often administered to the kidney failure patient for cardiac surgery (0.3 µg/kg) to stimulate the release of von Willebrand factor from the endothelium. In spite of this, often kidney failure patients require multiple blood products including platelets to control bleeding. Care should be taken when positioning the patient for cardiac surgery to avoid compression and injury of the arteriovenous fistula used for dialysis access.

Anesthetic management of the patient with kidney disease often includes a ride on the hemodynamic roller coaster. Patients fresh from dialysis may be volume depleted making central venous access difficult and the patient hypotensive. Volume loading and cardioplegia solution during CPB may result in a hyperkalemic and volume overloaded patient with cardiac distention and heart failure. Volume status can be corrected while the patient is on CPB through hemofiltration (see Chapter 17).

Various drugs including natriuretic peptides (nesiritide) and fenoldopam have been suggested as treatments to improve or prevent acute kidney injury in heart surgery patients. However, a trial of 667 patients with early acute kidney injury following cardiac surgery were randomized to receive either fenoldopam or a placebo. No difference in mortality or need for renal replacement therapy was demonstrated; however, the fenoldopam group experienced increased hypotension.[28] Maintenance of adequate kidney perfusion perioperatively is the best approach to prevent perioperative kidney injury; however, the causes of perioperative kidney injury are multifactorial including ischemia, reperfusion injury, and inflammation. The management of newly acquired postoperative kidney dysfunction and its possible prevention are more extensively discussed in Chapter 14.

REFERENCES

1. DeRose J, Toumpoulis I, Balaram S, et al. Preoperative prediction of long-term survival after coronary artery bypass grafting in patients with low left ventricular ejection fraction. *J Thorac Cardiovasc Surg.* 2005;129:314-321.

2. Maslow A, Regan M, Panzica P, et al. Precardiopulmonary bypass right ventricular function is associated with poor outcome after coronary artery bypass grafting in patients with severe left ventricular systolic dysfunction. *Anesth Analg.* 2002;95:1507-1518.

3. Appoo J, Norris C, Merali S, et al. Long term outcome of isolated coronary artery bypass surgery in patients with severe left ventricular dysfunction. *Circulation.* 2004;110(suppl II):II-13-II-17.

4. Groban L, Butterworth J. Perioperative management of chronic heart failure. *Anesth Analg.* 2006;103: 557-575.

5. Christenson JT, Simonet F, Badel P, et al. Evaluation of preoperative intra-aortic balloon pump support in high risk coronary patients. *Eur J Cardiothorac Surg.* 1997;11:1097-1103.

6. Yancy CW, Jessup M, Bozkurt B. et al. 2013 ACCF/AHA guideline for the management of heart failure: a report of the American College of Cardiology Foundation/American Heart Association Task Force on Practice Guidelines. *J Am Coll Cardiol.* 2013;62:e147-239.

7. Apostolakes E, Baikoussis, N, Parissis H, et al. Left ventricular diastolic dysfunction of the cardiac surgery patient; a point of view for the cardiac surgeon and cardio-anesthesiologist. *J Cardiothorac Surg.* 2009;4:67.

8. Nagueh SF, Smiseth OA, Appleton CA et al. Recommendations for the evaluation of left ventricular diastolic function by echocardiography: an update from the American Society of Echocardiography and European Association of Cardiovascular Imaging. *J Am Soc Echocardiogr.* 2016;29:277-314.

9. Eriksson H, Jalonen J, Heikkinen L. Levosimendan facilitates weaning from cardiopulmonary bypass in patients undergoing coronary artery bypass grafting with impaired left ventricular function. *Ann Thorac Surg.* 2009;87:448-454.

10. Butterworth J. Dobutamine: too dangerous for "routine" administration? *Anesthesiology.* 2008;108(6): 973-974.

11. Fellahi J, Parienti J, Hanouz J, et al. Perioperative use of dobutamine in cardiac surgery and adverse cardiac outcome: propensity-adjusted analyses. *Anesthesiology.* 2008;108(6):979-987.

12. Christenson J, Schmuziger M, Simonet F. Reoperative coronary artery bypass procedures: risk factors for early mortality and late survival. *Eur J Cardiothorac Surg.* 1997;11:129-133.

13. Sabik J, Blackstone E, Houghtaling P, et al. Is reoperation still a risk factor in coronary artery bypass surgery. *Ann Thorac Surg.* 2005;80;1719-1727.

14. McNeil M, Buth K, Brydie A, et al. The impact of diffuseness of coronary artery disease on the outcomes of patients undergoing primary and reoperative coronary artery bypass grafting. *Eur J Cardiothorac Surg.* 2007;31:827-833.

15. Ngaage D, Cowen M, Griffin S, et al. The impact of symptom severity on cardiac reoperative risk: early referral and reoperation is warranted. *Eur J Cardiothorac Surg.* 2007;32:623-628.

16. Carvalho G, Moore A, Qizilbash B, et al. Maintenance of normoglycemia during cardiac surgery. *Anesth Analg.* 2004;99:319-324.

17. Ouattara A, Lecomte P, Le Manach Y, et al. Poor intraoperative blood glucose control is associated with a worsened hospital outcome after cardiac surgery in diabetic patients. *Anesthesiology.* 2005;103(4):687-694.

18. Van den Berghe G, Wouters P, Weekers F, et al. Intensive insulin therapy in critically ill patients. *NEJM.* 2001;345:1359-1367.

19. Gandhi G, Nuttall G, Abel M, et al. Intensive intraoperative insulin therapy versus conventional glucose management during cardiac surgery. *Ann Internal Med.* 2007;146:223-243.

20. Pezzella A, Holmes S, Pritchard G, et al. Impact of perioperative glycemic control strategy on patient survival after coronary bypass surgery. *Ann Thorac Surg.* 2014;98:1281-1285.

21. Hartman G, Yao F, Bruefach M, et al. Severity of aortic atheromatous disease diagnosed by transesophageal echocardiography predicts stroke and other outcomes associated with coronary artery surgery: a prospective study. *Anesth Analg.* 1996;83:701-708.

22. Gold J, Torres K, Maldarelli W, et al. Improving outcomes in coronary surgery: the impact of echo directed aortic cannulation and perioperative hemodynamic management in 500 patients. *Ann Thorac Surg.* 2004;78:1579-1585.

23. Aronson S. Management of blood pressure in the patient requiring cardiothoracic surgery: what's the correct end point? In: Cohen NH (ed). *Medically Challenging Patients Undergoing Cardiothoracic Surgery.* Baltimore, MD: Lippincott Williams & Wilkins; 2009:29.

24. Aronson S, Fontes M, Miao Y, et al. Risk index for perioperative renal dysfunction/failure: critical dependence on pulse pressure hypertension. *Circulation.* 2007;115:733-742.

25. Fontes M, Aronson S, Mathew J, et al. Pulse pressure and risk of adverse outcome in coronary artery bypass surgery. *Anesth Analg.* 2008;107:1122-1129.

26. Ochroch E, Oware A, Ellis J. Carotid stenosis and coronary disease: understanding the disease processes and defining how to approach them. In: Cohen NH (ed). *Medically Challenging Patients Undergoing Cardiothoracic Surgery.* Baltimore, MD: Lippincott Williams & Wilkins; 2009:69.

27. Fatehi P, Liu K, Cohen NH. Perioperative management of the patient with dialysis dependent renal failure requiring cardiac surgery. In: Cohen NH (ed). *Medically Challenging Patients Undergoing Cardiothoracic Surgery.* Baltimore, MD: Lippincott, Williams & Wilkins; 2009:129.

28. Bove T, Zangrillo A, Guarracino F, Alvaro G, et al. Effect of fenoldopam on use of renal replacement therapy among patients with acute kidney injury after cardiac surgery: a randomized clinical trial. *JAMA* 2014;312(21):2244-2253.

Aortic Valve Disease

TOPICS

The aortic valve (AV) is the gateway through which the stroke volume is ejected from the left ventricle (LV) into the systemic circulation. Should the gateway be narrowed as in aortic stenosis (AS), the LV hypertrophies concentrically and ejects the stroke volume through the reduced aortic valve orifice. The thickened heart muscle and the increased work of ventricular ejection augments the oxygen demand of the ventricle, which if not met, results in myocardial ischemia. On the other hand, if the valve is incompetent resulting in aortic insufficiency or regurgitation (AR), the left ventricle dilates and develops eccentric hypertrophy to accommodate the increased volume filling the LV cavity during diastole. When the AV is incompetent, diastolic pressure falls and coronary perfusion pressure (CPP) decreases, increasing the risk of ischemia. Providing anesthesia for patients with AV disease undergoing aortic valve surgery or noncardiac procedures can be challenging.

OVERVIEW

The American Heart Association Task Force on Practice Guidelines reports the current recommendations for the management of patients with AV disease.[1] In the past, valvular diseases were most likely the consequence of rheumatic heart disease. Currently, with an increasingly aging population, degenerative diseases of the valves are most frequently diagnosed.[2] More than one in eight individuals older

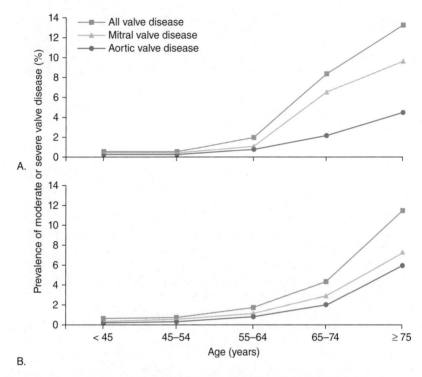

Figure 6–1. The increasing prevalence of valvular heart disease associated with age in population-based studies (A) and in one U.S. county. (B) Anesthesiologists are increasingly likely to encounter patients with valvular disease as the population ages. [Reproduced with permission from Nkomo VT, Gardin JM, Skelton TN, et al: Burden of valvular heart diseases: a population-based study, *Lancet.* 2006 Sep 16;368(9540):1005-1011.]

than 75 years of age have moderate or severe valvular heart disease of one type or another.[2] Life span is reduced in patients with severe valvular disease (Figures 6–1 and 6–2). Additionally, elderly women may have underdiagnosed valvular heart diseases.[2] Consequently, it is likely that as the population ages, AV disease will become ever more prevalent in cardiac surgical and noncardiac surgical patients alike. Sometimes, anesthesiologists are the first to diagnose a heart murmur during preoperative assessment.[3] Van Klei et al. in a study from the Netherlands found during routine preoperative examination a prevalence of 2.4% for AS in patients greater than 60 years of age scheduled for noncardiac surgery.[3]

THE CLINICAL SIGNS AND SYMPTOMS OF AV DISEASE

The aortic valve is normally tricuspid, with semilunar cusps and an aortic valve area (AVA) of 2.5 to 3.5 cm^2. The most common causes of AS are degenerative changes of a normal trileaflet valve (Figure 6–3) or of a congenital bicuspid valve (Figure 6–4 and **Videos 6–1 and 6–2**).[4] Other congenital malformations

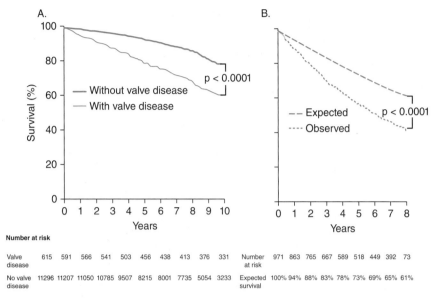

Number at risk

| Valve disease | 615 | 591 | 566 | 541 | 503 | 456 | 438 | 413 | 376 | 331 |
| No valve disease | 11296 | 11207 | 11050 | 10785 | 9507 | 8215 | 8001 | 7735 | 5054 | 3233 |

| Number at risk | 971 | 863 | 765 | 667 | 589 | 518 | 449 | 392 | 73 |
| Expected survival | 100% | 94% | 88% | 83% | 78% | 73% | 69% | 65% | 61% |

Figure 6–2. Survival graphs after detection of moderate or severe valvular heart disease demonstrate decreased survival in population-based (A) and community (B) studies of patients with valvular heart disease. Graph A: survival in population-based studies. Graph B: expected versus observed survival in one U.S. county of 971 residents diagnosed with valve disease between 1990 and 1995 compared with the expected survival of an age- and sex-matched population. [Reproduced with permission from Nkomo VT, Gardin JM, Skelton TN, et al: Burden of valvular heart diseases: a population-based study, *Lancet.* 2006 Sep 16;368(9540):1005-1011.]

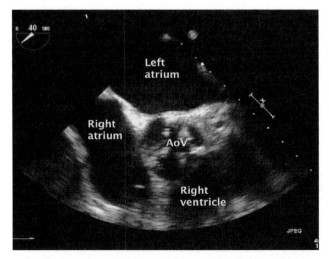

Figure 6–3. A calcified and stenotic aortic valve is seen in this midesophageal short-axis aortic valve view. Calcification of the aortic valve is usually associated with senile degeneration. However, congenitally abnormal (bicuspid) and rheumatic presentations also occur.

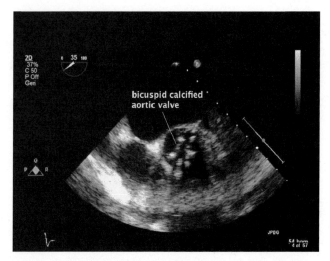

Figure 6-4. A congenitally bicuspid valve is seen in this midesophageal aortic valve short-axis view.

of the AV, such as unicuspid and quadricuspid valves, although uncommon, can lead to aortic stenosis even in the adolescent population. However, the majority of patients will develop AS as a consequence of inflammation, lipid accumulation, and calcification of normal trileaflet valves associated with aging.[5] Degenerative processes also contribute to the development of AR.

Aortic Stenosis

Severe AS is associated with an aortic valve area of less than 1.0 cm². Calcification of the AV progresses with time, which leads to the presentation of clinical symptoms including: angina, syncope, and dyspnea. With progressive stenosis, a pressure gradient develops across the valve and a systolic murmur results from the turbulent ejection of blood through the narrowed orifice. Over time, ventricular function can become impaired reducing the force of left ventricular ejection and paradoxically reducing the intensity of the murmur even as the stenosis itself remains unchanged or progresses. Patient survival following the onset of symptoms is fairly limited (2-5 years).[6]

Chronic Aortic Regurgitation

Aortic regurgitation (Video 6–3) may occur as a consequence of any number of etiologies including: infectious endocarditis, rheumatic heart disease, connective tissue diseases producing aortic root dilatation, Marfan syndrome, vasculitis, and syphilis.[1] Irrespective of the cause of AR the end result is the same. Namely, the leaflets of the aortic valve fail to coapt, allowing the retrograde flow of blood from the aorta into the left ventricular outflow track (LVOT) during diastole. The heart becomes volume overloaded from the incompetent valve and develops eccentric hypertrophy and increased end-diastolic pressure.[7] Patients frequently develop diastolic hypotension and a widened pulse pressure secondary to the runoff of blood through the AV into the heart during diastole and the augmented ejection of blood volume during ventricular systole. Clinically, the patient with chronic AR frequently becomes dyspneic. Over time, the volume overloaded LV fails and heart failure ensues.

Acute Aortic Regurgitation

Unlike the patient with chronic AR, the acute AR patient often presents with pulmonary edema in the setting of acute congestive heart failure. The heart of the patient with chronic AR generally adapts to volume overload with time. The heart of the patient with acute AR is presented with a large, regurgitant volume challenge at the time of disease onset and does not have the opportunity to compensate. Such patients often present in cardiogenic shock. Conditions leading to acute AR include aortic dissection, traumatic aortic injury, and endocarditis.

Increasingly surgeons are repairing the aortic valve in patients with aortic insufficiency. A classification system has been developed to identify the conditions leading to aortic regurgitation. Dilatation of the proximal aorta results in central aortic insufficiency. Conversely, restriction or prolapse of the aortic valve leaflets can produce eccentric jets of aortic regurgitation on echocardiographic examination. The nature of the repair to be undertaken depends upon the precipitating source of aortic insufficiency. For example, in patients with intact valve cusp motion but a dilated aorta (type 1a), placement of an aortic graft would likely restore competency of the leaky aortic valve (Figure 6–5).

Combined Aortic Stenosis and Regurgitation

At times patients will manifest both AS and AR. Echocardiography can frequently help to discern the dominant physiologic derangement.

PHYSIOLOGIC COMPENSATORY MECHANISMS OF AV DISEASE

The heart of the patient with AV disease attempts to compensate for the additional pressure and/or volume work challenges presented to it by either a stenotic or an incompetent aortic valve.[8]

The LV of the patient with worsening AS generates ever-increasing ventricular systolic pressures to force blood through the narrowed aortic valve. Increased ventricular wall tension develops leading to an increased myocardial oxygen demand. Recall, LaPlace's law:

Wall tension = (Ventricular pressure × Ventricular radius)/2 × Myocardial wall thickness

By increasing LV wall thickness, the heart compensates for the increased pressure necessary to overcome obstruction to systolic ejection. Increased wall thickness decreases wall tension. Although LV hypertrophy can over time compensate for worsening AS, compensatory adaptations have limits. Myocardial ischemia may

AI Class	Type I Normal cusp motion with FAA dilatation or cusp perforation				Type II Cusp prolapse	Type III Cusp restriction
	Ia	Ib	Ic	Id		
Mechanism	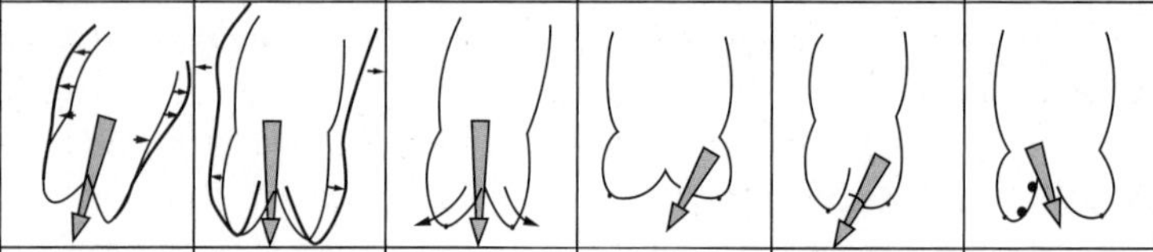					
Repair techniques (primary)	STJ remodeling Ascending aortic graft	Aortic valve sparing: Reimplantation or Remodeling with SCA	SCA	Patch repair Autologous or bovine pericardium	Prolapse repair Plication Triangular resection Free margin Resuspension patch	Leaflet repair Shaving decalcification patch
(Secondary)	SCA		STJ Annuloplasty	SCA	SCA	SCA

Figure 6–5. Repair-oriented functional classification of aortic insufficiency (AI) with description of disease mechanisms and possible repair techniques. FAA = functional aortic annulus; SCA = subcommissural annuloplasty; STJ = sinotubular junction. [Reproduced with permission from Boodhwani M, de Kerchove L, Glineur D, et al: Repair-oriented classification of aortic insufficiency: impact on surgical techniques and clinical outcomes, *J Thorac Cardiovasc Surg.* 2009 Feb;137(2):286-294.]

develop secondary to inadequate blood supply to the thickened myocardium. The AS patient may also have concurrent coronary artery disease. Moreover, as wall tension increases and the heart becomes unable to compensate by increasing wall thickness, myocardial oxygen demands increase evermore. The thickened ventricle is also at risk for diastolic dysfunction because the hypertrophied LV is relatively noncompliant.[9] Often the noncompliant ventricle tolerates volume challenges poorly and is heavily dependent upon atrial contraction to effectively load the LV during diastole. Particularly, the loss of the "atrial kick" through the development of atrial fibrillation greatly reduces the CO.

AR challenges the heart by overwhelming it with volume. Compensatory mechanisms increase the heart's ability to accommodate an increased diastolic blood volume.[10] The heart dilates to accommodate ever greater amounts of diastolic volume. By dilating, over time, the heart can increase its diastolic capacity with minimal change in left ventricular end-diastolic pressure (LVEDP). Whereas the AS ventricle becomes noncompliant, the AR ventricle becomes increasingly compliant.[1] The LV hypertrophies eccentrically to respond to both volume and pressure work challenges. The increased volume load of the LV produces an increase in stroke volume (SV) and can contribute to an increase in systolic pressure. Over time the LV can no longer dilate sufficiently to accommodate the regurgitant volume. As LV compliance becomes impaired, the heart is no longer able to increase diastolic volume with minimal increases in diastolic pressure. Left ventricular end-diastolic pressure increases thereby reducing CPP. Heart failure ensues. As time passes, the heart no longer compensates for the challenges presented to it, resulting in subclinical ischemia, myocyte cell death, LV fibrosis, and ventricular systolic and diastolic dysfunction.[8]

The patient with acute AR lacks the time for any compensatory remodeling of the heart's structure. In such instances, a rapid increase in left ventricular end-diastolic volume produces a dramatic rise in left ventricular end-diastolic pressure (LVEDP). Cardiogenic shock with systemic hypoperfusion and pulmonary edema develop. The anesthetic management of these patients can be very challenging as they frequently present to the operating room hypotensive and hypoxemic secondary to pulmonary edema.

ECHOCARDIOGRAPHY AND AV DISEASE

Basic views and diagnostic approaches to the AV were presented in the introduction to echocardiography at the start of this text and should be briefly reviewed before proceeding with this section. The role of echocardiography in the management of these patients cannot be underestimated.[1]

Aortic Stenosis

The aortic valve is examined in the midesophageal short-axis (ME AVSAX) and long-axis views (ME AVLAX) of the aortic valve. The ME AVSAX provides an ideal opportunity to examine the three leaflets of the valve. By using color flow Doppler, turbulent flow across the AV can be seen. Planimetry (Figure 6–6) of the stenotic valve permits a rough estimate of the valve area. Planimetry of the

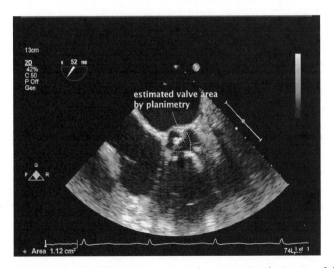

Figure 6–6. The aortic valve short-axis view seen here permits planimetry of the aortic valve. By freezing the image, the aortic valve orifice can be traced estimating its valve area. Often planimetry is not accurate as calcifications in the valve can make tracing its true outline difficult.

AV is performed in the ME AVSAX view. Once the leaflets are imaged, the *freeze* button is pressed. Using the *trace* function, the valvular orifice is highlighted at mid-systole. Estimates of AV orifice area by planimetry may be unreliable due to acoustic shadowing in the presence of calcifications, difficulty in visualizing the leaflet edges in the same plane, flow variability, and temporal variability in AV area during ejection.[11]

Stenotic orifice area can be calculated using the "continuity equation" which follows the conservation of flow or mass. As water flows down a river, its velocity is slow where the river is wide and its velocity is fast where it is narrow—the rapids!!! The flow of blood through the LVOT and the aortic valve obeys the same conservation law.

Because flow duration through the LVOT and AV is the same, the LVOT V_{max} and the AV V_{max} approximate their respective time velocity integrals (TVI):

$$LVOT\ flow = AV\ flow$$
$$LVOT\ flow = LVOT\ CSA \times LVOT\ V_{max}$$
$$AV\ flow = AV\ CSA \times AV\ V_{max}$$

Therefore,

$$AV\ CSA = (LVOT\ CSA \times LVOT\ V_{max})/AV\ V_{max}$$
$$CSA = cross\text{-}sectional\ area$$
$$V_{max} = maximal\ velocity$$

So if the velocity of blood in the LVOT is known and the cross-sectional area of the LVOT is also known, then the flow through the LVOT can be calculated. Obtaining the velocity of flow through the stenotic AV permits calculation of the stenotic valve area.

According to the conservation of mass, the same volume of blood that goes through the LVOT will traverse the AV:

$$LVOT\ volume = AV\ volume$$
$$LVOT\ volume = LVOT\ CSA \times LVOT\ VTI$$

Recall that the VTI (velocity-time integral) represents the distance that the blood travels during systole as the result of the machine integrating the velocities with the systolic ejection time. The LVOT VTI is measured in the deep transgastric long-axis view, by placing the pulsed wave sample gate in the LVOT and tracing the spectral envelope obtained (Figure 6–7). The VTI is expressed in centimeters.

CSA is estimated by approximating the LVOT with a cylinder. CSA in this setting is estimated for that of a circle or πr^2, where r is the radius of the circle. By measuring the LVOT diameter (d) (Figure 6–8), the CSA of the LVOT can be calculated:

$$LVOT\ CSA = 0.785 \times d^2\ (cm^2)$$

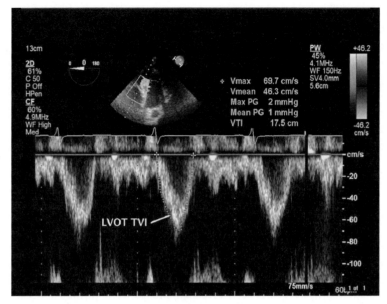

Figure 6–7. Pulse waved Doppler is employed to determine the time-velocity integral (TVI) of the left ventricular outflow tract. A deep transgastric view is used to best align the Doppler beam with the direction of blood flow to minimize the angle of incidence between the two. Pulse wave Doppler is used because the maximal velocity is slow—under 60 cm/s. Tracing the velocity flow envelope allows the machine to calculate the time-velocity integral. Note that in this image there is no pressure gradient in the LVOT as would normally be expected.

Knowing both the CSA and the VTI of the LVOT permits calculation of the volume of blood going across the LVOT during systole.

Next, using the deep transgastric long-axis view, the Doppler beam is aligned in parallel with flow across the stenotic aortic valve and continuous wave Doppler is used to obtain the maximal velocity and the VTI across the AV (Figure 6–9). Limitations regarding the use of the continuity equation for AV area calculation include: misalignment of the Doppler beam with the blood flow, assumptions regarding the circular shape of the LVOT, and error introduced in the measurement of the LVOT diameter. Three-dimensional echocardiography permits planimetry of the LVOT and thus reduces any error in calculation of the aortic valve area from assuming that the LVOT has a circular rather than an elliptical shape.

With these three elements it is possible to calculate the orifice area of the AV valve.

$$\text{LVOT volume} = \text{AV volume}$$
$$\text{LVOT volume} = \text{LVOT CSA} \times \text{LVOT VTI}$$
$$\text{AV volume} = \text{AV CSA} \times \text{LVOT VTI}$$

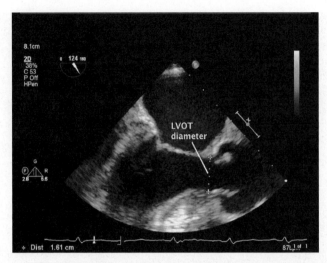

Figure 6–8. In this midesophageal long-axis view of the aortic valve is seen the anterior leaflet of the mitral valve, the aortic valve, the left ventricular outflow track, and the mitral valve. The image has been frozen permitting measurement of the diameter of the LVOT. This measurement is essential for use in the continuity equation to determine the area of the aortic valve.

Therefore,

$$AV\ CSA = LVOT\ CSA \times LVOT\ VTI/AV\ VTI$$

Pressure gradients across a narrowed aortic valve are also used as an estimate of the severity of AS. Here, too, echocardiography is essential in determining the peak and mean pressure gradients across a narrowed orifice. The peak pressure gradient can be calculated using the Bernoulli equation, but the mean pressure gradient is calculated by the machine through an automated function by averaging the instantaneous gradients over the ejection period from the traced velocity curve.

Recall from the introductory chapter Bernoulli's equation:

$$Pressure\ gradient = 4V^2$$

where V is the maximal velocity.

Generally, flow within the heart proceeds at a velocity < 1.2 m/s. In areas of narrowing, the velocity can increase to upward of 5 to 6 m/s. Using Bernoulli's equation, it is clear that a 5-m/s velocity would be associated with a 100 mm Hg peak pressure gradient. When flow in the LVOT is greater than 1.5 m/s, the simple Bernoulli equation above cannot be used. In this instance

$$Pressure\ gradient = 4(V_2^2 - V_1^2)$$

where V_2 is the velocity of flow at the aortic valve and V_1 reflects the velocity in the LVOT.

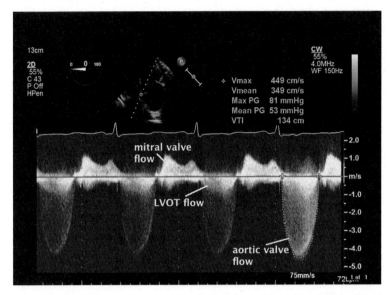

Figure 6–9. The TVI of the aortic valve is calculated using continuous wave Doppler. Recall that pulse wave Doppler is useful for measurements at lower blood velocities. Here continuous wave Doppler has been aligned parallel to that aortic valve flow as imaged using the deep transgastric view. Of note, the blood velocity across the aortic valve is greater than 4 m/s.

It must be remembered that a low-pressure gradient does not exclude a narrowed aortic valve. The ventricle must be capable of doing sufficient pressure work to generate pressures of this degree. As heart failure ensues, the gradient can fall simply because the LV can no longer generate such dramatic intracavitary pressures. The LVOT VTI/AV VTI ratio or velocity ratio (V_{LVOT} / V_{AV}) can also be used to identify aortic stenosis. A ratio less than 0.25 is significant for severe aortic stenosis. Baumgartner et al. provide a summary to grade the severity of aortic stenosis (Table 6–1).

Table 6–1. Recommendations for Grading of AS Severity

	Aortic sclerosis	Mild	Moderate	Severe
Peak velocity (m/s)	≤ 2.5 m/s	2.6–2.9	3.0–4.0	≥ 4.0
Mean gradient (mm Hg)	–	< 20	20–40	≥ 40
AVA (cm²)	–	> 1.5	1.0–1.5	< 1.0
Indexed AVA (cm²/m²)	–	> 0.85	0.60–0.85	< 0.6
Velocity ratio	–	> 0.50	0.25–0.50	< 0.25

Reproduced with permission from Baumgartner H, Hung J, Bermejo J, et al: Recommendations on the Echocardiographic Assessment of Aortic Valve Stenosis: A Focused Update from the European Association of Cardiovascular Imaging and the American Society of Echocardiography, *J Am Soc Echocardiogr.* 2017 Apr;30(4):372-392.

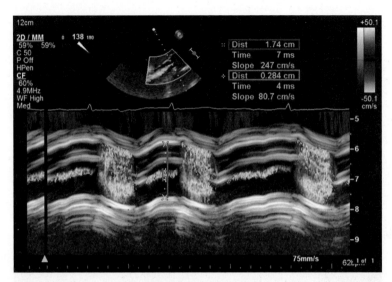

Figure 6–10. Color M-mode applied in the midesophageal aortic valve long-axis view measures the width of the aortic regurgitant jet (0.28 cm) and the width of the left ventricular outflow tract (1.74 cm). In this case, the width of the aortic regurgitant jet occupies 16% of the left ventricular outflow tract width.

Aortic Regurgitation

Echocardiography is likewise essential in the evaluation of AR.[12,13] There are a number of approaches available to determine just how leaky is the AV. Anesthesiologists use everything from visual estimates of the regurgitant jet to more quantitative approaches.

AR can be evaluated in both ME AVSAX and ME AVLAX views of the aortic valve. Application of color flow Doppler in both views provides an image of the regurgitant flow during diastole. Both qualitative and quantitative methods are used to assess the severity of chronic AR.

One of the parameters is the width of the regurgitant jet below the AV relative to the width of the LVOT. Severe AR is associated with jets that occupy greater than 65% of the LVOT width.[11] Unfortunately, the AR regurgitant jet can be subject to many factors unrelated to the severity of AR, such as aortic diastolic pressure, LVEDP, and eccentricity of the jet, making it a less reliable estimate for AR severity (Figure 6–10).

Another semi-quantitative parameter is the "vena contracta" width. Figure 6–11 demonstrates the vena contracta of a regurgitant jet. The vena contracta width is the smallest diameter of the regurgitant jet measured at the level of the aortic valve. The vena contracta area corresponds to the area of the effective regurgitant orifice (EROA). Simply, vena contracta measurements permit an estimation of how big is the leak through the aortic valve. A vena contracta width greater than 6 mm is

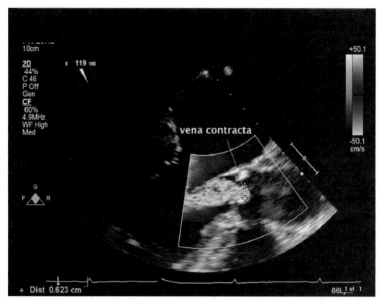

Figure 6-11. This color flow Doppler image of the midesophageal aortic valve long-axis view demonstrates measurement of the vena contracta of aortic regurgitation. The vena contracta represents the smallest diameter of the regurgitant jet at the level of the aortic valve. A vena contracta of 6.2 mm grades the aortic regurgitation in this case as severe.

considered indicative of severe AR. An EROA greater than 0.30 cm^2 is considered severe.

Calculation of the EROA requires determination of the regurgitant volume of the aortic valve regurgitant volume (AVRV):

$$AVRV = LVOT\ SV - RVOT\ SV$$

where,

LVOT SV = stroke volume in the LVOT including AV regurgitant volume

RVOT SV = systemic stroke volume across the right ventricular outflow tract (RVOT) assuming no other shunts or regurgitant lesions

$$AVRV = [(0.785)(\text{diameter } LVOT)^2(LVOT\ VTI)]$$
$$- [(0.785)(\text{diameter } RVOT)^2(RVOT\ VTI)]$$
$$AVRV = (EROA)(AVR\ VTI)$$
$$EROA = AVRV/AVR\ VTI$$

where,

AVRV = AV regurgitant volume

EROA = effective regurgitant orifice area

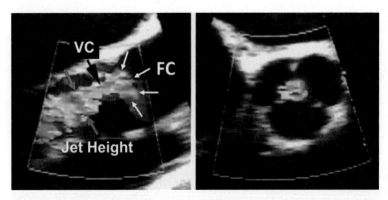

Figure 6–12. Color flow Doppler of AR in the parasternal long- and short-axis views. The three components of the jet are shown with arrows: flow convergence (FC), VC, and jet height (or width) in the LV outflow. [Reproduced with permission from Zoghbi WA, Adams D, Bonow RO, et al: Recommendations for Noninvasive Evaluation of Native Valvular Regurgitation: A Report from the American Society of Echocardiography Developed in Collaboration with the Society for Cardiovascular Magnetic Resonance, *J Am Soc Echocardiogr.* 2017 Apr;30(4):303-371.]

AVR VTI = velocity time integral of the AV regurgitant jet
  VTI = velocity time integral or stroke distance (the distance the blood travels during a heartbeat)

$$\text{Area (cm}^2) \times \text{Distance (cm)} = \text{Volume (cm}^3)$$

The flow convergence or PISA (proximal isovelocity surface area) method can also be employed to estimate EROA and AV RV. As blood accelerates to pass through the EROA during diastole, it accelerates producing an area of flow convergence (Figure 6–12).

The flow convergence appears as a hemisphere on color flow Doppler. Flow can be determined proximal to the EROA by measuring the radius of the PISA hemisphere, calculating the area of the hemisphere and then noting aliasing velocity from the Nyquist limit (Figure 6–13). Multiplying the EROA by the time velocity integral of the regurgitant flow (VTI) calculates the regurgitant volume.

Another measure of the severity of aortic regurgitation is pressure half-time (PHT), which represents the time necessary for the pressure gradient between the ascending aorta and the left ventricle to decrease by 50%. PHT is measured in the deep transgastric view using continuous wave Doppler and measuring the slope of the Doppler envelope. A steep slope indicates more significant regurgitation and a shorter PHT, as LVEDP rises more rapidly with severe regurgitation. A pressure half-time < 200 ms is considered severe aortic regurgitation. Conditions that increase left ventricular end-diastolic pressure shorten the pressure half-time potentially leading to an overestimation of the severity of aortic regurgitation. Conversely, a dilated highly compliant left ventricle will increase the PHT potentially

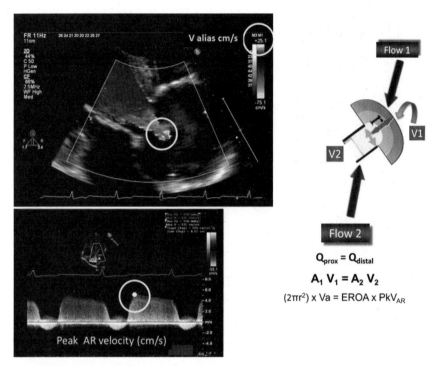

Figure 6–13. Flow convergence or PISA can be performed for obtaining the EROA in patients with AR. Zooming in on the LVOT in either the parasternal or apical long-axis views is the best way to record the proximal flow convergence area. Adjust the Nyquist limit using the baseline shift control to obtain and measure the flow convergence radius (arrow). Regurgitant flow rate is calculated as $2\pi r^2 V_{alias}$ [r = the radius of the flow convergence in early diastole (arrow), and V_{alias} is the Va in cm/s]. EROA and R_{vol} can then be calculated as EROA = regurgitant flow rate/peak AR velocity in early diastole in cm/s. R_{vol} = EROA × VTI of the AR. For the aortic valve, severe regurgitation is an EROA greater than 0.30 cm² and an R_{vol} greater than 60 mL. [Reproduced with permission from Zoghbi WA, Adams D, Bonow RO, et al: Recommendations for Noninvasive Evaluation of Native Valvular Regurgitation: A Report from the American Society of Echocardiography Developed in Collaboration with the Society for Cardiovascular Magnetic Resonance, *J Am Soc Echocardiogr.* 2017 Apr;30(4):303-371.]

underestimating the severity of the regurgitation. In practice, multiple methods are employed to discern the severity of aortic insufficiency (Figure 6–14).

Zoghbi et al. have summarized the grading of chronic aortic regurgitation with echocardiography (see Table 6–2).

Most patients encountered by the cardiac anesthesiologist will already have their diagnosis and a surgical plan prior to surgery. Survival is improved in patients with severe aortic stenosis who undergo valve replacement (Figure 6–15). Occasionally, moderate aortic stenosis is detected during the course of coronary artery bypass surgery. The recent guidelines of the American Heart Association provide definitions

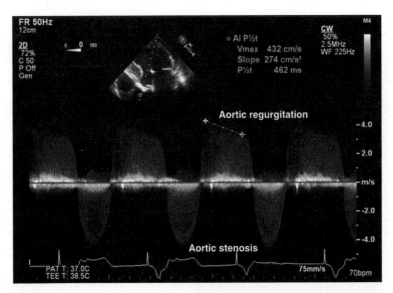

Figure 6–14. PHT aortic regurgitation: spectral Doppler waveforms obtained by applying continuous wave Doppler in the deep transgastric five-chamber view. Above the baseline the aortic regurgitation jet has a pressure half-time of 462 ms (moderate aortic regurgitation) and below the baseline the aortic stenosis flow has a maximum velocity of 4 m/s (severe aortic stenosis).

for mild, moderate, and severe AV disease.[1] Moreover, they provide guidelines for indications for AV replacement (AVR). Although incidentally discovered, severe AS will generally be addressed by the surgeon. The risks and benefits of surgical intervention in the setting of incidentally discovered moderate disease should be considered by the surgeon in consultation with the patient's cardiologist. Patients with moderate AS may progress rapidly thus supporting replacement of a moderately stenotic, incidentally discovered aortic valve at the time of coronary bypass surgery.[14] However, the increasing availability of catheter-delivered aortic valve replacement no longer places the patient at risk for repeat sternotomy should the decision be made not to replace moderately stenotic valves incidentally discovered at the time of coronary artery bypass surgery.

SURGICAL AND CATHETER-MEDIATED AV REPLACEMENT

Once it has been determined that the AV requires replacement, the type of intervention must be determined. Bioprosthetic and mechanical valves are both employed in AVR. It is a surgical/patient decision as to the type of valve that is placed. The patient's tolerance for anticoagulation influences the choice of a mechanical or bioprosthetic valve. There is some evidence that in patients aged 50 to 70 years, a mechanical valve may offer advantages.[15] Even patients with significantly reduced left ventricular ejection fractions are increasingly seen as candidates for valve replacement.[16] Likewise, in patients with severe, asymptomatic AS, AVR

Table 6–2. Grading the Severity of Chronic AR with Echocardiography

	AR severity		
	Mild	**Moderate**	**Severe**
Structural parameters			
Aortic leaflets	Normal or abnormal	Normal or abnormal	**Abnormal/flail, or wide coaptation defect**
LV size	**Normal***	Normal or dilated	Usually dilated[†]
Qualitative Doppler			
Jet width in LVOT, color flow	**Small in central jets**	Intermediate	**Large in central jets;** variable in eccentric jets
Flow convergence, color flow	**None or very small**	Intermediate	**Large**
Jet density, CW	**Incomplete or faint**	Dense	Dense
Jet deceleration rate, CW (PHT, msec)[‡]	Incomplete or faint Slow, > 500	Medium, 500-200	**Steep, < 200**
Diastolic flow reversal in descending aorta, PW	**Brief, early diastolic reversal**	Intermediate	**Prominent holodiastolic reversal**
Semiquantitative parameters[§]			
VCW (cm)	< 0.3	0.3-0.6	> 0.6
Jet width/LVOT width, central jets (%)	< 25	25-45 46-64	≥ 65
Jet CSA/LVOT CSA, central jets (%)	< 5	5-20 21-59	≥ 60
Quantitative parameters[§]			
RVol (mL/beat)	< 30	30-44 45-59	≥ 60
RF (%)	< 30	30-39 40-49	≥ 50
EROA (cm²)	< 0.10	0.10-0.19 0.20-0.29	≥ 0.30

PHT, Pressure half-time; *PW*, pulsed wave Doppler.
Bolded qualitative and semiquantitative signs are considered specific for their AR grade. Color Doppler usually performed at a Nyquist limit of 50-70 cm/sec.
*Unless there are other reasons for LV dilation.
[†]Specific in normal LV function, in absence of causes of volume overload. Exception: acute AR, in which chambers have not had time to dilate.
[‡]PHT is shortened with increasing LV diastolic pressure and may be lengthened in chronic adaptation to severe AR.
[§]Quantitative parameters can subclassify the moderate regurgitation group.
Reproduced with permission from Zoghbi WA, Adams D, Bonow RO, et al: Recommendations for Noninvasive Evaluation of Native Valvular Regurgitation: A Report from the American Society of Echocardiography Developed in Collaboration with the Society for Cardiovascular Magnetic Resonance, *J Am Soc Echocardiogr.* 2017 Apr;30(4):303-371.

has long-term benefit.[17] Elderly patients too are increasingly seen as acceptable candidates for AVR.[18] Consequently, it is likely that cardiac anesthesiologists will encounter patients for AVR who are older and have reduced ventricular function.

Various catheter-delivered aortic valves have also recently been employed in the management of patients with severe aortic valvular disease and significant comorbidities[19] (Figure 6–16). Percutaneous aortic valve implantation techniques take

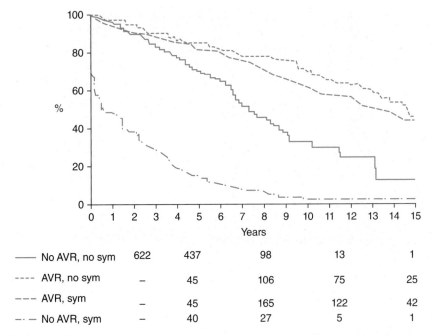

—— No AVR, no sym	622	437	98	13	1
---- AVR, no sym	–	45	106	75	25
--- AVR, sym	–	45	165	122	42
—·— No AVR, sym	–	40	27	5	1

Figure 6–15. Survival of patients with severe aortic stenosis with and without aortic valve replacement. Survival curves of patients with severe aortic stenosis by echocardiographic examination who were symptomatic (sym) or not symptomatic (no sym) and if they underwent aortic valve replacement. Survival clearly favors valve replacement. [Reproduced with permission from Brown ML, Pellikka PA, Schaff HV, et al: The benefits of early valve replacement in asymptomatic patients with severe aortic stenosis, *J Thorac Cardiovasc Surg.* 2008 Feb;135(2):308-315.]

many different forms. The transcatheter aortic valve replacement (TAVR) can be deployed through different approaches, depending on the patient's vascular anatomy and severity of atherosclerotic disease: femoral, aortic, axillary, transapical and very rarely transcarotid.[20] Prior to valve deployment, a balloon valvuloplasty may be performed to increase native cusps excursion and ensure adequate cardiac output at the time the transcatheter delivery system traverses the native valve and before deployment (Figure 6–17). Balloon valvuloplasty is performed with rapid ventricular pacing, and ventilation is also held.

After balloon valvuloplasty, deployment of the transcatheter valve is performed either during rapid ventricular pacing (balloon expandable valves) or over the course of multiple cardiac beats (self-expandable valves) (Figure 6–18).

Risks of catheter-mediated valve placement include perivalvular leaks and stroke from embolic material as the cusps of the native valve are pressed toward the aortic root walls by expansion of the catheter-delivered prosthetic valve. Valve migration, occlusion of coronary artery ostia, and aortic annulus rupture can also complicate the procedure. It is likely that the use of catheter-mediated valves in patients with intermediate surgical risk will increase. Additionally, catheter-delivered valves

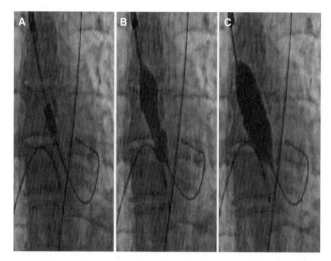

Figure 6–16. A balloon-mounted aortic valve being deployed. [Reproduced with permission from Webb JG, Chandavimol M, Thompson CR, et al: Percutaneous aortic valve implantation retrograde from the femoral artery, *Circulation.* 2006 Feb 14;113(6):842-850.]

are suggested as a treatment for stenosis of previous bioprosthetic aortic valves. Osnabrugge et al. estimate that there are currently 290,000 elderly patients at high surgical risk who could possibly benefit from catheter-delivered aortic valve replacement in Europe and North America alone.[21] A sutureless aortic prosthetic valve deployed on cardiopulmonary bypass (CPB) has been suggested as an alternative to catheter-delivered valves to reduce procedure times and ease valve implantation during "minimally invasive" AV replacements.[22]

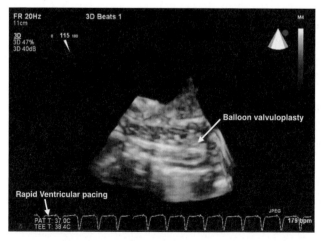

Figure 6–17. 3-D dataset of an expanded balloon through the aortic valve seen in long axis during balloon valvuloplasty and rapid ventricular pacing and 180 beats/min.

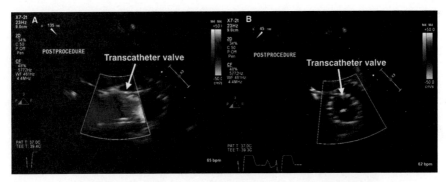

Figure 6-18. TAVR_{deployed}: Self-expandable transcatheter valve seen in long axis (panel A) and short axis (panel B). Trace intravalvular regurgitation is seen in short axis.

Traditional AV valve surgery is accomplished by the surgeon correctly sizing the valve and sewing it into position in the aortic annulus.[23] Placement of too small a valve can lead to elevated transvalvular pressure gradients even with a perfectly working prosthetic valve. The effective orifice area (EOA) of the prosthetic valve divided by the body surface area (BSA) indicates if patient prosthetic mismatch is likely to be present. Severe mismatch should be suspected when EOA/BSA is less than 0.65 cm^2/m^2. In such instances, ventricular dysfunction can progress in spite of surgery. At times surgeons will enlarge the aortic root to permit the placement of a larger valve. AVR surgery can be done through a full sternotomy, a partial sternotomy, or a mini thoracotomy.

The cardiac anesthesiologist must be familiar with the surgery as well as the valve placed and most importantly with its echo patterns. Video 6–4 demonstrates a bileaflet mechanical aortic valve. Video 6–5 shows a bioprosthetic valve in the aortic position. Perivalvular leaks, aorto-atrial fistulas, and aortic ruptures and dissections can occur and complicate AV replacement. TEE is useful in detecting these developments during the perioperative period. Oversewing of a coronary artery or coronary ostium, a rare complication, can likewise present during AV replacement resulting in ischemia and infarction. TEE can often be employed to demonstrate continuation of blood flow through the left main coronary artery (and occasionally the right coronary artery) following AVR (Video 6–6). Occlusion of a coronary artery should be suspected whenever there is a new, unexpected ventricular wall motion abnormality following AVR. Although other etiologies can similarly impair ventricular function, attempts to visualize flow in the coronary arteries by TEE can be helpful.

ANESTHETIC IMPLICATIONS OF AV DISEASES

Anesthetic management of the AV surgery patient is formulated based upon the answers to the following questions:

• What is the dominant valvular pathology: AS or AR?
• What other cardiac pathologies are manifest?

- How well compensated is the patient?
- How are those compensatory mechanisms likely to be affected following the induction of anesthesia?

The patient with critical AS is at significant risk during anesthesia induction. The hypertrophied LV is in need of sufficient coronary blood flow to prevent myocardial ischemia. Moreover, the LV of the patient with AS is often noncompliant leading to an increase in LVEDP. Induction of anesthesia can reduce coronary perfusion pressure (CPP) resulting in myocardial ischemia. Maintenance of vascular tone with a vasoconstrictor at the time of induction can reduce the severity of hypotension associated with anesthesia induction. The fixed obstruction of the stenotic valve prevents the AS patient from sufficiently augmenting CO to offset reduced vascular tone at the time of induction. Consequently, patients very quickly deteriorate and become profoundly hypotensive. Maintenance of sinus rhythm is essential as the atrial contraction contributes as much as 40% to the LV filling in the context of LV hypertrophy and diastolic dysfunction. Should the patient have coexisting coronary artery disease (and most patients probably do), the possibility of peri-induction hemodynamic collapse increases.

The choice of particular anesthetic agents for the AS patient matters less than managing the consequences of the loss of vascular tone or sinus rhythm. Should the patient experience hemodynamic collapse, various vasoconstrictors can be employed including phenylephrine, norepinephrine, and vasopressin. Vasopressin restores vascular tone until the patient is placed on CPB. At times patients with severe AS arrest during anesthetic induction simply because their cardiac reserve is such that loss of vascular tone leaves them too hypotensive to generate an effective CPP. In this instance, resuscitative measures are taken, but efforts should be directed toward the rapid institution of CPB. Consequently, it is prudent to have both the surgeon and perfusionist readily available at the time of anesthetic induction in patients with limited cardiac reserve and severe aortic stenosis.

Anesthetic management of the AR patient is often dependent upon the degree of compensation and the time course of the patient's disease. The chronic AR patient often has had adequate time to develop compensatory mechanisms to maintain an adequate cardiac output. The dilated heart of the AR patient can generate a sufficient stroke volume in spite of a relatively low ejection fraction simply because of the size of the LV cavity. Moreover, the vasodilation and mild tachycardia, which often accompany anesthesia induction and maintenance, promote forward blood flow and reduce diastolic time—thereby reducing the degree of AR.

On the other hand, in those patients with long-standing AR and a noncompliant LV, the induction of anesthesia can produce problems similar to those encountered in the AS patient. In AR patients with poor ventricular compliance, LVEDP is increased. Anesthesia induction reduces the already low diastolic blood pressure producing dramatic reductions in CPP with resultant ischemia and hemodynamic collapse.

The acute AR patient will likely be in or close to cardiogenic shock. Such patients present with acidosis, tissue ischemia, low cardiac output, and pulmonary edema.

Frequently they are supported with many vasoactive agents and arrive emergently to the operating room for an attempt at salvage. Anesthetic management centers on resuscitative efforts and successful institution of CPB.

Following valve replacement, separation of the AV patient from CPB may be challenging. The thickened myocardium of the AS patient at times is not optimally protected by cardioplegia administration during CPB resulting in dysfunction and difficulty weaning from bypass. Likewise, the patient with a newly competent AV following long-standing AR can have a profoundly dysfunctional left ventricle. Intra-coronary air can also complicate the weaning process leading to ischemia and fibrillation in the immediate post-bypass or postoperative period. Patients experience both systolic and diastolic dysfunction. Strategies to weaning patients with poor LV function from CPB are discussed in Chapter 5.

Increasingly, selected patients for transcatheter aortic valve replacement (TAVR) are managed with sedation. Other patients are anesthetized with general anesthesia. Patient cooperation and ability to lie flat should be considered when planning sedation versus general anesthesia for TAVR.[24]

CLINICAL SCENARIO: THE PATIENT WITH MIXED AS/AR AND THE EMERGENCY INSTITUTION OF CPB

A 55-year-old man presents to the hospital following a syncopal episode. He is found to have aortic stenosis with a valve area of 0.7 cm^2 and 50% occlusion of the left main coronary artery. Additionally, he reports that following surgery for an appendix 3 years earlier he required admission to the ICU secondary to traumatic intubation. He reports that he was told never to have anesthesia without warning the staff that it is impossible to place a breathing tube in him!!

What are the anesthesia issues at play here? What other information would be helpful?

The patient has tight AS and is at great risk for myocardial ischemia during anesthesia induction. The AS and 50% left main occlusion place him at great jeopardy for hemodynamic collapse at the time of anesthesia induction. However, the airway issue has to be the first concern. Awake fiber-optic or video-assisted intubation can be performed in the patient at risk for cardiac collapse. Frequently it is useful to assign one anesthesiologist to monitor and manage the patient's hemodynamics while another focuses on securing the airway. Because tachycardia associated with awake intubation could exacerbate myocardial ischemia, some degree of sedation and analgesia should be considered. It is important to understand that during the performance of an awake intubation the patient could arrest and collapse hemodynamically. Consequently, hemodynamic management is directed at avoiding tachycardia and maintaining systemic pressure. If the patient's airway is considered at such risk that airway or hemodynamic collapse is thought likely, then the patient could be placed on femoral CPB using local anesthesia and sedation.

The anesthesiologist also learns that the patient has a decreased ejection fraction of 25%. Following successful awake intubation, anesthesia is induced. How should one proceed?

Again, the choice of anesthetic agents is secondary to maintaining vascular tone and providing for a sufficiently long diastolic time to load the noncompliant heart of the AS patient.

Bypass proceeds uneventfully, and the surgeon places the valve seen on TEE in Video 6–6. What type of valve is this?

A bioprosthetic valve has been placed.

Bubbles are seen on the TEE examination and the patient experiences VF arrest. What should be done?

If the patient remains connected to the CPB machine and no protamine has been given, the patient can be placed back on bypass. Additionally, the surgeon can attempt to defibrillate using internal paddles. Should the patient have already been given protamine, an additional full dose of heparin is required before returning to bypass should the VF be refractory to multiple shocks. Surgeons initiate open chest massage while they attempt to replace the CPB cannula. Once back on CPB, vasoconstrictors are used to increase mean arterial pressure to eliminate any trapped air from the coronary vasculature. Additionally, the surgeons attempt to further remove air from the heart. An intraaortic balloon pump is placed, and the patient is successfully weaned from CPB and recovers uneventfully.

REFERENCES

1. Nishimura RA, Otto CM, Bonow RO, et al. 2014 AHA/ACC guideline for the management of patients with valvular heart disease: executive summary: a report of the American College of Cardiology/American Heart Association Task Force on Practice Guidelines. *Circulation* 2014;129:2440-2492.
2. Nkomo VT, Gardin JM, Skelton TN, et al. Burden of valvular heart diseases: a population based study. *Lancet*. 2006;368:1005-1011.
3. Van Klei WA, Kalkman CJ, Tolsma M. Pre-operative detection of valvular heart disease by anaesthetists. *Anaesthesia*. 2006;61:127-132.
4. Lester SJ, Heilbron B, Dodek A, et al. The natural history and rate of progression of aortic stenosis. *Chest*. 1998;113:1109-1114.
5. Mohler ER, Gannon F, Reynolds C, et al. Bone formation and inflammation in cardiac valves. *Circulation*. 2001;103:1522-1528.
6. Iivanainen AM, Lindroos M, Tilvis R, et al. Natural history of aortic valve stenosis in the elderly. *Am J Cardiol*. 1996;78:97-101.
7. Enriquez-Sarano M, Tajik AJ. Aortic regurgitation. *NEJM*. 2004;351(15):1539-1546.
8. Paul S, Mihaljevic T, Rawn JD, Cohn LH, and Byrne J. Aortic valve replacement in patients with severely reduced left ventricular function. *Cardiology*. 2004;101:7-14.
9. Aurigemma GP, Zile MR, Gaasch WH. Contractile behavior of the left ventricle in diastolic heart failure: with emphasis on regional systolic function. *Circulation*. 2006;113:296-304.
10. Carabello BA, Crawford FA. Valvular heart disease. *NEJM*. 1997;337(1):32-40.
11. Friedrich AD, Shekar PS. Interrogation of the aortic valve. *CCM*. 2007;35(8):s365-s371.
12. Tribouilloy CM, Enriquez-Sarano M, Bailey KR, et al. Assessment of severity of aortic regurgitation using the width of the vena contracta: a clinical color Doppler imaging study. *Circulation*. 2000;102:558-564.

13. Detaint D, Maalouf J, Tribouilloy C, et al. Congestive heart failure complicating aortic regurgitation with medical and surgical management: a prospective study of traditional and quantitative echocardiographic markers. *J Thorac Cardiovasc Surg.* 2008;136(6):1549-1557.

14. Du X, Soon J. Mild to moderate aortic stenosis and coronary bypass surgery. *J Cardiology.* 2011;57(1):31-35.

15. Brown ML, Schaff HV, Lahr BD, et al. Aortic valve replacement in patients aged 50 to 70 years: improved outcome with mechanical valves versus biologic prostheses. *J Thorac Cardiovasc Surg.* 2008;135(4):878-884.

16. Chukuemeka A, Rao V, Armstrong S, et al. Aortic valve replacement: a safe and durable operation in patients with impaired left ventricular systolic function. *Eur J Cardiothorac Surg.* 2006;29:133-138.

17. Brown ML, Pellikka PA, Schaff HV, et al. The benefits of early valve replacement in asymptomatic patients with severe aortic stenosis. *J Thorac Cardiovasc Surg.* 2008;135(2):308-315.

18. Filsoufi F, Rahmanian PB, Castillo JG, et al. Excellent early and late outcomes of aortic valve replacement in people aged 80 and older. *JAGS.* 2008;56:255-261.

19. Lichtenstein SV, Cheung A, Ye, J, et al. Transapical transcatheter aortic valve implantation in humans: initial clinical experience. *Circulation.* 2006;113:591-596.

20. Webb JG, Chandavimol M, Thompson C, et al. Percutaneous aortic valve implantation retrograde from the femoral artery. *Circulation.* 2006;113:842-850.

21. Osnabrugge R, Mylotte D, Head S, et al. Aortic stenosis in the elderly. *J Am Coll Cardiol.* 2013;62:1002-1012.

22. Santapino G, Pfeiffer S, Jessl J, et al. Sutureless replacement versus transcatheter valve implantation in aortic valve stenosis: a propensity-matched analysis of 2 strategies in high risk patients. *J Thorac Cardiovasc Surg.* 2014;147:561-567.

23. Mohty-Echahidi D, Malouf JF, Girard SE, et al. Impact of prosthesis-patient mismatch on long-term survival in patients with small St. Jude medical mechanical prostheses in the aortic position. *Circulation.* 2006;113:420-426.

24. Neuburger PJ, Patel PA. Anesthetic techniques in transcatheter aortic valve replacement and the evolving role of the anesthesiologist. *J Cardiothorac Vasc Anesth.* 2017;31(6):2175-2182.

REVIEWS

Baumgartner H, Hung J, Bermejo J, et al. Recommendations on the echocardiographic assessment of aortic valve stenosis: a focused update from the European Association of Cardiovascular Imaging and the American Society of Echocardiography. *J Am Soc Echocardiogr.* 2017;30:372-392.

Nishimura RA, Otto CM, Bonow RO, et al. 2017 AHA/ACC Focused Update of the 2014 AHA/ACC Guideline for the Management of Patients with Valvular Heart Disease. *Circulation.* 2017;135:e1159-e1195.

Zoghbi W, Adams D, Bonow RO, et al. Recommendations for noninvasive evaluation of native valvular regurgitation: a report of the American Society of Echocardiography developed in collaboration with the Society for Cardiovascular Magnetic Resonance. *J Am Soc Echocardiogr.* 2017;30(4):303-371.

Mitral Valve Disease

TOPICS

Whereas the aortic valve serves as the gateway to the systemic circulation, the mitral valve (MV) is the doorway to the left ventricle (LV). Should the valve be too tight as in mitral stenosis (MS), the LV is under loaded reducing the stroke volume (SV) **(Video 7–1A-C)**. Moreover, the narrowed MV prevents adequate drainage of the left atrium (LA) and the pulmonary circulation. With time, the LA dilates and pulmonary arterial (PA) pressures increase, leading to atrial fibrillation, pulmonary edema, and right ventricular failure. Consequently, these conditions make the anesthetic management of the MS patient for MV replacement most challenging.

When the MV becomes incompetent, it no longer functions to ensure the one-way, forward flow of blood during each cardiac cycle. As the LV contracts during systole, blood can be ejected forward through the aortic valve (AV) into the systemic circulation, or the blood can flow backward into the LA via the leaky MV. Like aortic regurgitation (AR), mitral regurgitation (MR) can develop both acutely or exist chronically. Patients with chronic MR develop compensatory mechanisms, which permit them to eject a sufficient SV into the systemic circulation to maintain circulatory function. Conversely, the patient with acute MR lacks adequate compensatory mechanisms. Acute MR frequently presents secondary to papillary muscle dysfunction or rupture following myocardial infarction or due to the destruction of the valve by mechanical trauma or infectious processes. As such, the acute MR patient usually presents in cardiogenic shock as the SV ejected into the systemic circulation is inadequate to meet the patient's metabolic demands. Additionally, acutely increased pulmonary artery pressures contribute to the development of pulmonary edema in the MR patient.

THE CLINICAL SIGNS AND SYMPTOMS OF MV DISEASES

Mitral Stenosis

The normal area of the MV is 4 to 6 cm^2. Isolated narrowing of the MV is frequently associated with rheumatic heart disease and degenerative calcification of the MV.[1] Rheumatic MS is characterized by commissural fusion, chordal shortening, leaflet thickening, and reduced leaflet mobility. It can occur at any age > 5 years. Degenerative calcification of the MV occurs more frequently in advanced age and is characterized by calcification of the MV annulus which extends progressively into the leaflet bases, gradually reducing diastolic excursion of the MV leaflets. Calcification of the MV leading to MS can also occur in renal failure, disorders of calcium metabolism, and after radiation of the chest. As the disease process progresses, the valve area declines leading to an increased pressure gradient between the LA and the LV during diastole. This increased gradient drives diastolic filling of the LV through the stenotic MV orifice.

As the gradient progressively increases and MV area falls below 1.5 cm^2, patients become increasingly symptomatic. Such patients frequently become dyspneic as high LA pressures are transmitted to the pulmonary vasculature leading to pulmonary edema. Patients with MS may be asymptomatic at rest, but when diastolic time is decreased (such as during exercise, stress, or pregnancy), the LA may not have sufficient time to empty into the LV—reducing the SV and increasing LA pressure. Increased LA pressure is transmitted to the pulmonary vasculature and the patient becomes dyspneic. Likewise, as the LA becomes distended secondary to MS, the patient can develop atrial fibrillation. Atrial fibrillation, especially when accompanied by a rapid ventricular rate, reduces diastolic filling time, which in conjunction with the lack of atrial contraction at the end of diastole further decreases LV filling and increases LA pressure leading to the patient becoming clinically symptomatic.

Chronic Mitral Regurgitation

Many disease processes can acutely or chronically disrupt the integrity of the MV apparatus. For the valve not to leak, the valve annulus, leaflets, chordae, and papillary muscles must function properly (Video 7–2). Should the heart dilate secondary to cardiomyopathy, the annulus can become enlarged preventing the coaptation of the anterior and posterior valve leaflets during systole—resulting in regurgitation (Figure 7–1 and Video 7–3). Should the papillary muscles or chordae be dysfunctional, torn, or stretched, the leaflets can prolapse or flail into the LA during systole—again resulting in regurgitation (Figure 7–2 and Videos 7–4A and B). Similarly, should a leaflet become tethered and restricted, it will not be able to effectively close during systole (Figure 7–3 and Video 7–5). Finally, a disease process that destroys or damages the leaflets, such as endocarditis, will also cause the regurgitation of blood into the LA during ventricular systole.

Various diseases including coronary artery disease, cardiomyopathies, and rheumatic heart disease may lead to chronic MR. Patients can tolerate mild to moderate

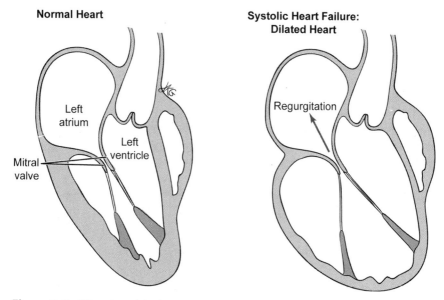

Figure 7–1. Dilatation of the heart results in the leaflets of the mitral valve failing to coapt resulting in central mitral regurgitation.

chronic MR for many years until they become increasingly dyspneic with exertion. As chronic MR is often secondary to other cardiac diseases such as coronary artery disease, it may be difficult to differentiate between the symptoms of the chronic MR and those of the underlying cardiac disease.

American Heart Association/American College of Cardiology (AHA/ACC) guidelines for the management of patients with valvular heart disease note that it

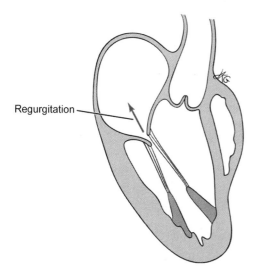

Figure 7–2. Mitral regurgitation can also occur when there is too much motion of the leaflets of the mitral valve as depicted here. The anterior leaflet of the mitral valve has too much movement compared to the posterior leaflet resulting in failure to coapt and mitral regurgitation.

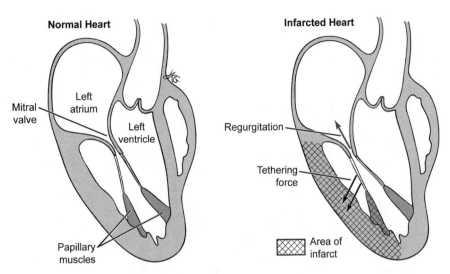

Figure 7–3. Mitral regurgitation also occurs where the movement of a mitral valve is restricted such as can occur following myocardial infarction.

is important to distinguish between chronic primary MR and chronic secondary MR (Table 7–1). In primary MR the structures of the valve components result in the mitral valve becoming incompetent. For example, a prolapsing MV leaflet produces MR. Repair of the valve itself corrects the pathological condition and cures the disease. Conversely, the valve components in patients with chronic secondary MR are themselves normal; however, the heart is dilated secondary to other disease processes (e.g., ischemic heart failure). AHA/ACC guidelines note that since MR is but one component of disease, reestablishing mitral valve competence is not necessarily curative. Consequently, therapeutic recommendations differ between primary and secondary MR. Additionally, the Carpentier classification is used to

Table 7–1. Etiology of Primary and Secondary MR

Primary MR (leaflet abnormality)	
MVP myxomatous changes	Prolapse, flail, ruptured or elongated chordae
Degenerative changes	Calcification, thickening
Infectious	Endocarditis vegetations, perforations, aneurysm
Inflammatory	Rheumatic, collagen vascular disease, radiation, drugs
Congenital	Cleft leaflet, parachute MV
Secondary MR (ventricular remodeling)	
Ischemic etiology secondary to coronary artery disease	
Nonischemic cardiomyopathy	
Annular dilation	Atrial fibrillation, restrictive cardiomyopathy

Reproduced with permission from Zoghbi WA, Adams D, Bonow RO, et al: Recommendations for Noninvasive Evaluation of Native Valvular Regurgitation: A Report from the American Society of Echocardiography Developed in Collaboration with the Society for Cardiovascular Magnetic Resonance, *J Am Soc Echocardiogr.* 2017 Apr;30(4):303-371.

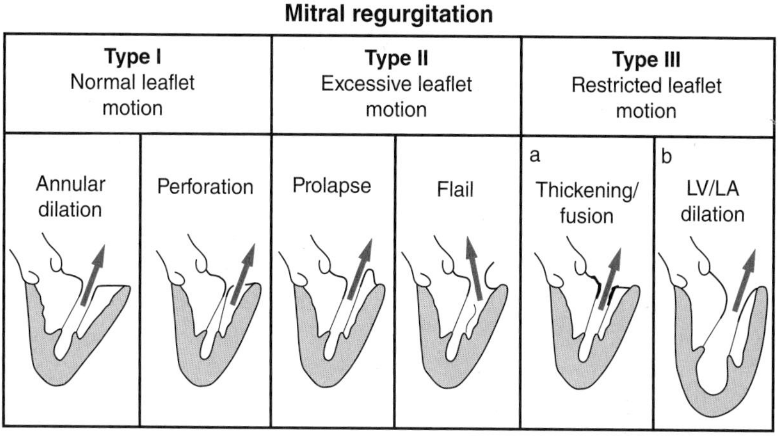

Mitral regurgitation

Type I Normal leaflet motion		Type II Excessive leaflet motion		Type III Restricted leaflet motion	
Annular dilation	Perforation	Prolapse	Flail	a Thickening/ fusion	b LV/LA dilation

Figure 7–4. The Carpentier classification for mechanisms of mitral regurgitation. [Reproduced with permission from Zoghbi WA, Adams D, Bonow RO, et al: Recommendations for Noninvasive Evaluation of Native Valvular Regurgitation: A Report from the American Society of Echocardiography Developed in Collaboration with the Society for Cardiovascular Magnetic Resonance, *J Am Soc Echocardiogr.* 2017 Apr;30(4):303-371.]

identify normal or abnormal leaflet motion as the mechanism of regurgitation (Figure 7–4).

Acute Mitral Regurgitation

Acute MR occurs when the mitral apparatus becomes acutely dysfunctional. Patients may present in shock in the setting of an acute myocardial infarction with papillary muscle ischemia. Similarly, endocarditis can lead to loss of MV integrity resulting in acute MR and cardiogenic shock (**Video 7–6**). Patients are often dyspneic and in congestive heart failure. Such cases usually require emergent surgery if they are to be salvaged. Intra-aortic balloon pump (IABP) placement may be temporarily needed to reduce LV afterload so to minimize regurgitation. Patients may also be supported with a percutaneous placed ventricular assist device (see Chapter 11).

PHYSIOLOGIC COMPENSATORY MECHANISMS OF MV DISEASES

The patient with MV disease attempts to compensate for the inability of the MV to ensure efficacious loading of the LV and ejection of an adequate SV into the systemic circulation. The LV of the patient with MS is chronically underloaded, while that of the patient with MR is either acutely or chronically volume overloaded.

MR can occur either from a primary defect in the structure of the MV or secondary to abnormalities in the structure and geometry of the LV. As the LV dilates secondary to cardiomyopathy or ischemia, the leaflets are being tethered by the papillary muscles displaced apically and are prevented from closing effectively. Annular dilatation contributes to MV.

The LV of the patient with MR must compensate for the incompetency of the mitral valve.[2-5] In the patient with an incompetent MV, during ventricular systole the SV is not fully ejected out through the AV into the systemic circulation. Rather, a variable percentage of the SV enters the LA. To compensate, the LV hypertrophies eccentrically and dilates allowing for a greater left ventricular end-diastolic volume (LVEDV) to augment the forward flowing SV. This dilatation can further worsen MR. At the same time, the LA dilates to accommodate the regurgitant volume. The increase in LVEDV is often accomplished without an increase in left ventricular end-diastolic pressure (LVEDP). Consequently, patients can tolerate chronic MR for many years because they maintain the forward SV by increasing the size of the LV.

Unfortunately, as with all ventricular remodeling compensatory mechanisms there are limits to their ability to maintain near-normal physiologic function in the setting of abnormal structure. As the disease progresses, the heart increasingly dilates and contractile function deteriorates. LV compliance becomes decreased, thereby reducing the ability of the heart to accommodate increased LVEDV with only minimal changes in LVEDP. Additionally, ventricular remodeling increases the ratio of ventricular radius to ventricular wall thickness.[4] This increased ratio together with an increase in LVEDP will result in an increase in wall stress according to the LaPlace law:

$$\text{LV wall stress} = (\text{LV pressure} \times \text{LV radius})/2(\text{LV thickness})$$

This increase in wall stress ultimately leads to an increase in myocardial oxygen demand.

The increased LVEDP is transmitted to the LA raising the left atrial pressure (LAP). Patients become progressively dyspneic and fatigued, as the heart can no longer eject a near normal SV into the systemic circulation.

The patient with acute MR does not have time to develop compensatory mechanisms for the reduction in forward flowing SV. When the MV becomes acutely incompetent, a part of the total SV is ejected in a retrograde manner in to the LA during systole.

$$\text{Total SV} = \text{Forward SV} + \text{Retrograde SV}$$

In the chronic MR patient, the total SV is increased secondary to dilation of the LV to partially compensate for that fraction of the total SV, which flows retrograde. Consequently, the forward SV remains relatively unaffected until the heart's compensatory mechanisms are overwhelmed at which time the patient becomes symptomatic.

The patient with acute MR cannot increase the total SV because there is no time for such compensatory mechanisms to develop. Therefore, the forward flowing SV is reduced. The patient often presents in cardiogenic shock secondary to a reduced forward cardiac output. Concurrently, the LA cannot accommodate the regurgitant volume resulting in increased pulmonary pressures and pulmonary congestion.

The heart of the patient with MS must compensate for the chronic underloading of the LV and a reduced SV. Additionally, the pulmonary vasculature must mitigate the effects of increased LAP to prevent pulmonary congestion.

In patients with MS, a pressure gradient develops between the LA and LV during diastole. Recall, the SV is loaded into the LV during diastole. The stenotic MV impedes the delivery of blood to the LV. As the MV area decreases, an increased LAP develops as blood is forced to flow through the narrowed MV orifice. This increased LAP is transmitted to the pulmonary veins. Should atrial fibrillation develop or the patient become tachycardic for any reason, the patient will experience a decrease in diastolic time—further reducing the time that blood can pass through the narrowed orifice of the MV into the LV. Left atrial pressure further increases leading to pulmonary congestion. At the same time, the SV is progressively reduced as the LV is inadequately loaded. Patients become increasingly inactive, as the SV cannot meet the needs of the patient to conduct normal life activities.

The pulmonary vasculature tries to mitigate the increase in LAP to protect against the development of pulmonary edema. Pulmonary arteriolar changes may protect the pulmonary capillary bed by making it less leaky in the setting of high pulmonary venous pressures.[1] Although such compensatory mechanisms may retard the development of pulmonary edema, they produce over time profound pulmonary hypertension (Chapter 8). Increasing resistance in the pulmonary arteries requires the right ventricle (RV) to do increased pressure work to pump the SV through the pulmonary vasculature. Although the RV responds with compensatory mechanisms to this pressure challenge, in time, RV failure ensues leading to peripheral edema, ascites, and hepatic failure. Consequently, the compensatory responses of the heart and pulmonary vasculature to MS can produce profound pulmonary hypertension and RV failure. Additionally, the chronically underloaded LV may itself have impaired contractility.

ECHOCARDIOGRAPHY AND MV DISEASES

Transthoracic echocardiography (TTE) is an initial step in the cardiologist's diagnosis of the MV patient. Perioperatively, TEE is most likely to be employed to assist the surgeon/cardiologist performing the MV repair or replacement.[6] Three-dimensional TEE is becoming more commonly available and is used increasingly to examine the mitral valve perioperatively (**Video 7–7**). The basic TEE views of the normal mitral valve were discussed in the introduction to echocardiography and should be briefly reviewed before proceeding with this section (Figure 7–5).

Mitral Stenosis

The anterior and posterior leaflets of the MV appear thickened and poorly mobile in patients with MS. Rheumatic MS manifests as commissural fusion, chordal shortening, leaflet thickening, and reduced leaflet mobility, which involves predominantly the leaflet tips with relative sparing of the mitral annulus and leaflet bases. In degenerative MS, calcification of the MV annulus extends progressively into the leaflets, resulting in decreased diastolic excursion. As the patient's valve becomes stenotic, the orifice narrows obstructing diastolic filling of the LV.

When performing a perioperative TEE examination in the MS patient, it is also critical to look for additional echo findings associated with MS such as a dilated LA with stagnant blood (Video 7–8). The smoky appearance or spontaneous echo contrast is indicative of decreased blood velocities in the LA. The two-chamber view demonstrates both the MV and the beak-like left atrial appendage (LAA). The LAA is often the site of clot formation; the clot can be removed at the time of surgery and the LAA subsequently ligated. Left and right ventricular function is often impaired in the MS patient secondary to LV under loading, pulmonary hypertension, and RV failure. The RV is frequently pressure overloaded secondary to pulmonary hypertension.

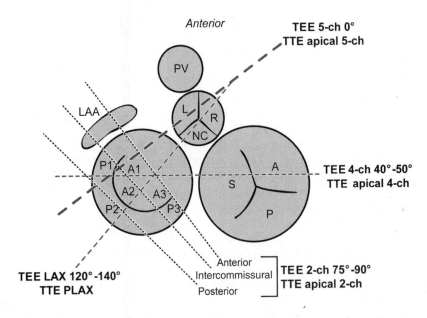

Figure 7–5A. Ultrasound sector scans using transesophageal (TEE) and transthoracic echocardiography (TTE) are presented in the schematic. The mitral valve is a part of the fibrous architecture of the heart. The anterior leaflet is immediately adjacent to the structures of the aortic valve. The posterior leaflet scallops are designated P1, P2, and P3 using the Carpentier system. The regions of the anterior mitral valve directly associated with the corresponding posterior scallops are designated A1, A2, and A3. The orientation of the anterior and posterior leaflets can be appreciated in relation to the left (L), right (R), and noncoronary (NC) cusps of the aortic valve. The left atrial appendage (LAA) is near the P1 scallop. The septal (S), anterior (A), and posterior (P) leaflets of the tricuspid valve and the pulmonic valve (PV) are depicted. The pulmonic valve is located most anteriorly and farthest from the transesophageal echocardiography probe. [Reproduced with permission from Condado JA, Vélez-Gimón M: Catheter-based approach to mitral regurgitation, *J Interv Cardiol.* 2003 Dec;16(6):523-534.]

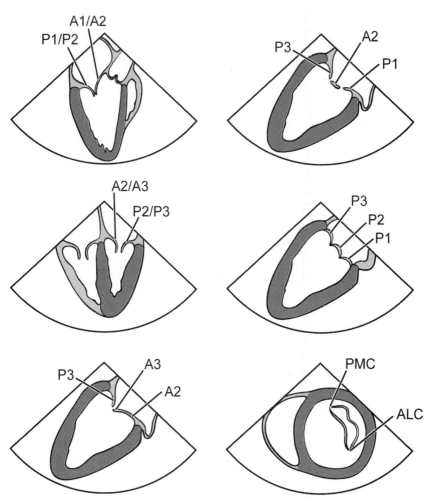

Figure 7–5B. Identification of the scallops using two-dimensional echocardiography can be difficult depending upon how the echocardiography scan cuts through the valve structures. At times distinguishing between A1 and A2 can be problematic depending on the views obtained. The basal short-axis view sketched above also reveals the postero-medial and anterolateral mitral valve commissures. [Adapted with permission from Lambert AS, Miller JP, Merrick SH, et al: Improved evaluation of the location and mechanism of mitral valve regurgitation with a systematic transesophageal echocardiography examination, *Anesth Analg.* 1999 Jun;88(6):1205-1212.]

Echocardiographers employ both TTE and TEE to examine and quantify the mitral valve.[7,8] Perioperatively, the valve area and pressure gradient across the MV will have already been determined before the patient is referred for surgery. Nonetheless, it is important to be able to assess the pressure gradient and esti-mate valve area in the operating room. Doppler measurements and the Bernoulli

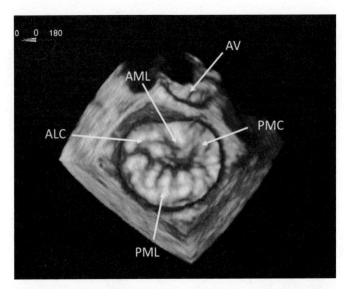

Figure 7–5C. Three-dimensional echocardiography of the mitral valve demonstrates: the anterior leaflet (AML), the posterior leaflet (PML), the anterolateral commissure (ALC) and the posteromedial commissure (PMC). The aortic valve (AV) is also seen.

equation are used to determine the transmitral pressure gradient between the LA and the LV.

$$\text{Peak pressure gradient} = 4V^2$$

where V is the peak velocity of flow between the LA and the LV across the stenotic MV. Recall, that in areas of stenosis, blood flows faster (the rapids!!) indicating a greater pressure gradient between the two heart chambers. Mean pressure gradients greater than 10 mm Hg are associated with severe MS and a valve area less than 1.0 cm^2.

There are several techniques, which can estimate the valve area of the stenotic MV. Although the cardiologist will have performed these prior to surgery, it is useful to understand the concepts especially when MS is detected unexpectedly during a perioperative TEE examination.

The pressure half-time (PHT) method can estimate the degree of MS (Figure 7–6). Using continuous wave Doppler, as discussed in the introductory chapter, the blood velocity across the stenotic mitral valve is measured, and by using the Bernoulli equation the atrioventricular pressure gradient is calculated. PHT is the time required for the atrioventricular peak pressure gradient to decrease from the initial maximal value to one-half of that value, or for the peak velocity across the MV to decrease to about two-thirds of that value (0.7 × peak velocity). PHT is obtained from the spectral Doppler display of the blood flow across the mitral valve by tracing the slope from the maximal to the minimal velocity in the Doppler envelope.

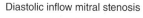

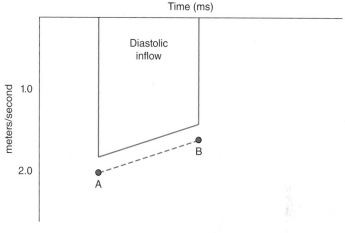

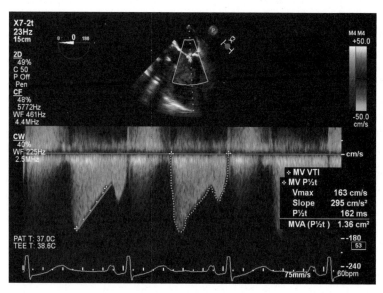

Figure 7–6. Pressure half-time (PHT) measurement in a patient with mitral stenosis. Using PHT measurement for calculating mitral valve area (MVA) in this patient (MVA = 220/PHT), MVA is 1.36 cm^2.

In patients with greater degrees of stenosis, it takes longer for the pressures between the LA and LV to equilibrate resulting in a longer pressure half-time. The stenotic valve area can be estimated from the PHT calculation as follows:

$$MV \text{ valve area} = 220/PHT$$

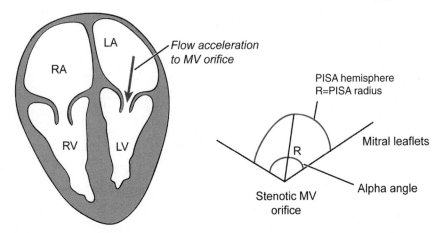

Figure 7–7. The PISA method also is employed to estimate mitral valve area in mitral stenosis. As blood passes through the tight mitral valve orifice, it accelerates generating a flow convergence hemisphere, which can be visualized using color flow Doppler.

Hence, any PHT greater than 220 milliseconds is associated with a mitral valve area of less than 1 cm^2 area and as such with severe MS. The PHT method is useful for assessment of native valves areas but not prosthetic valves areas.

The proximal isovelocity surface area (PISA) method can likewise be used to estimate valve area in MS (Figure 7–7).

The blood flow across the mitral valve can be visualized by using color flow Doppler. As blood rushes toward the narrowed orifice of the stenotic mitral valve, it accelerates, with the formation of multiple shells of hemispheric shape of increasing blood velocity as displayed by color flow Doppler. The area of a flow convergence hemisphere is known as proximal isovelocity surface area, and the velocities at points on the surface of this hemisphere are assumed to be the same. According to the conservation of mass principle, the flow at the surface of a hemispheric shell is the same as the flow through the stenotic mitral valve. Generally, the Nyquist limit determines the velocity on the color flow map where the blood flow appears to change direction known as "aliasing." By noting the Nyquist limit of the color flow Doppler map, the flow velocity at the hemispheric surface where the flow is "aliasing" can be known. The radius of the hemisphere where the flow is "aliasing" is measured. The maximum velocity of the blood at the level of the stenotic valve is also measured. Thus, it is possible to estimate valve area by knowing the velocity of blood flow at the point of the stenosis, the area of the PISA hemisphere, and the velocity of flow at the PISA hemisphere.

$$\text{PISA area} = 2\pi R^2$$

where R is the radius of the PISA (cm).

$$\text{PISA velocity} = \text{Nyquist limit (cm/s)}$$

The velocity of blood flow through the stenotic valve is measured with continuous wave Doppler at the level of the mitral valve in diastole. So,

MV area = (PISA area × Nyquist limit/maximal MV flow velocity) × α/180

The angle correction α/180 is added to the calculation to adjust for the reality that the PISA is not a complete hemisphere. The alpha (α) angle reflects that the mitral valve leaflets do not sit as a straight line but are angled from the baseline.

The continuity equation can likewise be employed to estimate the area of a stenotic mitral valve assuming that mitral/aortic valve regurgitation is absent.

Thus, the SV at the LVOT must equal the SV at the mitral valve:

$$SV \ LVOT = (Area \ LVOT)(VTI \ LVOT)$$
$$SV \ MV = (Area \ MV)(VTI \ MV)$$

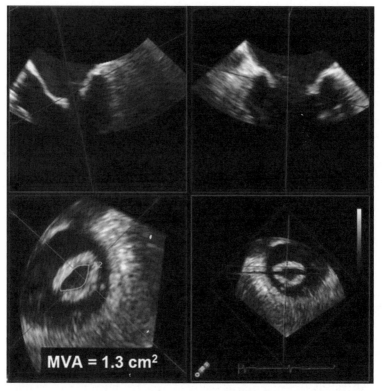

Figure 7–8. Multiplanar reconstruction of a three-dimensional dataset used to measure through planimetry in short axis the area of the mitral valve. [Reproduced with permission from Lang RM, Badano LP, Tsang W, et al: EAE/ASE recommendations for image acquisition and display using three-dimensional echocardiography, *Eur Heart J Cardiovasc Imaging.* 2012 Jan;13(1):1-46.]

Therefore,

$$\text{Area MV} = (\text{Area LVOT}) \, (\text{VTI LVOT})/(\text{VTI MV})$$

Where,

$$\text{VTI} = \text{velocity-time integral}$$

Three-dimensional echocardiography can also be employed to assess the area of the stenotic mitral valve (Figure 7–8).

Mitral Regurgitation

Both acute and chronic MR can be diagnosed with the aid of either TTE or TEE. Knowledge of MV anatomy is necessary to determine the mechanism and the significance of MR in the perioperative period.

The anterior and posterior mitral leaflets are joined at both the anterolateral and posteromedial commissures. The posterior leaflet has been described as consisting of three scallops: anterolateral (P1), medial (P2), and posteromedial (P3). These three posterior leaflet scallops coapt with their respective areas of the anterior leaflet of the MV (A1, A2, and A3). The various TEE views of the MV allow the visualization of these scallops. As such, it is possible to identify areas of valvular prolapse or restriction and thus use the TEE to identify the mechanism of regurgitation. The mitral valve fails to coapt during systole secondary to one of the following possible mechanisms:

1. The mitral annulus is dilated such that the leaflets do not come together sufficiently to fully close. In this instance, the color flow Doppler jet of MR is usually centrally directed.

2. The leaflets of the mitral valve move too much and prolapse or flail above the point of coaptation. This likely results in an eccentric jet by color flow Doppler directed away from the prolapsing/flail valve leaflet.

3. The mitral valve leaflets are restricted in closing during systole. Restriction of movement of one or more of the leaflets prevents the valve from coapting resulting similarly in an eccentric regurgitant jet directed toward the restricted leaflet.

Often disease processes of the papillary muscles and chordae can lead to the development of acute MR secondary to ruptured chordae and/or ischemic papillary muscles resulting in a "flail" mitral leaflet (Video 7–9).

TEE allows the determination of both the location and cause of MR as well as an estimation of its severity. Using the Carpentier nomenclature of the mechanisms of MR as outlined above, it is possible to identify the source of leaflet pathology. Mastery of this takes some time, and only those with the appropriate training and certification in perioperative TEE should undertake to guide surgery by the identification of MV pathology. Still, it is quite possible to readily discern if leaflets are restricted, flail, prolapsed, intact, or unable to coapt secondary to annular dilatation.

There are a number of TEE techniques that can be employed to assess the severity of MR including:[9]

Jet Area: The area of the regurgitant color flow jet is compared with that of the area of the LA. If the area is greater than 40%, the MR is thought severe. There are many potential errors associated with this method to determine severity of MR.[10] Also, if the jet hugs the wall of the LA, this method will underestimate the severity of MR **(Video 7–10)**.

Vena Contracta Width (VCW): The vena contracta is the narrowest part of the regurgitant jet as it passes through the valve. A vena contracta width greater than 0.7 cm is thought to be associated with significant MR **(Video 7–11)**. VCW less than 0.3 cm is associated with mild MR. Three-dimensional TEE is useful in measuring the vena contracta especially when multiple small vena contracta jets are present. However, the width of the multiple jets should not be added for a total vena contract width.[11,12]

Vena Contracta Area (VCA): The VCA can be determined using 3-D echocardiography. Once identified, the VCA is traced to measure and the area determined. An area greater than 0.4 cm² is associated with severe MR. When multiple jets are present, they should be traced independently and then added. Figure 7–9 demonstrates measurement of VCA.

Effective regurgitant orifice area (EROA): The concept of PISA was described in an earlier section, and it is here used to calculate the EROA. As the LV contracts during systole, blood accelerates in the LV toward the incompetent mitral valve

3D Quantitation in Primary and Secondary MR

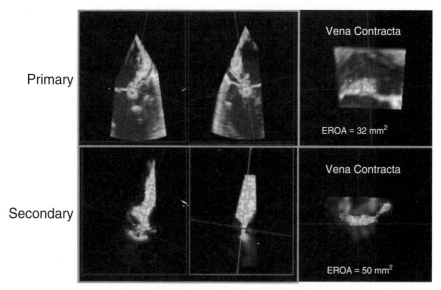

Figure 7–9. Two cases showing evaluation and quantitation of VCA with 3-D echocardiography and multiplanar reconstruction. A case of primary MR (*upper panels*) with a circular VCA and hemispheric PISA and another with secondary MR (*lower panels*) with elliptical VCA and nonhemispheric PISA. [Reproduced with permission from Zoghbi WA, Adams D, Bonow RO, et al: Recommendations for Noninvasive Evaluation of Native Valvular Regurgitation: A Report from the American Society of Echocardiography Developed in Collaboration with the Society for Cardiovascular Magnetic Resonance, *J Am Soc Echocardiogr.* 2017 Apr;30(4):303-371.]

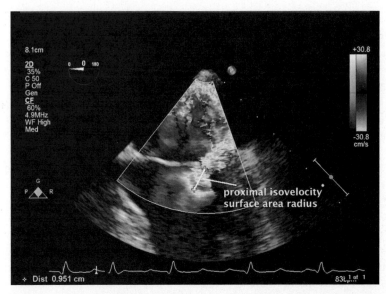

Figure 7–10. A PISA is seen in this patient with mitral regurgitation. In patients with mitral stenosis, the PISA sphere is seen in the LA during diastole as flow accelerated to pass through the narrowed mitral orifice into the LV. However, during mitral regurgitation the 0.951-cm PISA radius is seen on the ventricular side of the mitral valve as flow accelerates to pass through the leaky mitral valve during systole.

forming multiple shells of hemispheric shape as seen using color flow Doppler (Figure 7–10). Using the PISA formula previously described, the EROA can be calculated by knowing the Nyquist limit or velocity where the regurgitant flow is aliasing, the radius of the hemisphere where the flow is aliasing, and the maximal velocity of the regurgitant flow at the level of the regurgitant orifice.

EROA = effective regurgitant orifice area

PISA = $2\pi R^2$, where R is the radius of the PISA sphere using color flow Doppler

Nyquist limit = aliasing velocity at the level of the hemispheric shell

Maximal flow velocity = velocity of regurgitant blood flow as it passes through the EROA

The PISA approach once again employs the continuity principle. Therefore,

PISA × Nyquist limit = EROA × Maximal flow velocity

EROA = (PISA × Nyquist limit)/(Maximal flow velocity)

An EROA greater than 0.4 cm^2 is considered severe.

As previously illustrated, knowing the area through which the blood passes (cm^2) and the distance the blood travels (cm), it is possible to calculate the volume delivered per beat (cm^3).

The mitral regurgitant jet velocity time integral can be traced (MR VTI) to determine the stroke distance.

Thus,

$$\text{Regurgitant volume (RV)} = \text{EROA} \times \text{MR VTI}$$

An RV greater than 60 cm^3 (mL) is considered severe.

If a 5-m/s MR regurgitant jet is present and the aliasing velocity is set at 40 cm/s (by adjusting the Nyquist limit or baseline shifting the color flow Doppler), the EROA can be calculated in a simplified manner

$$\text{EROA} = R^2/2$$

Zogbhi et al. in the guidelines for noninvasive assessment of regurgitant lesions caution that when using techniques such as PISA EROA, VCW, and VCA, which rely on single frame measurements, that the severity of regurgitation might be overestimated in patients where MR is not holosystolic.

Pulmonary vein flow Doppler: Blood flows from the pulmonary veins into the LA both in systole and in diastole. The systolic flow in the pulmonary vein is normally greater than that of diastolic flow (Figure 7–11A). When severe MR is present, because of greatly increased LA pressure the systolic pulmonary vein flow is often blunted or reversed (Figure 7–11B).

Table 7–2 summarizes echocardiographic evaluation of MR.

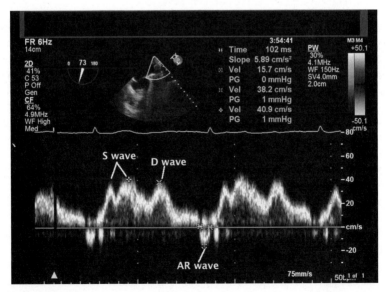

Figure 7–11A. The normal pulmonary vein pattern is seen above. Pulse wave Doppler (PWD) is used in the left upper pulmonary vein. Flow is normally toward the left atrium throughout systole (S) and diastole (D). There is reversal of flow during atrial contraction at the end of diastole (AR).

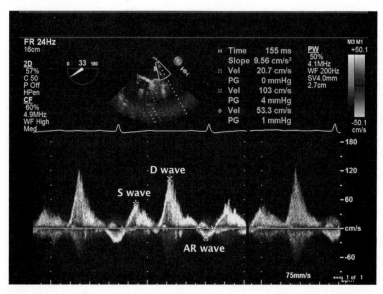

Figure 7–11B. In patients with severe mitral regurgitation, the S wave is often blunted or reversed in comparison to the D wave during pulse wave Doppler interrogation of the pulmonary vein.

SURGICAL AND CATHETER-MEDIATED APPROACHES TO THE REPAIR AND REPLACEMENT OF THE MV

The decision regarding repair or replacement of the MV is dependent upon discussions between the patient, surgeon, and cardiologist. Cardiac anesthesiologists are closely involved not only in providing for perioperative management but also in guiding and assessing the immediate results of surgical manipulations. Perioperative echocardiography is used extensively in both surgical and catheter-based procedures.

MS patients with appropriate valve morphology may be candidates for percutaneous mitral balloon valvotomy.[1] Other patients are likely to be referred for MV replacement. Valvotomy is not indicated if there is concomitant MR or LA thrombus or if the valve morphology does not appear favorable for that technique. Following puncture of the interatrial septum, a balloon catheter is introduced and expanded thereby opening the stenotic valve. Postprocedure echocardiographic assessments can detect the degree of induced MR as well as assess postprocedure valve area and pressure gradients.

Patient survivability after MV replacement due to MS is dependent upon patient age, ventricular function, presence of pulmonary hypertension, and the absence of coronary artery disease. Preservation of the mitral apparatus during MV replacement has been shown to improve LV function and patient survival.[13] Patient prosthetic mismatch can occur also in valves placed in the mitral position (EOA/BSA < 1.2 cm^2/m^2).

Patients presenting with MR will frequently undergo mitral valve repair. MV repair offers the advantage of eliminating the need for systemic long-term

Table 7–2. Grading the Severity of Chronic MR by Echocardiography

	MR severity*		
	Mild	**Moderate**	**Severe**
Structural			
MV morphology	**None or mild leaflet abnormality** (e.g., mild thickening, calcifications or prolapse, mild tenting)	Moderate leaflet abnormality or moderate tenting	**Severe valve lesions** (primary: flail leaflet, ruptured papillary muscle, severe retraction, large perforation; secondary: severe tenting, poor leaflet coaptation)
LV and LA size[†]	Usually normal	Normal or mild dilated	Dilated[‡]
Qualitative Doppler			
Color flow jet area[§]	**Small, central, narrow, often brief**	Variable	Large central jet (> 50% of LA) or eccentric wall-impinging jet of variable size
Flow convergence[∥]	**Not visible, transient or small**	Intermediate in size and duration	**Large throughout systole**
CWD jet	Faint/partial/parabolic	Dense but partial or parabolic	Holosystolic/dense/**triangular**
Semiquantitative			
VCW (cm)	< 0.3	Intermediate	≥ 0.7 (> 0.8 for biplane)[¶]
Pulmonary vein flow[#]	**Systolic dominance** (may be blunted in LV dysfunction or AF)	Normal or systolic blunting[#]	Minimal to no systolic flow/**systolic flow reversal**
Mitral inflow[**]	**A-wave dominant**	Variable	E-wave dominant (> 1.2 m/s)
Quantitative[††,‡‡]			
EROA, 2D PISA (cm²)	< 0.20	0.20-0.29	0.30-0.39	≥ 0.40 (may be lower in secondary MR with elliptical ROA)
RVol (mL)	< 30	30-44	45-59[††]	≥ 60 (may be lower in low flow conditions)
RF (%)	< 30	30-39	40-49	≥ 50

ROA, Regurgitant orifice area.
Bolded qualitative and semiquantitative signs are considered specific for their MR grade.
*All parameters have limitations, and an integrated approach must be used that weighs the strength of each echocardiographic measurement. All signs and measures should be interpreted in an individualized manner that accounts for body size, sex, and all other patient characteristics.
[†]This pertains mostly to patients with primary MR.
[‡]LV and LA can be within the "normal" range for patients with acute severe MR or with chronic severe MR who have small body size, particularly women, or with small LV size preceding the occurrence of MR.
[§]With Nyquist limit 50-70 cm/sec.
[∥]Small flow convergence is usually < 0.3 cm, and large is ≥ 1 cm at a Nyquist limit of 30-40 cm/s.
[¶]For average between apical two- and four-chamber views.
[#]Influenced by many other factors (LV diastolic function, atrial fibrillation, LA pressure).
[**]Most valid in patients > 50 years old and is influenced by other causes of elevated LA pressure.
[††]Discrepancies among EROA, RF, and RVol may arise in the setting of low or high flow states.
[‡‡]Quantitative parameters can help subclassify the moderate regurgitation group.
Reproduced with permission from Zoghbi WA, Adams D, Bonow RO, et al: Recommendations for Noninvasive Evaluation of Native Valvular Regurgitation: A Report from the American Society of Echocardiography Developed in Collaboration with the Society for Cardiovascular Magnetic Resonance, *J Am Soc Echocardiogr.* 2017 Apr;30(4):303-371.

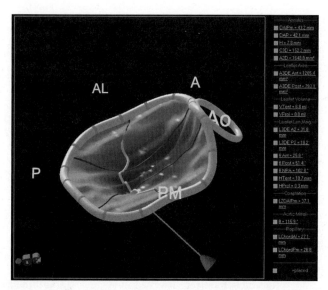

Figure 7-12. Parametric model of the mitral valve represents a static reconstruction of the mitral valve illustrating the topography of the mitral valve and displaying specific parameters of the mitral annulus and leaflets geometry.

anticoagulation and additionally spares the mitral apparatus leading to improved ventricular function (**Videos 7–12 and 7–13**). When complete, the repaired/replaced MV should have no residual MR (**Videos 7–14, 7–15, and 7–16**). Residual regurgitation *must* be reported to the surgical team so that they can determine if the repair is inadequate and MV re-repair or replacement is warranted. Increasingly, 3-D TEE is employed to examine the mitral valve perioperatively to model and to discern approaches to mitral valve repair (Figure 7–12). In patients with ischemic cardiomyopathy, ventricular dilatation secondary to remodeling results in the coaptation point of the valve leaflets being located more apically in the LV.[14] This creates a tent-like area between the mitral valve annulus and the point of leaflet coaptation. The angles between the planes of the annulus and the anterior and posterior leaflets identify the degree of restricted leaflet movement that contributes to the development of ischemic MR. Increased leaflet restriction augments the angle resulting in the leaflet coaptation point positioned more apically. Post-processing of the 3-D dataset of the mitral valve provides estimates of the tenting volume and tenting height of the valve (Figure 7–13). These volumetric measures may assist in guiding valve therapy in patients with ischemic MR.

A tenting height equal to or greater than 11 mm or a tenting area > 2.5 cm^2 is associated with a risk of significant MR following annuloplasty. Additionally, perioperative echocardiography can be used to identify patients at risk for dynamic outflow tract obstruction secondary to systolic anterior motion of the mitral valve. If the coaptation point between the anterior and posterior leaflets occurs more anteriorly, there is greater potential for dynamic outflow obstruction of the left ventricular outflow (Figure 7–14) (see Chapter 10).

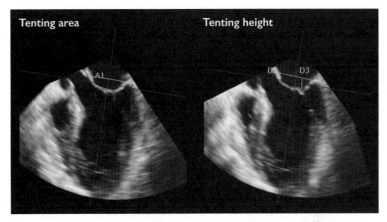

Figure 7–13. Tenting height and tenting area measure the degree of tenting of the mitral valve leaflets and apical displacement of the coaptation point. It is generally measured in the midesophageal long-axis view at end-systole.

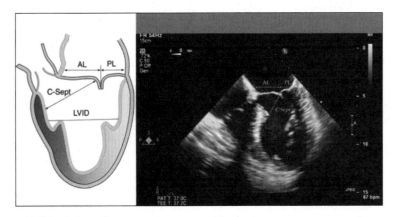

Figure 7–14. C-Sept distance measurement. These measurements are made in the pre-cardiopulmonary bypass period to assess for the risk of postrepair SAM and dynamic LVOT obstruction. *C-Sept:* the shortest distance between the coaptation point at end-systole and the interventricular septum. Any distance < 2.75 cm implies a relative anterior displacement of the coaptation point and, hence, susceptibility to SAM after repair and annuloplasty. *Anterior-leaflet/posterior-leaflet ratio:* This ratio represents the relative heights of both the leaflets. A ratio < 1.5 implies a relatively taller posterior leaflet with an anterior displacement of the coaptation point. This also is a guide during surgical repair to shorten the posterior leaflet height before placement of an annuloplasty ring to further reduce the risk of dynamic LVOT obstruction. Smaller left ventricular cavity size also is a risk factor for dynamic LVOT obstruction after mitral valve repair. *LVID* = left ventricular internal diameter; *SAM* = systolic anterior motion. [Reproduced with permission from Mahmood F, Matyal R: A quantitative approach to the intraoperative echocardiographic assessment of the mitral valve for repair, *Anesth Analg.* 2015 Jul;121(1):34-58.]

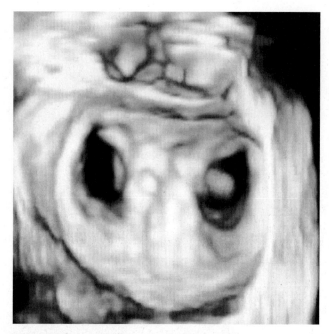

Figure 7-15. The double-orifice appearance of the mitral valve following catheter mediated edge-to-edge clipping of the mitral valve leaflets.

Various catheter-mediated approaches to MR have also been proposed.[15,16] Regurgitation secondary to annular dilatation is surgically corrected by placement of an annuloplasty ring to restore competency of the valve. Catheter-based devices have been introduced into the coronary sinus to "cinch" the mitral annulus and improve valve competency. Catheter-based techniques can also repair the MV by clipping together the anterior and posterior leaflets of the valve to restore valve coaptation creating a double orifice mitral valve (Figures 7–15 and 7–16). Development of catheter-delivered prosthetic mitral valves similar to those found in the aortic position have lagged due to the complex interactions between the valve leaflets, chords, annulus, and ventricle. Still, it is likely that anesthesiologists will, with increasing frequency, be called to care for patients in the catheterization laboratory/hybrid OR for mitral valve repair or replacement.[17,18]

SURGICAL APPROACHES TO THE MANAGEMENT OF ATRIAL FIBRILLATION

The MV disease patient is at risk for the development of atrial fibrillation (AF). Patients with MS are particularly at risk for developing hemodynamic instability associated with AF with a rapid ventricular response. Reduced diastolic time allows less than adequate loading of the LV and increases left atrial pressure (LAP).

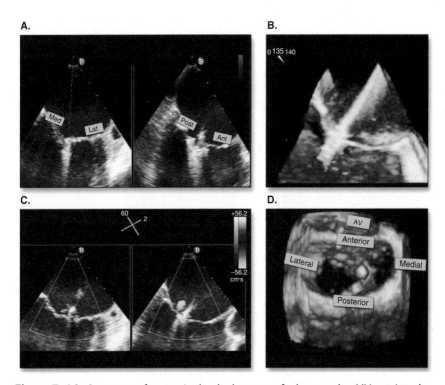

Figure 7-16. Sequence of events in the deployment of edge-to-edge MV repair technique (MitraClip). (A) Simultaneous biplane imaging at 60° and 150° demonstrates the exact location of the MitraClip within the MV structure. Once the position is confirmed, grasping of the MV leaflet occurs. (B) Live 3-D zoomed view of the delivery catheter and MitraClip grasping the A2 and P2 scallops of the MV. (C) Similar to part A, simultaneous biplane imaging at 60° and 150° demonstrates trivial to mild (1+) MR after MitraClip grasps the MV leaflets. (D) The MitraClip system is finally released from the delivery system and seen in the center of the new figure 8. Ant = anterior; Post = posterior; Med = medial; Lat = lateral; AV = aortic valve. [Reproduced with permission from Cavalcante JL, Rodriguez LL, Kapadia S, et al: Role of echocardiography in percutaneous mitral valve interventions, *JACC Cardiovasc Imaging*. 2012 Jul;5(7):733-746.]

MS patients quickly develop pulmonary edema and cardiogenic shock when in rapid AF. Up to 40% of patients with symptomatic MS will develop AF.[1] Medical therapy is aimed at controlling the ventricular response through the use of beta-blockers, calcium antagonists, or amiodarone. Additionally, anti-coagulants are administered to prevent thrombus development. In the setting of acute hemodynamic decompensation, synchronized cardioversion is indicated. However, patients who have been in AF for a period of hours may develop left atrial thrombus. The presence of LA thrombus should be ruled out by TEE examination before proceeding with elective cardioversion as restoration of sinus rhythm might provoke systemic thromboembolism.

At the time of MV repair or replacement, surgeons may also undertake the Cox-Maze procedure, the gold standard for surgical treatment of AF.[19] The Maze procedure interrupts pathways of electrical conduction in the atria to reduce the incidence of atrial fibrillation postoperatively. Numerous interruptions in the atrial conduction pathways are performed sometimes using radio frequency or cryoablation. (TEE probes are disconnected from the machine and withdrawn at the time of the maze to avoid the potential for aberrant conduction through the probe and possible esophageal injury.) Patients are placed on amiodarone therapy intraoperatively. Management of AF in the electrophysiology laboratory is discussed in Chapter 15.

ANESTHETIC IMPLICATIONS OF MV DISEASES

Mitral stenosis patients can be among the most challenging faced by anesthesiologists for either cardiac or noncardiac surgery. The stenotic valve prevents adequate loading of the LV. A slow heart rate and sufficient diastolic time are needed for adequate diastolic filling. Tachycardia reduces diastolic time and, hence, results in increased LAP and decreased SV. Because cardiac output (CO) = SV × HR, the low SV reduces CO. Because BP = CO × SVR, maintenance of BP is predicated upon sufficient systemic resistance. Unfortunately, surgery and anesthesia can both result in tachycardia, hypovolemia, and reduction in vascular tone rendering the patient potentially hemodynamically unstable during anesthesia and surgery. Moreover, the MS patient may have a degree of pulmonary hypertension and RV failure. Inadequate ventilation and hypercarbia, or simply application of positive pressure ventilation, can further increase PA pressures and exacerbate RV failure. The failing RV may inadequately load the left heart, additionally contributing to a diminished systemic CO. The mere institution of positive pressure ventilation can reduce RV output with concomitant RV and LV failure. Rhythm disturbances associated with anesthetics (e.g., nodal rhythm) can similarly impair LV filling, further worsening the patient's hemodynamic performance.

Ideally for the MS patient, anesthetic management is adjusted to mitigate the various potential perturbations of hemodynamic stability described above. In practice, this may be more complicated than might be initially apparent. As always, the choice of anesthetic agents employed is less significant than managing the hemodynamic consequences of those choices. Patients for noncardiac surgery with significant MS should have invasive monitoring of blood pressure. Patients coming for MV surgery will, of course, be fully monitored including TEE guidance. TEE can also be employed in the patient with MV disease coming for noncardiac surgery. Additionally, should a PA catheter be included in the plans for hemodynamic management, the wedge position is best avoided in patients with pulmonary hypertension to avoid PA rupture.

Vasodilatation encountered at the time of anesthetic induction can be managed through the administration of vasopressors (e.g., vasopressin, norepinephrine, phenylephrine). RV failure as a consequence of increased PA pressure can be treated by administering inotropic agents. Inotropes such as dobutamine and milrinone may improve myocardial contractility with the caveat that they can also result in systemic hypotension as well as tachycardias. Inhaled nitric oxide (NO) can be very useful in the patient who has pulmonary hypertension and RV dysfunction. Reducing pulmonary vascular resistance with NO or other pulmonary vasodilators can improve RV function and consequently better volume load the LV with a resultant increase in the SV. However, pulmonary vasodilators should be used carefully in patients with untreated significant mitral valve disease and/or left ventricular dysfunction as they may precipitate elevation in pulmonary venous pressure and pulmonary edema. Postprocedure, after the MV disease has been surgically addressed, pulmonary vasodilators should be used if needed to facilitate adequate RV function.

Using echocardiography and invasive pressure monitoring, the anesthesiologist must adjust volume delivery, pulmonary vascular resistance, systemic vascular tone, and myocardial contractility to the degree possible to optimize hemodynamic performance. Management of the pregnant patient with severe MS is particularly challenging due to the volume shifts and tachycardia associated with delivery.[20]

The patient with acute MR often presents to the OR in the setting of myocardial infarction in cardiogenic shock. These patients are frequently hypotensive, requiring multiple vasoactive infusions, and are often supported with an intraaortic balloon pump or percutaneous left ventricular assist device (Chapter 11). Management is largely resuscitative in nature until the patient is supported on cardio pulmonary bypass (CPB). Anesthetics other than muscle relaxants are administered as hemodynamically tolerated. Bispectral index (BIS) monitoring, although subject to much debate, is suggested for use in this and all cardiac patients as hemodynamic instability frequently requires the use of small amounts of anesthetic agents. Consequently, these patients are at increased risk of awareness intraoperatively and should be assessed for awareness postoperatively.

Patients with chronic MR generally have time to compensate for their leaky MV, and routine anesthetic management is aimed at promoting forward blood flow by avoiding bradycardia and by lowering systemic resistance. Induction of anesthesia often results in both vasodilatation and tachycardia making the chronic MR patient somewhat more manageable perioperatively up to a point. However, over time compensatory mechanisms fail and the patients develop ventricular dysfunction, increased ventricular wall stress, dysrhythmias, pulmonary hypertension, and RV failure. These patients can be as hemodynamically unstable as patients with severe MS during anesthesia.

In those patients with severely impaired LV function, RV failure, and pulmonary hypertension coming for valve repair or replacement, anesthetic management up to the initiation of CPB can be stormy. The anesthesiologist must manipulate volume administration, inotropes, vasoconstrictors, and anesthetic agents to make the patient as hemodynamically "stable" as possible. It is important to understand that hemodynamic stability might be an elusive goal in the prebypass period and some patients will need emergent institution of CPB.

Patients following valve repair may be challenging to wean from CPB. The patient following MV replacement or repair may be unstable secondary to left, right, or biventricular failure. Inotropes, vasopressors, pulmonary vasodilators, and

IABP counterpulsation are often necessary to facilitate separation from cardiopulmonary bypass.

CASE SCENARIO

A 61-year-old woman presents to her cardiologist with a complaint of dyspnea and irregular rhythm. She is found to be in atrial fibrillation, and a TEE examination is performed.

What lesion is present in **Video 7–1A**?

Mitral stenosis.

How can the severity of MS be determined by echocardiography?

The severity of MS can be determined intraoperatively by measuring the transmitral pressure gradient. Additionally, the valve area can be estimated using both the PISA and pressure half-time methods. Three-dimensional echocardiography can also be employed to determine the orifice area of the stenotic mitral valve.

A mean pressure gradient of 15 mm Hg is determined and a valve area of 1 cm^2 is noted. What other findings should be considered upon reviewing the echo examination?

RV and LV function are assessed, and the atrium is examined for the presence of LAA thrombus.

No thrombus is found; however, RV function appears reduced. After uneventful surgery, the MV is replaced.

A bileaflet mechanical valve is placed in the mitral position **(Video 7–14)**. There are no peri-valvular leaks around the valve and the normal washing jets, which prevent the buildup of clot on the valve surface, are present.

The patient is weaned from CPB using milrinone. Her BP is 60/40 mm Hg, PA 40/22, HR 100 bpm, CI 2.2 L/min/m^2.

What can be done to improve systemic BP?

Vasopressin 1 to 2 U/h by infusion is administered with improvement of the BP to 90/60 mm Hg.

However, her pulmonary arterial pressures rise to 70/50 mm Hg and she develops right ventricular dysfunction. What can be done?

Nitric oxide (NO) is administered by inhalation and her PA pressures somewhat decrease to 60/40 mm Hg.

Her systemic blood pressure is 75/45 mm Hg and her LV is poorly contractile as well despite increasing inotropic support. How can her function be improved?

An IABP is placed and effective counterpulsation decreases PA pressures to 45/29 mm Hg. Adding epinephrine as a second inotrope can be considered. Her systemic pressure improves as does her CI. She is safely transported to the ICU.

REFERENCES

1. Bonow RO, Carabello BA, Chatterjee K, and the writing committee to revise the 1998 guidelines for the management of patients with valvular heart disease. 2008 focused update incorporated into the ACC/AHA 2006 guidelines for the management of patients with valvular heart disease: a report of the American College of Cardiology/American Heart Association Task Force on Practice Guidelines. *JACC.* 2008;52(13):e1-e142.

2. Russo A, Suri RM, Grigioni F, et al. Clinical outcome after surgical correction of mitral regurgitation due to papillary muscle rupture. *Circulation.* 2008;118:1528-1534.

3. Carabello BA. Ischemic mitral regurgitation and ventricular remodeling. *JACC.* 2004;43(3):384-385.

4. Carabello BA. The current therapy for mitral regurgitation. *JACC.* 2008;52(5):319-326.

5. Bursi F, Enriquez-Sarano M, Jacobsen SJ, et al. Mitral regurgitation after myocardial infarction: a review. *Am J Med.* 2006;119:103-112.

6. Shernan SK. Perioperative transesophageal echocardiographic evaluation of the native mitral valve. *CCM.* 2007;35(8):s372-s383.

7. Enriquez-Sarano M, Tribouilloy C. Quantitation of mitral regurgitation: rational, approach, and interpretation in clinical practice. *Heart.* 2002;88(SIV):iv1-iv4.

8. Enriquez-Sarano M, Avierinos JF, Messika-Zeitoun D, et al. Quantitative determinants of the outcome of asymptomatic mitral regurgitation. *NEJM.* 2005;352:875-883.

9. Savage RM, Konstadt S. Con: Proximal isovelocity surface area should not be measured routinely in all patients with mitral regurgitation. *Anesth Analg.* 2007;105(4):944-946.

10. Lancellotti P, Moura L, Pierard L, et al. European Association of Echocardiography recommendations for the assessment of valvular regurgitation. Part 2: mitral and tricuspid regurgitation. *Eur J Echocardiog.* 2010;11:307-332.

11. Hyodo E, Iwata S, Tugcu A, et al. Direct measurement of multiple vena contract areas for assessing the severity of mitral regurgitation using 3D TEE. *JACC Cardiovasc Imaging.* 2012;5(7):669-676.

12. Thavendiranathan P, Phelan D, Collier P, et al. Quantitative assessment of mitral regurgitation: how best to do it. *JACC Cardiovasc Imaging.* 2012;5(11):1161-1175.

13. Condado JA, Velez-Gimon M. Catheter based approach to mitral regurgitation. *J Interv Cardiol.* 2003;16(6):523-534.

14. Shakil O, Jainandunsing J, Ilic R, et al. Ischemic mitral regurgitation: an intraoperative echocardiographic perspective. *J Cardiothorac Vasc Anesth.* 2013;27(3):573-585.

15. Feldman T, Wasserman HS, Herrmann HC, et al. Percutaneous mitral valve repair using the edge to edge technique. *JACC.* 2005;46(11):2134-2140.

16. Lozonschi L, Quaden R, Edwards NM, et al. Transapical mitral valved stent implantation. *Ann Thorac Surg.* 2008;86:745-748.

17. Mack MJ. Percutaneous treatment of mitral regurgitation: so near, yet so far! *J Thorac Cardiovasc Surg.* 2008;135(2):237-239.

18. Ghanbari H, Kidane AG, Burriesci G, et al. Percutaneous heart valve replacement: an update. *Trends Cardiovasc Med.* 2008;18(4):117-125.

19. Stulak JM, Sundt TM, Dearani J, et al. Ten year experience with the Cox-Maze procedure for atrial fibrillation: how do we measure success? *Ann Thorac Surg.* 2007;83:1319-1325.

20. Pan PH, D'Angelo R. Anesthetic and analgesic management of mitral stenosis during pregnancy. *Reg Anesth Pain Med.* 2004;29(6):610-615.

REVIEWS

Cavalcante J, Rodriguez L, Kapadia S, et al. Role of echocardiography in percutaneous mitral valve interventions. *JACC Cardiovasc Imaging.* 2012;5(7):733-746.

Lang R, Badano L, Tsang W, et al. EAE/ASE recommendations for image acquisition and display using three-dimensional echocardiography. *Eur Heart J Cardiovasc Imaging.* 2012;13(1):1-46.

Mahmood F, Matyal R. A quantitative approach to the intraoperative echocardiographic assessment of the mitral valve for repair. *Anesth Analg.* 2015;121(1):34-58.

Zoghbi W, Adams D, Bonow R, et al. Recommendations for noninvasive evaluation of native valvular regurgitation. *JASE.* 2017;30(4):303-371.

Baumgartner H, Hung J, Bermejo J, et al. Echocardiographic assessment of valve stenosis; EAE/ASE recommendation for clinical practice. *JASE*. 2009;22(1);1-23.

Nishimura RA, Otto CM, Bonow RO, et al. 2014 AHA/ACC guideline for the management of patients with valvular heart disease. *JACC.* 2014; 63(22):E57-E185.

Nishimura RA, Otto CM, Bonow RO, et al. 2017 AHA/ACC focused update of the 2014 AHA/ACC guideline for the management of patients with valvular heart disease: a report of the American College of Cardiology/American Heart Association Task Force on Clinical Practice Guidelines. *Circulation.* 2017;135:E1159-E1195.

Cherry SC, Jain P, Rodriguez–Blanco Y, Fabbro M. Noninvasive evaluation of native valvular regurgitation: a review of the 2017 American Society of Echocardiography Guidelines for the Perioperative Echocardiographer. *J Cardiothorac Vasc Anesth.* 2018;32:811-822.

Mahmood F, Matyal R, Mahmood F, Sheu R, et al. Intraoperative echocardiographic assessment of prosthetic valves: a practical approach. *J Cardiothorac Vasc Anesth.* 2018;32:823-837.

Right Heart Valves and Function

8

Much as the mitral valve (MV) and aortic valve (AV) direct blood flow into the systemic circulation, the tricuspid valve (TV) and the pulmonic valve (PV) direct flow into the pulmonary circulation. The right ventricle (RV) ensures loading of the left ventricle (LV) by pumping blood through the normally low pressure pulmonary vasculature. Perioperative RV failure is frequently associated with pulmonary artery hypertension and systemic hypoperfusion. Treatment is directed at reducing pulmonary arterial resistance to promote the forward flow of blood into the pulmonary vasculature. Inotropes and ventricular assist devices are also used to support right heart function perioperatively.

THE CLINICAL SIGNS AND SYMPTOMS OF TRICUSPID VALVE DISEASES

The tricuspid valve (TV) can develop both stenotic and regurgitant lesions. Tricuspid stenosis (TS) is most often secondary to rheumatic heart disease. Less encountered causes are carcinoid and endomyocardial fibrosis. Obstructing cardiac masses can also occlude the TV.[1]

Tricuspid regurgitation (TR) can be primary or secondary. Primary TR is rare (approximately 15% of TR cases) and results from endocarditis, connective tissue diseases, carcinoid syndrome, anorectic drugs (fenfluramine), Ebstein anomaly, pergolide, or chest radiation. Ebstein anomaly is due to apical displacement of the tricuspid valve leaflets, especially the septal leaflet, and is associated with TR and RV dysfunction. Secondary TR is the result of left heart disease or intrinsic lung disease, which increase pulmonary artery pressures and pulmonary vascular resistance (PVR). Examples of disease processes that produce secondary TR are mitral stenosis, severe mitral regurgitation, severe left ventricular dysfunction, pulmonary embolism, primary pulmonary hypertension, or lung disease.

Patients with TS frequently present with other valvular diseases associated with rheumatic heart disease (e.g., mitral stenosis, aortic stenosis) or carcinoid disease (e.g., pulmonary valve stenosis). Consequently, their clinical features often represent the combined impact of these lesions.

The patient with TR secondary to pulmonary hypertension is likely to present with signs of right heart failure and systemic venous engorgement. Peripheral edema, hepatic dysfunction, and ascites frequently occur. Systolic pulmonary pressures greater than 55 mm Hg[1] will likely result in TR even with normal valve structure. Transvenous pacemaker wires or catheters can both cause a mild degree of TR. Additionally, many patients have echocardiographically detected mild TR without clinical significance.

RV FUNCTION

The interaction between the right and left heart is critical to maintaining healthy cardiovascular function. Although patients can survive with only a single ventricle devoted to the systemic circulation (e.g., Fontan circulation—Chapter 12), a functioning right heart effectively loads the LV so that the stroke volume (SV) is ejected systemically. When the RV fails, the LV may be inadequately loaded reducing SV.

RV failure develops both acutely and chronically. Acute RV failure can occur with sudden increases in PVR (e.g., during a protamine reaction) or secondary to myocardial ischemia and infarction. Chronic RV failure presents secondary to progressive increases in pulmonary hypertension (e.g., from mitral stenosis or lung diseases) or as a consequence of volume overload (e.g., intracardiac left-to-right shunts or primary TR).

Both acute and chronic RV failure progress to RV dilatation and TR. Moreover, as the RV dilates, the intraventricular septum is flattened distorting the LV cavity and impeding its filling and geometry. Consequently, failure of the RV reduces LV function often resulting in decreased cardiac output and systemic hypotension. Acute RV failure during protamine administration for heparin reversal is a dramatic, life-threatening occurrence. As PA pressures increase, the RV distends and is unable to overcome the elevated pulmonary vascular resistance. The patient develops TR, and the LV is severely underloaded. Systemic hypotension can be severe, and circulatory collapse often is imminent. At times, it may become necessary to reheparinize the patient and reinstitute emergent cardiopulmonary bypass.

Therapy for RV failure is directed at its etiology and reducing PVR to improve RV forward output. There are no specific inotropic agents that directly target the right ventricle. Milrinone, dobutamine, levosimendan[2-5] can all be employed to improve RV contractility. These agents have inotropic effects upon both the left and the right ventricle and will likewise vasodilate both the systemic and pulmonary circulations. Reduction of pulmonary vascular resistance can improve RV function, LV function, and RV-LV interaction. Vasodilators including sodium nitroprusside and nitroglycerin will lower both systemic and pulmonary vascular resistance and can be useful, assuming the impact upon systemic pressure does not outweigh any benefit resulting from the diminution of pulmonary vascular resistance.

Nitric oxide (NO) is the molecule by which both nitroprusside and nitroglycerin ultimately produce vasodilatation. NO is present only minimally in the circulation and produces an increase in cGMP in vascular smooth muscle.[6-8] A more appealing method of delivering pulmonary vasodilators is the inhaled route, either as a gas (inhaled NO) or as an aerosolized solution (inhaled epoprostenol or inhaled milrinone). Inhaled NO produces selective pulmonary vasodilation and a decrease in pulmonary artery pressure and PVR by augmenting cGMP, with minimal systemic circulatory effects.

Patients with long-standing pulmonary arterial hypertension (PAH) also present for surgery. Patients are often managed with multiple agents to take advantage of different mechanistic pathways to promote pulmonary vasodilation. The endothelin pathway contributes to the development of PAH, and endothelin receptor antagonists (e.g., Bosentan) have shown the ability to improve exercise tolerance in PAH patients.[9] Long-established agents such as sildenafil slow cGMP degradation increasing vascular dilatation. Soluble guanylate cyclase stimulators (sGC) increase cGMP production. Patients treated with riociguat, an sGC stimulator, have improved exercise tolerance. Prostacyclin analogues are likewise used to dilate the pulmonary vasculature.

Unique right heart cardiomyopathies can also complicate perioperative management. Arrhythmogenic right cardiomyopathy[10] develops when the right heart undergoes fatty infiltration. Patients are at risk for sudden death from ventricular dysrhythmias. Often these patients will have been treated with an implantable cardioverter/defibrillator device. Hypertrophic cardiomyopathy (HCM) can likewise present with involvement of the right ventricle although to a far lesser degree than that seen in the LV. A pressure gradient can develop across the right ventricular outflow tract leading to RV failure. These patients are also at risk for sudden cardiac death (SCD).

THE PULMONIC VALVE

Like all other heart valves, the pulmonic valve can develop both stenotic and regurgitant lesions; however, it is the least likely valve to be affected by acquired heart disease.[1] Pulmonary stenosis (PS) may be congenital or acquired as seen in carcinoid syndrome. PS results in RV failure and under loading of the LV. Pulmonary regurgitation is also unusual but may occur due to annular dilatation as a result of pulmonary hypertension, following balloon valvuloplasty of a stenotic pulmonary valve or following repair of tetralogy of Fallot.

ECHOCARDIOGRAPHY OF RIGHT HEART STRUCTURES AND RIGHT VENTRICULAR FUNCTION

Right heart structures are located anteriorly and therefore away from the transesophageal echocardiography (TEE) probe. Consequently, they are less well visualized than those of the LV. Nonetheless, TEE can assist in the perioperative discernment of both RV function and valvular integrity. The basic views of the right heart and its structures were discussed in the introduction to TEE.

Additional TEE views of the right heart have been recommended to improve right heart assessment.[11] Right heart evaluation is an essential element of a comprehensive TEE exam especially since pulmonary hypertension and right ventricular dysfunction contribute to overall hemodynamic instability. TEE windows of right heart structures are presented in Figure 8–1.

RV function is not as easy to characterize on TEE as is that of the LV. Video 8–1 reveals a normally contracting RV. In contrast, Video 8–2 presents a dilated, dysfunctional RV. In this instance, the RV has dilated to overcome the increased resistance presented to it by chronic pulmonary hypertension eventually resulting in RV dilation and leftward movement of the intraventricular septum into the LV (Figures 8–2 and 8–3). Acute, perioperative RV failure can be identified through the use of TEE. For example, Video 8–3 shows acute pulmonary embolism as another cause of acute RV function deterioration.

Similar to the LV, the RV musculature is oriented in a complex multilayered fashion. However, longitudinal orientation of fibers predominate; therefore, RV contractility is primarily longitudinal during systolic ejection phase.[12] Tricuspid annular plane systolic excursion (TAPSE) provides a good estimate of right ventricular function. In transthoracic echocardiography (TTE), TAPSE can be measured by using M-mode and aligning the lateral annulus of the TV with the Doppler beam in the apical four-chamber view (Figures 8–4A and 8–4B). Aligning the M-mode cursor with the TV annulus could be challenging with TEE. An alternative method frequently used by TEE is to calculate the difference between the lateral annulus of the TV and RV apex distance measured by calipers at end-diastole (ED) and at end-systole (ES) in the mid- esophageal four-chamber view (ME four-chamber). Normal TAPSE is greater than 17 mm toward the apex of the heart.[13]

RV function can also be assessed by fractional area change by tracing the ED and ES area of the RV in the ME four-chamber view (Figure 8–5). An RV fractional area change < 35% is considered abnormal.

Tissue Doppler can also be employed to assess right ventricular function by measuring myocardial velocities during systole (S') at the lateral annulus of the TV. An S' less than 10 cm/s is consistent with RV dysfunction (Figure 8–6). Doppler-based assessments of right heart function are less accurate using TEE as it may not be possible to align the Doppler signal with the direction of motion of the tricuspid annulus.

Speckle tracking is also employed to assess myocardial performance for both the left and right ventricles. Speckle tracking imaging permits the quantification of myocardial deformation by tracking frame by frame the speckles created through

Standard Views	Required Structures	Additional Views	Required Structures

S-I. Mid-esophageal four-chamber view 0–20°

Left atrium, right atrium, left ventricle, right ventricle, interatrial and interventricular septum, mitral valve, tricuspid valve

A-I. Transgastric right ventricular basal short-axis view 0–40°

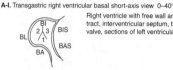

Right ventricle with free wall and outflow tract, interventricular septum, tricuspid valve, sections of left ventricular cavity

S-II. Mid-esophageal long-axis view 120–160°

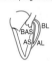

Left atrium, left ventricle with outflow tract, mitral valve, aortic valve, ascending aorta, parts of the right ventricle

A-II. Transgastric right ventricular apical short-axis apical view 0–40°

Right ventricle with free wall, interventricular septum, sections of left ventricular cavity

S-III. Mid-esophageal right ventricular inflow-outflow view 60–90°

Right atrium, right ventricle with inflow and outflow tract and free wall, tricuspid valve, pulmonary valve, proximal pulmonary artery, aortic valve

A-III. Transgastric right ventricular inflow-outflow view 0°

Right ventricular inflow and outflow tracts and parts of the free wall, tricuspid valve, pulmonary valve, main pulmonary artery, aortic root

S-IV. Transgastric mid short-axis view 0°

Left ventricle with >50% of the circumference and visible endocardium, papillary muscles sections of the right ventricle

A-IV. Deep transgastric right ventricular inflow-outflow view 120–160°

Right ventricular inflow and outflow tracts and parts of the free wall, tricuspid valve, pulmonary valve, main pulmonary artery, aortic root

S-V. Transgastric right ventricular inflow view 100–120°

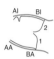

Parts of the right atrium and right ventricle, tricuspid valve, tricuspid subvalvular apparatus

A-V. Deep transgastric right ventricular outflow view 40–50°

Right ventricle with free wall and outflow tract, pulmonary valve

S-VI. Mid-esophageal ascending aortic short-axis view 0–60°

Ascending aorta, vena cava superior, pulmonary artery

S-VII. Upper esophageal aortic arch short-axis view 90°

Aortic arch, pulmonary artery, pulmonary valve

Figure 8–1. Seven standard (S) transesophageal echocardiographic views and five additional (A) views studied in 60 patients. Five basal segments: BA = basal anterior; BAS = basal anteroseptal; BI = basal inferior; BIS = basal inferoseptal; BL = basal lateral. Four apical segments: AA = apical anterior; AI = apical inferior; AL = apical lateral; AS = apical septal. Tricuspid valve: 1 = anterior cusp; 2 = posterior cusp; 3 = septal cusp. Pulmonary valve: 4 = anterior cusp; 5 = right cusp; 6 = left cusp. [Reproduced with permission from Kasper J, Bolliger D, Skarvan K, et al: Additional cross-sectional transesophageal echocardiography views improve perioperative right heart assessment, *Anesthesiology*. 2012 Oct;117(4):726-734.]

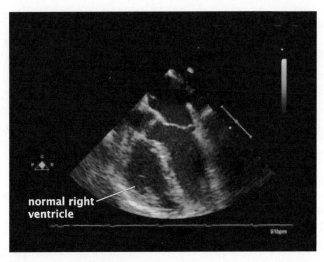

Figure 8–2. A normal RV is presented in this image. The RV does not extend to the apex of the heart nor does the septum flatten into the LV cavity.

the interaction of the myocardium with ultrasound.[14] Strain is the relative change in length of a structure compared with its baseline where

$$\text{Strain } (\varepsilon) = (L_1 - L_0)/L_0$$

where the strain rate is the change in strain with time $(\varepsilon/\Delta t)$.

Speckle tracking can detect radial, circumferential, and longitudinal deformation of the myocardium. For evaluating the RV, the longitudinal component of the

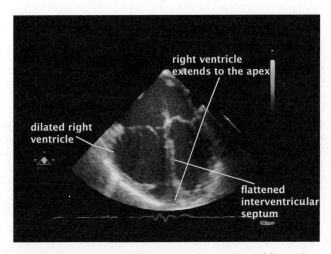

Figure 8–3. In this image, the RV is dilated assuming a spherical form. The ventricular septum is flattened, and the RV extends to the apex of the heart.

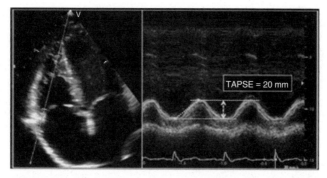

Figure 8–4A. Measurement of tricuspid annulus plane systolic excursion (TAPSE) using M-mode in the apical four-chamber view by transthoracic echocardiography. [Reproduced with permission from Lang RM, Badano LP, Mor-Avi V, et al: Reproduced with permission from Lang RM, Badano LP, Mor- Avi V, et al Recommendations for cardiac chamber quantification by echocardiography in adults: an update from the American Society of Echocardiography and the European Association of Cardiovascular Imaging, *J Am Soc Echocardiogr.* 2015 Jan;28(1):1-39.]

myocardial deformation is assessed. Because the myocardium shortens in systole, normal values for strain are negative. For the RV, a global longitudinal strain less than −20% (in absolute value) is considered abnormal.[14,15] TEE can likewise be used to assess strain (Figure 8–7).

ECHOCARDIOGRAPHIC EVALUATION OF THE TRICUSPID VALVE AND TRICUSPID REGURGITATION

Visualizing all three leaflets of the TV simultaneously is challenging. More than one 2-D TEE view is required to examine the entire TV apparatus, and it may necessitate subtle probe manipulations and nonstandard views. However,

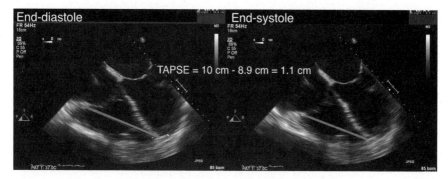

Figure 8–4B. Calculation of tricuspid annulus plane systolic excursion (TAPSE) through the difference between the lateral annulus of the tricuspid valve and the right ventricle apex distance measured by calipers at end-diastole (ED) and at end-systole (ES) in the mid-esophageal four-chamber view by transesophageal echocardiography.

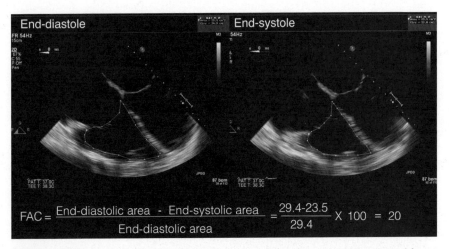

$$FAC = \frac{\text{End-diastolic area - End-systolic area}}{\text{End-diastolic area}} = \frac{29.4\text{-}23.5}{29.4} \times 100 = 20$$

Figure 8–5. Calculation of the fractional area change (FAC) in the midesophageal four-chamber view by tracing the end-diastolic and end-systolic areas of the right ventricle endocardial border.

3-D echocardiography permits the leaflets to be identified simultaneously (Figure 8–8).

TR is often found incidentally during perioperative TEE examination. Most frequently, TR is associated with dilatation of the RV. However, as mentioned above, other disease states can produce TR. The severity of TR is generally assessed using techniques previously employed to assess mitral regurgitation (Table 8–1) (see Chapter 7). The severity of TR is based upon the area of the regurgitant jet, vena contracta width of the regurgitant jet, vena contracta area to estimate the effective regurgitant orifice area (e.g., EROA > 0.4 cm^2 as cutoff for

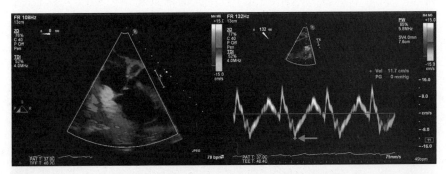

Figure 8–6. Tissue Doppler imaging of the tricuspid annulus and measurement of the systolic velocity (S'). These measurements should be interpreted with caution as error can be introduced through misalignment of the Doppler beam with the motion of the tricuspid annulus. Angle correction can be employed to reduce some of this error.

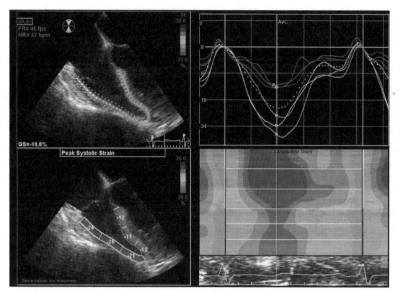

Figure 8–7. Speckle-tracking strain measurement of strain.

severe TR), or proximal isovelocity surface area (PISA) to quantitate the EROA and regurgitant volume of TR. Also, it is possible to use pulsed wave Doppler to interrogate the hepatic veins. Systolic reversal of hepatic vein flow in a manner similar to that of systolic reversal of pulmonary vein flow in mitral regurgitation is associated with severe TR (Figure 8–9).

Correction of less than severe TR in patients with pulmonary hypertension or tricuspid annular dilatation undergoing mitral valve surgery is increasingly recommended.[16]

TS is a relatively rare lesion. Its severity can be determined by measuring flow velocity across the stenotic valve to determine the peak and mean gradients across the TV. A mean pressure gradient higher than 5 mm Hg is considered significant.

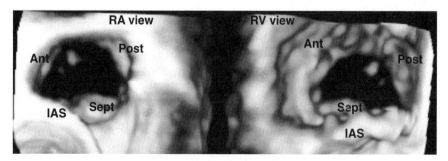

Figure 8–8. Three-dimensional dataset displaying the tricuspid valve leaflets from a right atrial (RA) and a right ventricle (RV) perspective. Ant, anterior leaflet; IAS, interatrial septum; Post, posterior leaflet; Sept, septal leaflet.

Table 8–1. Grading the Severity of Chronic TR by Echocardiography

Parameters	Mild	Moderate	Severe
Structural			
TV morphology	**Normal or mildly abnormal leaflets**	Moderately abnormal leaflets	**Severe valve lesions** (e.g., flail leaflet, severe retraction, large perforation)
RV and RA size	Usually normal	Normal or mild dilatation	Usually dilated[*]
Inferior vena cava diameter	Normal < 2 cm	Normal or mildly dilated 2.1-2.5 cm	Dilated > 2.5 cm
Qualitative Doppler			
Color flow jet area[†]	**Small, narrow, central**	Moderate central	**Large central jet** or eccentric wall-impinging jet of variable size
Flow convergence zone	**Not visible, transient or small**	Intermediate in size and duration	**Large throughout systole**
CWD jet	**Faint/partial/ parabolic**	Dense, parabolic or triangular	Dense, often triangular
Semiquantitative			
Color flow jet area (cm^2)[†]	Not defined	Not defined	**> 10**
VCW (cm)[†]	< 0.3	0.3-0.69	**≥ 0.7**
PISA radius (cm)[‡]	≤ 0.5	0.6-0.9	**> 0.9**
Hepatic vein flows[§]	Systolic dominance	Systolic blunting	**Systolic flow reversal**
Tricuspid inflow[§]	**A-wave dominant**	Variable	E-wave >1.0 m/s
Quantitative			
EROA (cm^2)	< 0.20	0.20-0.39[‖]	**≥ 0.40**
RVol (2D PISA) (mL)	< 30	30-44[‖]	≥ 45

RA, Right atrium.
Bolded signs are considered specific for their TR grade.
[*]RV and RA size can be within the "normal" range in patients with acute severe TR.
[†]With Nyquist limit > 50-70 cm/s.
[‡]With baseline Nyquist limit shift of 28 cm/s.
[§]Signs are nonspecific and are influenced by many other factors (RV diastolic function, atrial fibrillation, RA pressure).
[‖]There are little data to support further separation of these values.
Reproduced with permission from Zoghbi WA, Adams D, Bonow RO, et al: Recommendations for Noninvasive Evaluation of Native Valvular Regurgitation: A Report from the American Society of Echocardiography Developed in Collaboration with the Society for Cardiovascular Magnetic Resonance, *J Am Soc Echocardiogr.* 2017 Apr;30(4):303-371.

A pressure half-time of greater than or equal to 190 ms likely reflects severe tricuspid stenosis.

Examination of the PV is difficult using TEE because the PV is the most anteriorly situated of the heart valves with respect to the TEE probe (**Video 8–4**).

For this reason assessments of PV perioperatively are problematic using TEE. Figure 8–10 demonstrates a pulmonary artery catheter passing through the pulmonic valve. Using the midesophageal ascending aorta short-axis view, the main PA can be identified as it divides into left and right pulmonary arteries (Figure 8–11).

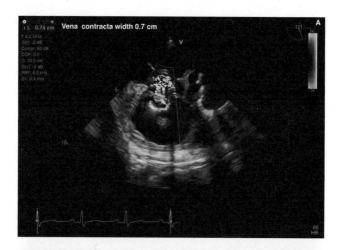

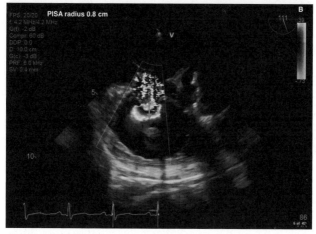

Figure 8–9. (A) A tricuspid regurgitation (TR) jet seen in the midesophageal modified bicaval view. The vena contracta width measures 0.7 cm. (B) The proximal isovelocity surface area (PISA) radius measures 0.8 cm. (C) Continuous wave Doppler interrogation of the TR jet measures a peak velocity (TR Vmax) of 300 cm/s. Using an aliasing velocity of 40 cm/s at the level of the PISA hemisphere and a radius of 0.8 cm renders an effective regurgitant orifice area (EROA) of 0.53 cm². (D) Pulsed wave Doppler interrogation of the hepatic veins shows the S (systolic) wave, V wave, D (diastolic) wave, and AR (atrial reversal) wave. The S wave is blunted (in relationship to the D wave) in the presence of elevated right atrial pressure due to significant TR.

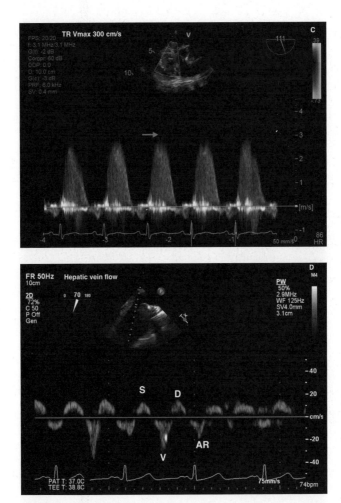

Figure 8–9. (Continued)

Usually the left pulmonary artery is difficult to visualize due to the interposition of the left main bronchus.

Zoghbi et al. highlight the echocardiographic assessment for pulmonary regurgitation. A pressure half-time of less than 100 ms of the regurgitant jet is associated with severe PR. Regurgitant jet vena contracta width/PV annulus diameter is also used to assess PR severity. A ratio greater than 0.7 correlates with severe PR.

Pulmonic stenosis (PS) is relatively rare and usually of congenital origin. Carcinoid disease is the most common source for acquired pulmonic stenosis. A peak jet velocity across the stenotic valve greater than 4 m/s is associated with severe stenosis, which correlates to a pressure gradient of greater than 64 mm Hg by the Bernoulli equation. Additionally, right ventricular hypertrophy is likewise associated with severe PS.

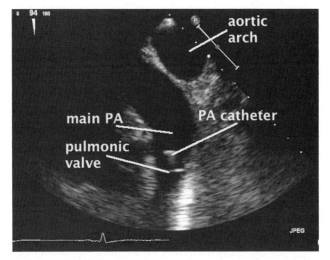

Figure 8-10. A pulmonary artery catheter is seen passing through the pulmonic valve in this image.

SURGICAL APPROACHES TO TV DISEASES

TR often occurs secondary to pulmonary hypertension associated with other cardiac lesions. Consequently, TR is frequently surgically addressed in combination with other interventions (e.g., mitral valve repair or replacement).[17] Ring annuloplasty is performed to restore integrity to the valve assuming leaflet structure is normal. Valve replacement is employed when the tricuspid leaflets no longer permit repair. Pulmonic valve surgery is relatively rare and is directed at restoring competency of the PV. The Ross procedure for correction of AV disease involves harvesting of the patient's pulmonic valve for placement into the aortic position and subsequent use

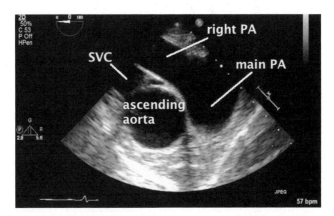

Figure 8-11. The main pulmonary artery divides into the left and right pulmonary arteries.

of a homograft to replace the pulmonic valve. Otherwise, operations on the PV in the adult patient are unusual.

ANESTHETIC IMPLICATIONS OF TV DISEASES, PULMONARY HYPERTENSION, AND RV FAILURE

RV failure may occur acutely during any cardiac surgical procedure. Classic protamine reactions will readily produce pulmonary hypertension and RV dysfunction. Should they occur, management is directed at restoration of RV function. Inotropic agents, such as epinephrine, dobutamine, and milrinone, can be used to increase RV contractility and produce pulmonary vasodilatation. Inhaled NO or other pulmonary vasodilators, if available, can be employed to dilate the pulmonary vasculature. If necessary, the patient can be reheparinized and cardiopulmonary bypass can be reinstituted. Mechanical assist devices can also be used to support right ventricular function if needed (see Chapter 11).

In patients with chronic pulmonary disease and long-standing pulmonary hypertension, RV function may be worsened with the institution of positive pressure ventilation, high inflation pressures, and high positive end-expiratory pressure. PA pressures might also increase in the setting of light anesthesia, hypoxemia, hypercarbia, or hypothermia. Perioperative volume overload can readily distend a poorly compliant RV. As a dysfunctional RV is likely to have an elevated RV end-diastolic pressure, it is paramount to maintain systemic blood pressure to maintain an adequate coronary perfusion pressure.

In patients with right-sided valvular lesions it might not be possible or prudent to place pulmonary arterial catheters. If considered desirable, the PA catheter can be placed in the venous circulation and then advanced by the surgeon after completion of the surgical repair.

CASE SCENARIO: THE PATIENT WITH ENDOCARDITIS

Endocarditis should be suspected whenever a patient presents with a new-onset heart murmur, positive blood cultures, fever, and splinter hemorrhages.[1] Patients can present with endocarditis with negative blood cultures. Echocardiographic assessment is critical in identification of the valves affected and the hemodynamic consequence of the infection. Antibiotic therapy can be used when the lesions are without hemodynamic consequence; however, should patients develop hemodynamic compromise, surgery is indicated. Likewise, vegetations producing embolisms usually need to be addressed surgically. The 2008 American College of Cardiology/American Heart Association guidelines have updated recommendations on the use of antibiotics to prevent endocarditis in patients with structural heart disease.[18] Revising long-held prophylactic guidelines, the 2008 recommendations include the use of antibiotic prophylaxis prior to dental procedures in patients with: prosthetic valves or prosthetic materials in valve repairs; previous endocarditis; congenital heart disease (e.g., unrepaired cyanotic heart disease, repaired congenital heart disease with prosthetic material or device for 6 months following repair, repaired congenital heart disease with residual defect); and following cardiac transplantation with valve regurgitation due to an abnormally structured heart valve. Prophylaxis is not recommended for nondental procedures such as TEE or colonoscopy in the absence of active infection.

A 33-year-old with endocarditis presents for surgery. **Video 8–5** reveals the presence of vegetations on which valve/s?

A tricuspid valve vegetation is demonstrated.

The patient is taken for surgery and the valve replaced. Following administration of protamine the patient's systemic blood pressure is 60/40 mm Hg, and his PA pressure is 60/40 mm Hg. What is the most likely diagnosis?

This patient is experiencing a protamine reaction. His right heart has dilated, and his LV is underloaded.

What are the treatment options at this time?

The patient is treated with inotropic support (epinephrine bolus and infusion). The RV becomes more contractile, systemic blood pressure is restored to 90/70 mm Hg, and PA pressure is now 45/20 mm Hg.

Had he not responded to inotropic therapy, what other options are available to the anesthesia and surgery team?

The patient can be reheparinized and placed on cardiopulmonary bypass. Inhaled NO therapy or other pulmonary vasodilators can be administered to lower PA pressures and decrease RV afterload.

REFERENCES

1. Bonow RO, Carabello BA, Chatterjee K, et al. 2008 focused update incorporated into the ACC/AHA 2006 guidelines for the management of patients with valvular heart disease. *JACC.* 2008; 52(13):e1-e142.

2. Cicekcioglu F, Parlar AI, Altinay L, Yay K, Katircioglu SF. Tricuspid valve replacement and levosimendan. *Gen Thorac Cardiovasc Surg.* 2008;56:559-562.

3. Parissis JT, Farmakis D, Nieminen M. Classical inotropes and new cardiac enhancers. *Heart Fail Rev.* 2007;12:149-156.

4. Cicekcioglu F, Parlar AI, Ersoy O, Yay K, Hijazi A, Katircioglu SF. Levosimendan and severe pulmonary hypertension during open heart surgery. *Gen Thorac Cardiovasc Surg.* 2008;56:563-565.

5. Mebazaa A, Nieminen M, Packer M, et al. Levosimendan vs. dobutamine for patients with acute decompensated heart failure: the SURVIVE randomized trial. *JAMA.* 2007;297(17):1883-1890.

6. Khazin V, Kaufman Y, Zabeeda D, et al. Milrinone and nitric oxide: combined effects on pulmonary artery pressures after cardiopulmonary bypass in children. *J Cardiothorac Vasc Anesth.* 2004;18(2):156-159.

7. Solina A, Papp D, Ginsberg S, et al. A comparison of inhaled nitric oxide and milrinone for the treatment of pulmonary hypertension in adult cardiac surgery patients. *J Cardiothorac Vasc Anesth.* 2000;14(1):12-17.

8. Rich GF, Murphy GD, Roos CM, Johns RA. Inhaled nitric oxide: selective pulmonary vasodilation in cardiac surgical patients. *Anesthesiology.* 1993;78:1028-1035.

9. Galie N, Corris P, Frost A. et al. Updated treatment algorithm of pulmonary arterial hypertension. *J Am Coll Cardiol.* 2013;62:D60-72.

10. Corrado D, Basso C, Nava A, Thiene G. Arrhythmogenic right cardiomyopathy: current diagnostic and management strategies. *Cardiol Rev.* 2001;9(5):259-265.

11. Kasper J, Bolliger D, Skarvan K, et al. Additional cross-sectional transesophageal echocardiography views improve perioperative right heart assessment. *Anesth.* 2012;117(4):726-734.

12. Tan C, Harley I. Perioperative transesophageal echocardiography assessment of the right heart and associated structures: a comprehensive update and technical report. *J Cardiothorac Vasc Anesth.* 2014;28(4):628-635.

13. Bartels K, Karhausen J, Sullivan B, Mackensen G. Update on perioperative right heart assessment using transesophageal echocardiography. *Sem Cardiothorac Vasc Anesth.* 2014;18(4):341-351.

14. Lang RM, Badano LP, Mor-Avi V, et al. Recommendations for cardiac chamber quantification by echocardiography in adults: an update from the American Society of Echocardiography and the European Association of Cardiovascular Imaging. *J Am Soc Echocardiogr.* 2015;28:1-39.

15. Chong A, Maclaren G, Chen R. Perioperative applications of deformation (myocardial strain) imaging with speckle tracking echocardiography. *J Cardiothorac Vasc Anesth.* 2014;28(1):128-140.

16. Maus T. Right heart three dimensional echocardiography: time for the limelight. *J Cardiothorac Vasc Anesth.* 2013;27(4):637-638.

17. Tang GHL, David TE, Singh SK, Maganti MD, Armstrong S, Borger MA. Tricuspid valve repair with an annuloplasty ring results in improved long-term outcomes. *Circulation.* 2006;114(suppl I):I577-I581.

18. Nishimura R, Carabello B, Faxon D, et al. ACC/AHA 2008 guideline update on valvular heart disease: focused update on infective endocarditis: a report of the American College of Cardiology/American Heart Association Task Force on Practice Guidelines. *J Am Coll Cardiol.* 2008;52:676-685.

REVIEWS

Zoghbi W, Bonow R, Enriquez- Sarano M, et al. Recommendations for noninvasive evaluation of native valve regurgitation: a report from the American Society of Echocardiography developed in collaboration with the Society for Cardiovascular Magnetic Resonance. *JASE.* 2017;30(4):303-371.

Nishimura R, Otto C, Bonow R, et al. 2014 AHA/ACC guideline for the management of patients with valvular heart disease. *JACC.* 2014;63(22):E57-E185.

Baumgartner H, Hung J, Bermejo J, et al. Echocardiographic assessment of valve stenosis; EAE/ASE recommendations for clinical practice. *JASE.* 2009;22(1):1-23.

Rao V, Ghadimi K, Keeyapaj W, et al. Inhaled nitric oxide (iNO) and inhaled epoprostenol (iPGI$_2$) use in cardiothoracic surgical patients: is there sufficient evidence for evidence-based recommendations? *J Cardiothorac Vasc Anesth.* 2018;32(3):1452-1457.

Anesthesia for Repair of Diseases of Thoracic Aorta

9

TOPICS

With each heartbeat, blood is ejected into the aorta generating multiple mechanical forces including pressure, radial stress and longitudinal stress. These forces increase aortic wall tension potentially leading to the development of aortic dissections and aortic aneurysms that may require surgical or endovascular repair.

The aorta ascends in the anterior mediastinum, curves backward into the aortic arch from which emanate the great vessels of the head and the upper extremities, descends into the posterior mediastinum and beyond the diaphragm continues into the abdomen providing blood to the spinal cord, gut, kidneys, ultimately dividing to deliver blood to the lower extremities (Figure 9–1).

Diseases that interfere with the delivery of blood to the tissues (e.g., aortic dissections, atherosclerosis, and emboli) place patients at great risk for organ ischemia. Other disease conditions (e.g., aneurysms) weaken the wall of the aorta and often result in aortic rupture and sudden death. Many patients with aortic disease present emergently secondary to acute dissection, aneurysm rupture, or following traumatic aortic injury. Others, with long-standing aortic aneurysms, present for elective surgical or, increasingly common, for endovascular repair.

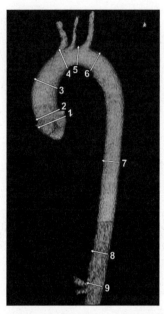

Figure 9–1. Normal anatomy of the thoracoabdominal aorta with standard anatomic landmarks for reporting aortic diameter as illustrated on a volume-rendered CT image of the thoracic aorta. CT indicates computed tomographic imaging. Anatomic locations: 1, aortic sinuses of Valsalva; 2, sinotubular junction; 3, mid ascending aorta (midpoint in length between numbers 2 and 4); 4, proximal aortic arch (aorta at the origin of the innominate artery); 5, mid aortic arch (between left common carotid and subclavian arteries); 6, proximal descending thoracic aorta (begins at the isthmus, approximately 2 cm distal to left subclavian artery); 7, mid descending aorta (midpoint in length between numbers 6 and 8); 8, aorta at diaphragm (2 cm above the celiac axis origin); 9, abdominal aorta at the celiac axis origin. [Reproduced with permission from Hiratzka LF, Bakris GL, Beckman JA, et al: ACCF/AHA/AATS/ACR/ASA/SCA/SCAI/SIR/STS/SVM Guidelines for the diagnosis and management of patients with thoracic aortic disease: Executive summary: A report of the American College of Cardiology Foundation/American Heart Association Task Force on Practice Guidelines, American Association for Thoracic Surgery, American College of Radiology, American Stroke Association, Society of Cardiovascular Anesthesiologists, Society for Cardiovascular Angiography and Interventions, Society of Interventional Radiology, Society of Thoracic Surgeons, and Society for Vascular Medicine, *Anesth Analg.* 2010 Aug;111(2):279-315.]

DISEASES OF THE ASCENDING THORACIC AORTA

Patients with ascending thoracic aortic aneurysms present either acutely or electively (Figure 9–2). Crushing chest pain often heralds acute presentations. Some of these acute patients never undergo surgery as they develop lethal complications such as coronary ischemia, pericardial effusion and tamponade, or intrathoracic bleeding. In most cases, patients will present emergently for repair following diagnosis in the emergency room. Acute, contained ascending aortic aneurysm ruptures require immediate surgical correction. Radiographic (MRI, CT) and ultrasound

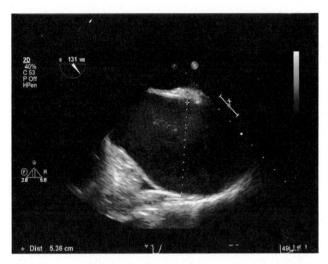

Figure 9–2. This long axis of the ascending aorta by transesophageal ecchocardiography demonstrates a 5.36-cm dilatation.

techniques are routinely employed to make the diagnosis of a thoracic aortic aneurysm. Rapid accumulation of blood in the pericardium results in a tamponade physiology necessitating emergency surgical treatment.

Nonemergent presentations occur when patients develop aneurismal dilatations over time and become symptomatic from anatomic compression of the trachea, the main bronchi, or the esophagus by the expanding aneurysm. At times, an ascending aneurysm widens the aortic root making the aortic valve leaflets no longer competent leading to severe aortic insufficiency (AI). These patients often present with the symptoms of aortic regurgitation. Echocardiography will readily demonstrate dilatation of the aortic root and aortic valvular incompetence. Often a widened mediastinum on routine radiological examination may signal the presence of an ascending thoracic aneurysm. Chronic aneurismal dilatations are regularly followed with repair suggested either when the patient becomes symptomatic or when the aneurysm becomes greater than 5 to 6 cm in diameter. Ascending aortic aneurysms are associated with genetic syndromes, inflammatory diseases, atherosclerosis, aortic stenosis, and infectious aortitis (Table 9–1).

Aortic dissections occur when a tear in the intimal layer of the aorta's wall permits blood under arterial pressure to create a false lumen in the wall of the aorta (Figures 9–3 and 9–4 and **Videos 9–1 and 9–2**). This false lumen can propagate along the entire length of the aorta. As the dissection expands, the false lumen compresses the true lumen and prevents blood from flowing down the aorta's many branches including the coronary, carotid, subclavian, spinal, mesenteric, and renal arteries. Consequently, an aortic dissection can readily result in severe end-organ ischemia producing myocardial infarction, stroke, paralysis, kidney injury, and visceral ischemia leading to ischemic bowel and possible sepsis. The aortic root becomes dilated distorting the aortic valve producing acute AI. Aortic dissections can also cause bleeding into the pericardium resulting in tamponade.

Table 9–1. Genetic Syndromes Associated with Thoracic Aortic Aneurysm and Dissection

Genetic syndrome	Common clinical features	Genetic defect	Diagnostic test	Comments on aortic disease
Marfan syndrome	Skeletal features (see text) Ectopia lentis Dural ectasia	*FBN1* mutations*	Ghent diagnostic criteria DNA for sequencing	Surgical repair when the aorta reaches 5.0 cm unless there is a family history of AoD at < 5.0 cm, a rapidly expanding aneurysm or presence or significant aortic valve regurgitation
Loeys-Dietz syndrome	Bifid uvula or cleft palate Arterial tortuosity Hypertelorism Skeletal features similar to MFS Craniosynostosis Aneurysms and dissections of other arteries	*TGFBR2* or *TGFBR1* mutations	DNA for sequencing	Surgical repair recommended at an aortic diameter of ≥ 4.2 cm by TEE (Internal diameter) or 4.4 to ≥ 4.6 cm by CT and/or MR (external diameter)
Ehlers-Danlos syndrome, Vascular form	Thin, translucent skin Gastrointestinal rupture Rupture of the gravid uterus Rupture of medium-sized to large arteries	*COL3A1* mutations	DNA for sequencing Dermal fibroblasts for analysis of type III collagen	Surgical repair is complicated by friable tissues Noninvasive imaging recommended
Turner syndrome	Short stature Primary amenorrhea Bicuspid aortic valve Aortic coarctation Webbed neck, low-set ears, low hairline, broad chest	45,X karyotype	Blood (cells) for karyotype analysis	AoD risk is increased in patients with bicuspid aortic valve, aortic coarctation, hypertension, or pregnancy

AoD indicates aortic dissection; *COL3A1*, type III collegen; CT, computed tomographic imaging; *FBN1*, fibrillin 1; MFS, Marfan syndrome; MR, magnetic resonance imaging; TEE, transesophageal echocardiogram; *TGFBR1*, transforming growth factor-beta receptor type I; and *TGFBR2*, transforming growth factor-beta receptor type II. *The defective gene at a second locus for MFS is *TGFBR2* but the clinical phenotype as MFS is debated. Reproduced with permission from Hiratzka LF, Bakris GL, Beckman JA, et al: ACCF/AHA/AATS/ACR/ASA/SCA/SCAI/ SIR/STS/SVM Guidelines for the diagnosis and management of patients with thoracic aortic disease: Executive summary: A report of the American College of Cardiology Foundation/American Heart Association Task Force on Practice Guidelines, American Association for Thoracic Surgery, American College of Radiology, American Stroke Association, Society of Cardiovascular Anesthesiologists, Society for Cardiovascular Angiography and Interventions, Society of Interventional Radiology, Society of Thoracic Surgeons, and Society for Vascular Medicine, *Anesth Analg.* 2010 Aug;111(2):279-315.

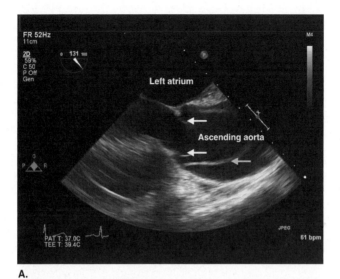

A.

B.

Figure 9–3. (A) Midesophageal aortic valve long-axis view showing dissection of the intimal flap (gray arrow) in the ascending aorta. The aortic valve cusps (white arrows) are seen in open (systolic) position, and the aortic root and ascending aorta seem dilated. (B) Midesophageal long-axis view with color flow Doppler showing aortic regurgitation. The intimal flap is identified in the ascending aorta by the gray arrow. (C) Nonstandard short-axis view of the aortic root. The intimal dissection flap is identified by the gray arrow. The left coronary artery seems to originate from the true lumen. (D) Intimal dissection flap (gray arrow) extended in the descending aorta seen in short axis.

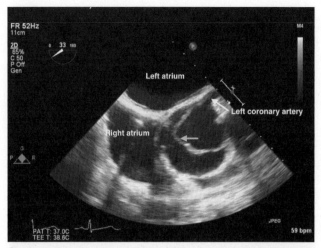

C.

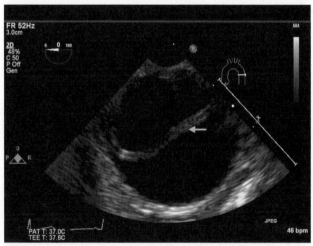

D.

Figure 9–3. (Continued)

There are two available classifications of aortic dissections. The DeBakey classification consists of three different types:

Type I: The intimal tear occurs in the ascending aorta, but the dissection extends all the way to the descending aorta.

Type II: The intimal tear occurs in the ascending aorta, and the dissection is limited to the ascending aorta.

Type III: The intimal tear occurs distal to the takeoff of the left subclavian artery with the dissection extending into the descending aorta for variable distances above (iiia) and below the diaphragm (iiib).[1]

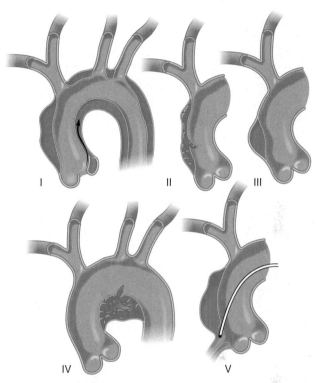

Figure 9–4. Classes of intimal tears. **I.** Classic dissection with intimal tear and double lumen separated by septum. Communication between lumens is typically in the descending aorta at sheared-off intercostal arteries or distal reentry site. **II.** Intramural hematoma (IMH). No intimal tear or septum is imaged but is usually found at surgery or autopsy. DeBakey types II and IIIa are a common extent of this lesion. **III.** Intimal tear without medial hematoma (limited dissection) and eccentric aortic wall bulge. Rare and difficult to detect by transesophageal echocardiography (TEE) or computed tomographic (CT) imaging. Patients with Marfan syndrome are prone to this type. It may result in aortic rupture or extravasation. **IV.** Penetrating atherosclerotic ulcer (PAU) usually to the adventitia with localized hematoma or saccular aneurysm. It may propagate to class I dissection, particularly when involving the ascending aorta or aortic arch. **V.** Iatrogenic (catheter angiography or intervention)/traumatic (deceleration) dissection. (Reproduced with permission from Cleveland Clinic Center for Medical Art & Photography © 2013-2018. All Rights Reserved.)

The Stanford Daily identifies two types of dissections:

Type A: This type of dissection involves the ascending aorta regardless of the location of the intimal tear or of the extension of the dissection into the descending aorta.

Type B: This type of dissection involves only the descending aorta distal to the takeoff of the left subclavian artery (Figure 9–5).[2]

Increasingly, type B dissections are managed with thoracic endovascular aortic repair (TEVAR).[3] Long-term survival of patients managed medically after type B

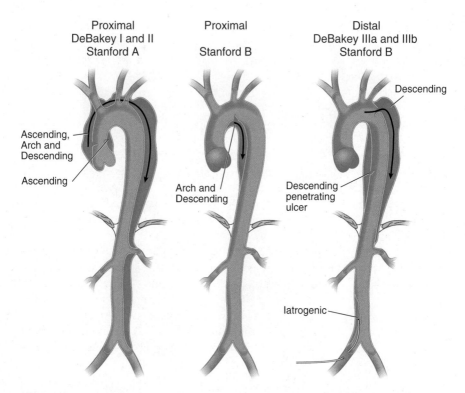

Figure 9-5. Aortic dissection classification: DeBakey and Stanford classifications. (Reproduced with permission from Cleveland Clinic Center for Medical Art & Photography © 2013-2018. All Rights Reserved.)

dissection is disappointing. Patients managed with endovascular stents have an enhanced outcome.[4] Endovascular repairs will be discussed subsequently. Repair of type A dissections requires surgical intervention.

Surgeons approach the ascending aorta through a median sternotomy much as they would do for a routine cardiac case. If the aortic arch and the great vessels to the head are not involved, the surgeon places an aortic cross clamp distal to the location of the aortic pathology and resects the diseased aorta using conventional cardiopulmonary bypass (CPB). Depending on the degree of aortic annulus dilatation and the severity of any AI, the aortic valve is either replaced or repaired. If the valve is competent, it may not require surgical intervention. If the aortic root (anatomical portion between the aortic annulus and the sinotubular junction) requires replacement, the right and left coronary arteries must be separated from the aorta and then sewn back into the new aortic graft.

Should the aortic pathology involve the entire ascending aorta up to the innominate artery, the intraoperative management of the patient is more complicated. Recall from Chapter 4 that during a routine cardiac surgery case with CPB, the surgeon generally places the aortic perfusion cannula in the ascending thoracic aorta.

An aortic cross clamp is placed below the perfusion cannula to isolate the heart from the systemic circulation. The coronary arteries at this point are no longer perfused and cardioplegia solution is administered via an anterograde cardioplegia cannula.

Therefore, if the aortic pathology involves the entire ascending aorta, the right axillary artery is typically cannulated. The cross clamp is placed beyond the diseased aorta but below the innominate artery so to perfuse the right carotid artery via the innominate artery. Cardioplegia is delivered in the aortic root or if significant AI is present, directly into the left and right coronary ostia after aortotomy. Moreover, retrograde cardioplegia can be administered in addition to or in lieu of antegrade cardioplegia (Chapter 17). Once a new aortic graft is sewn into place, the native coronary arteries are attached to the new aortic graft. When surgery is completed, the heart is de-aired, the cross clamp released, blood flows down the reattached right and left coronary arteries, and the patient hopefully is successfully weaned from CPB.

Unfortunately, this routine management scheme is not applicable when the disease involves the aortic arch including the innominate, the left subclavian, and the left carotid arteries. In these instances, aortic blood flow to these vessels must be interrupted while the aortic arch is reconstructed. For surgery to proceed, deep hypothermic circulatory arrest (DHCA) is used and selective retrograde (via the superior vena cava) or antegrade (via the right axillary artery) perfusion of the head vessels may be employed to possibly improve neurological outcomes during prolonged repairs (see following discussion).

DISEASES OF THE DESCENDING THORACIC AORTA

Descending thoracic aortic aneurysms occur distal to the takeoff of the left subclavian artery from the aortic arch. Aneurysms of the descending thoracic aorta are usually secondary to atherosclerosis, and these patients frequently have multiple other vascular diseases (e.g., carotid occlusion, coronary artery disease). Very seldom, presentation can be secondary to acute rupture with contained bleeding or after having been detected on routine examination.

The surgical approach to the descending thoracic aorta is via a left thoracotomy. Once the aorta is dissected free from surrounding tissues, cross clamps are placed above and below the lesion. The aneurysm is resected, and a tube graft is sewn into position. More recently, endovascular stents have been employed by surgeons and radiologists to exclude the aneurysmal walls from the circulation.[5] Using radiological guidance, a stent is positioned in the aorta such that blood flows through the aortic stent; therefore, arterial pressure does not contact the diseased aortic wall. Stents require areas of relatively normal aorta at their proximal and distal ends for proper anchoring. Additionally, when the stent is deployed, any artery, which takes off from the aorta in the stented area, will no longer receive aortic blood flow because the stent occludes it. Consequently, perfusion of the spinal cord, viscera, and kidneys may be impaired. Should the stent need to cover the left subclavian artery, a common carotid to left subclavian artery bypass is often performed to preserve vertebral artery blood flow (Figure 9–6).

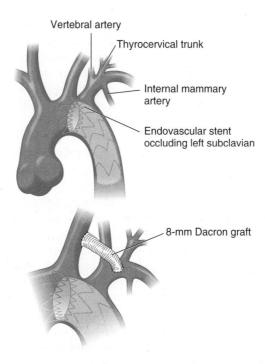

Vertebral artery

Thyrocervical trunk

Internal mammary artery

Endovascular stent occluding left subclavian

8-mm Dacron graft

Figure 9–6. Carotid-to-subclavian bypass graft with coil embolization of the origin of the subclavian artery is a technique used to revascularize the subclavian artery in patients with extent A or C thoracic aortic aneurysms undergoing thoracic endovascular aortic repair (TEVAR) that requires coverage of the subclavian artery. [Reproduced with permission from Ullery BW, Wang GJ, Low D, et al: Neurological complications of thoracic endovascular aortic repair, *Semin Cardiothorac Vasc Anesth.* 2011 Dec;15(4):123-140.]

During surgical repairs of the descending thoracic aorta, placement of aortic cross clamps often leads to significant hemodynamic changes with the development of hypertension above the proximal clamp and profound hypotension below the distal cross clamp. Insufficient arterial blood flow to the kidneys, viscera, and spinal cord can occur resulting in end-organ ischemia.

When performing descending thoracic artery surgery and using a simple cross-clamp technique, the surgeons attempt to complete their procedure as rapidly as possible to minimize the time of distal aortic hypoperfusion. Various mechanisms of distal aortic perfusion and spinal cord protection (see later section) have been advocated to mitigate injuries associated with distal aortic hypoperfusion and the occlusion of branching arteries.

ANESTHETIC MANAGEMENT OF THE PATIENT WITH DISEASE OF THE THORACIC AORTA

Anesthetic considerations in the management of the patient with surgical thoracic aortic disease take into account the location of the aortic pathology and the elective or emergent nature of the surgery.

Patients presenting with an isolated ascending aneurysm are usually scheduled for elective resection and are often managed in a manner similar to routine cardiac surgical patients as described in Chapter 4. Arterial line placement in the right radial artery can be useful to detect unwanted innominate artery occlusion by the aortic cross clamp. Hypertension should be carefully avoided during the peri-induction period as the aortic walls of the aneurysm are fragile. Surgery usually involves excision of the diseased ascending aorta and interposition of a synthetic graft between the aortic valve and the proximal aortic arch. Coronary ostia may need to be excised and reimplanted into the graft. When significant dilatation of the aortic annulus and AI is present, the aortic valve is also replaced together with the ascending aorta using a composite graft. Patients are weaned from CPB in the usual fashion if standard cannulation and bypass techniques are used.

Patients with acute ascending aortic dissections or contained aortic ruptures will present with a variety of pathological conditions. Documentation of baseline neurological function is necessary because some patients may have neurological injury secondary to inadequate perfusion of the carotid arteries preoperatively. Other patients with acute dissections or ruptures may develop myocardial ischemia (due to involvement of the coronary ostia), tamponade, and/or acute aortic regurgitation with heart failure. Such patients may be in heart failure upon their arrival in the operating room. These patients often will tolerate limited amounts of anesthetics (intravenous or otherwise), and their management prior to the initiation of CPB is largely resuscitative in nature. Unstable cardiac patients are at risk for intraoperative awareness and bispectral index monitoring is suggested, though it may have limited benefit. Older drugs, such as scopolamine may be useful in these situations to attenuate recall.

Should aortic pathology extend into the aortic arch, DHCA is employed to halt the circulation while the aortic arch is repaired. This is necessitated by the inability to cannulate and cross clamp in the ascending aorta. A cannula is placed in the right axillary artery to deliver arterial blood from the bypass machine into the systemic circulation.

During DHCA the patient's blood is cooled by the bypass machine and core temperature is reduced to less than 18°C. Although data regarding benefit is scant, the patient's head may be packed in ice bags to prevent rewarming of the scalp from ambient temperature. Adequate cooling of the brain can be confirmed by nasopharyngeal temperature monitoring or more accurately by electroencephalography (EEG) to ensure that isoelectric EEG has been reached prior to instituting DHCA. The bypass machine is turned off such that there is no flow from the machine back to the patient. Deep hypothermia reduces the risk of ischemic brain injury, and the surgeon attempts to replace the aorta with an aortic graft as quickly as possible. Following resection of the aneurysm, the distal anastomosis of the graft is performed. The vessels of the aortic arch are reattached to the graft as quickly as possible. The graft can be clamped now proximal to the innominate artery, and the flow to the descending aorta, aortic arch, and head reestablished by reinstituting CPB. Antegrade (through the right axillary cannula) or retrograde (through a cannula placed in the superior vena cava) cerebral perfusion is performed during the period of systemic circulatory arrest. If antegrade cerebral perfusion is performed, the perfusion pressure should be measured through a catheter placed in the right radial artery.

Also, in this case some surgeons choose to perform the systemic circulatory arrest at a more moderate degree of hypothermia (approximately 24°C). If retrograde cerebral perfusion is performed, the perfusion pressure should be monitored from the most proximal lumen of the central venous line, to avoid overflowing in the cerebral circulation.

Next, the proximal graft anatomosis is completed, flow is restored to the coronary arteries, and, after a long rewarming period, weaning from CPB is accomplished hopefully without any neurologic or visceral ischemic injury.

Patients with aortic dissections distal to the left subclavian artery have distal thoracic or thoracoabdominal disease and are sometimes managed medically but increasingly are treated with endovascular techniques. In surgical cases, anesthetic induction as with all cardiac surgery patients must be individualized based upon each patient's own hemodynamic behavior. A mixture of amnestics, analgesics, hypnotics, and muscle relaxants can generally be employed. However, at times during scheduled, nonemergent procedures, patients undergoing descending thoracic aneurysm surgery will be monitored with sensory and/or motor evoked potentials. Because spinal cord perfusion can be compromised during the cross-clamp period secondary to occlusion of the radicular arteries, surgeons attempt to detect spinal cord ischemia through the use of neurophysiological monitoring. Because muscle relaxants and inhalational agents interfere with monitoring evoked potentials, total intravenous anesthesia is generally required in these cases.

Descending thoracic aneurysm resections also require one-lung ventilation to improve surgical exposure via a thoracotomy incision. Either double-lumen endotracheal tubes or bronchial blockers can be employed to achieve isolation of the left lung. Bronchial blocker techniques may have the advantage of leaving a single lumen tube in place at the end of surgery. Because these are rather protracted cases on rather sick individuals, extubation at the immediate conclusion of surgery is not recommended. Double-lumen endotracheal tubes generally need to be changed to single-lumen tubes prior to the patient's transfer to the ICU. Unfortunately, many patients following descending thoracic aneurysm surgery frequently become edematous from perioperative fluid administration and head down position. Consequently, reintubation can be challenging making use of the bronchial blocker as a potentially more facile way of managing one-lung ventilation perioperatively. Additionally, guidelines for the diagnosis and management of patients with thoracic aortic disease note that routinely changing double-lumen endotracheal tubes at the end of surgical procedures associated with upper airway edema or hemorrhage is not recommended (class III risk ≥benefit).

After discussing the anesthetic and surgical plan with the surgical team, a lumbar cerebrospinal fluid drain is often placed when performing distal thoracic aneurysm resections.[6] During cross clamp of the distal aorta, blood flow to the spinal cord is reduced secondary to decreased perfusion of the radicular arteries. Thus, the spinal cord is at risk for ischemia. Removing cerebrospinal fluid is thought to improve spinal cord perfusion pressure by lowering CSF pressure. Before the lumbar drain is placed, the patient's coagulation status and medications should be confirmed and strict sterile technique must be employed.

DISTAL AORTIC PERFUSION AND SPINAL CORD PROTECTION DURING DESCENDING THORACIC ANEURYSM RESECTION AND ENDOVASCULAR STENTING

Much of what is unique in the management of the thoracic aortic aneurysm patient is centered upon reducing or preventing ischemic injury to the tissues secondary to inadequate perfusion during repair of the aorta.

Descending thoracic aortic aneurysms were originally performed with a "clamp and go" (Figure 9–7) technique.[7] In this approach, following cross clamping of the aorta the surgeon would simply attempt to sew in the aortic graft as quickly as possible. By minimizing ischemic time, injuries to the kidneys, viscera, and spinal cord hopefully might be prevented. Cross clamping the aorta produces systemic hypertension above the proximal clamp and profound hypotension below the distal clamp. Surgeons use various techniques to minimize the impact of cross clamping on hypoperfused organs including: CSF drainage, systemic patient cooling, distal aortic perfusion, and intercostal artery implantation. Monitoring of evoked potentials is also employed to alert surgeons of spinal cord ischemia. Spinal near-infrared spectroscopy (NIRS) probes have been placed over the T1-T3 vertebrate (baseline) and over the T8-T10 (at risk) vertebrae to provide an estimate of spinal cord perfusion and have been suggested to be useful as a herald of spinal cord ischemia.[8] CSF is drained to improve spinal cord perfusion pressure by keeping the CSF pressure to less than 10 mm Hg.[9] However, if CSF is drained too quickly, intracranial hypotension can develop which can lead to cerebral vein tearing and intracranial

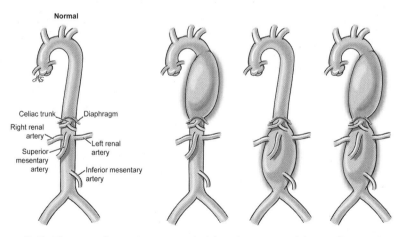

Normal

Celiac trunk
Right renal artery
Superior mesentary artery
Diaphragm
Left renal artery
Inferior mesentary artery

Figure 9–7. The normal aorta is compared with various types of descending aortic aneurysms. Surgical repair can impede flow to visceral, intercostal, and renal arteries resulting in gut ischemia, paralysis, and renal failure. In addition to the radicular arteries not depicted, the arterial supply to the viscera and kidneys is supplied from the descending aorta. Reimplantation of these vessels into the aortic graft conduit is necessary to prevent organ hypoperfusion.

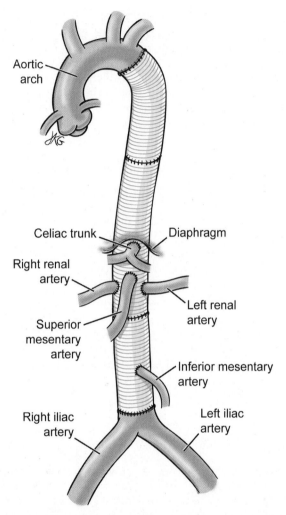

Aortic arch

Celiac trunk

Diaphragm

Right renal artery

Left renal artery

Superior mesentary artery

Inferior mesentary artery

Right iliac artery

Left iliac artery

Figure 9–7. *(Continued)*

hemorrhage. Individual protocols may limit the total amount of CSF drained (e.g., < 240 mL/d) to minimize this risk.[10] CSF catheter drainage may also place patients at risk for perioperative meningitis as the catheter remains in place for some time postoperatively.

Distal aortic perfusion may be provided during the time of distal aortic occlusion through the use of left atrial-to-femoral artery bypass. This approach uses a cannula placed in the left atrium to supply oxygenated blood, which is pumped into the distal aorta below the surgical field through a femoral artery cannula (Figure 9–8). A centrifugal type pump is used for this task. In this manner the viscera receive arterial flow while CSF is also drained to improve spinal cord perfusion pressure. Should monitoring of the evoked potentials indicate spinal cord

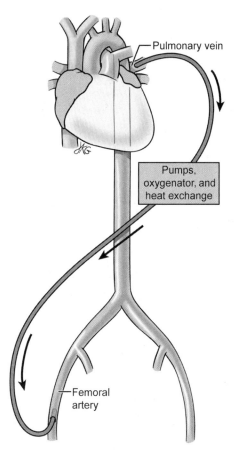

Figure 9–8. Distal aortic perfusion can be employed to provide oxygenated blood to the lower body during descending thoracic aneurysm repairs. Oxygenated blood can be drained from the left atrium and delivered to the femoral artery. Alternatively, partial bypass can take venous blood, oxygenate it, and likewise perfuse the arterial system distal to any aortic cross clamps.

ischemia, systemic blood pressure can be increased, distal perfusion increased, and additional CSF drained.

Close communication between surgical, anesthesia, and perfusion teams is advised before taking the patient to the operating room regarding the management of distal perfusion and spinal cord protection during the cross-clamp period.

Increasingly, descending thoracic arterial aneurysms are treated by endovascular techniques. These techniques ideally deploy the stent in such a manner as to avoid occlusion of vessels supplying the viscera or spinal cord. However, in patients with extensive aortic disease, coverage of significant branching arteries such as the intercostals may be unavoidable (Figure 9–9).[11]

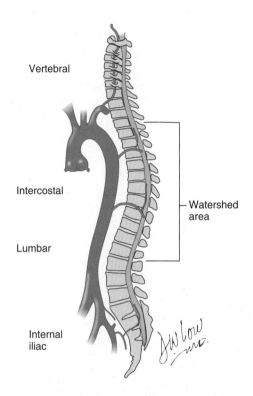

Figure 9–9. Branch vessels from the thoracoabdominal aorta form the collateral vascular network to supply the spinal cord. The vertebral arteries that branch off the subclavian arteries together with the cervical vascular network supply the upper portion of the collateral network in the region of the cervical and upper thoracic spinal cord. The thoracic intercostal and lumbar segmental arteries that may include a prominent midthoracic radicular artery together with the arteria magna radicularis (artery of Adamkewicz) supply the midportion of the collateral network in the region of the thoracic and lumbar spinal cord. The hypogastric vascular network formed from branches off the lumbar segmental arteries, middle sacral artery, lateral sacral arteries, and iliolumbar arteries supply the lower end of the collateral network in the region of the conus medullaris. Endovascular coverage or sacrifice of intercostal arteries, segmental arteries, and arteries supplying the hypogastric vascular network may cause a watershed infarction of the spinal cord in the region of T4 to the conus medullaris. [Reproduced with permission from Ullery BW, Wang GJ, Low D, et al: Neurological complications of thoracic endovascular aortic repair, *Semin Cardiothorac Vasc Anesth.* 2011 Dec;15(4):123-140.]

A hybrid procedure by which the aneurysm is stented after visceral vessels likely to be occluded by the stent are bypassed is being employed in some centers. Moreover, fenestrated stents are being developed to ensure flow to critical aortic branch vessels.

Risk factors for neurological complications following thoracic endovascular aortic repair (TEVAR) are presented in Table 9–2. Table 9–3 presents strategies to prevent and treat spinal cord ischemia associated with TEVAR. Efforts are directed to both detect early signs of ischemia through neurophysiological monitoring as

Table 9–2. Risk Factors Associated with Development of Spinal Cord Ischemia after TEVAR

Demographics	Age
	Male gender
	Lower body mass index
	Preoperative renal failure
	Prior abdominal aortic aneurysm repair
Anatomical	Prior distal aortic vascular graft
	Thoracic aortic pathology
	Extent of thoracic or thoracoabdominal aneurysm
	Number of patent lumbar arteries
Perioperative	
Preoperative	Emergency operation
Intraoperative	General anesthesia
	Procedure duration
	Endovascular stent coverage
	—Total length of aortic coverage
	—Extent of uncovered distal aorta
	—Coverage of left subclavian artery
	Number of thoracic stents used
	Concomitant open abdominal aortic surgery
	Hypotension
	Hypogastric artery occlusion
	Arterial access site injury
	Bleeding
Postoperative	Hypotension
	Postoperative renal failure

Abbreviations: TEVAR, thoracic endovascular aortic repair.
Reproduced with permission from Ullery BW, Wang GJ, Low D, et al: Neurological complications of thoracic endovascular aortic repair, *Semin Cardiothorac Vasc Anesth*. 2011 Dec;15(4):123-140.

well as to prevent ischemia by increasing spinal cord perfusion pressure and tissue oxygen delivery. Additionally, various neuroprotective pharmacological interventions have been suggested such as naloxone to reduce excitatory neurotransmitter neurotoxicity during periods of ischemia.

A systemic approach to managing spinal cord ischemia is presented in Figure 9–10.

DEEP HYPOTHERMIC CIRCULATORY ARREST

DHCA permits the surgeon to operate in a bloodless field without cross clamping the aorta. During DHCA the patient's temperature is reduced to 15°C to 18°C. At this point bypass flow is discontinued and the surgeon attempts to expeditiously place an aortic graft so that flow can be restored to the brain and other organs. Hypothermia protects the brain and viscera from ischemic injury; however, its effectiveness in each individual patient is unclear. There are multiple modalities, which have been advocated to either provide for the delivery of oxygenated blood to the brain during DHCA or to reassure practitioners that the brain is adequately oxygenated throughout the period of circulatory arrest.[12-14]

Table 9-3. Strategies for the Prevention and Treatment of Spinal Cord Ischemia after TEVAR

Increase spinal cord perfusion pressure
Lumbar CSF drainage (CSF pressure ≤ 10 mm Hg)
Arterial blood pressure augmentation (MAP ≥ 85 mm Hg)
—Intravascular volume expansion
—Vasopressor medications
Reduce central venous pressure
Resume antihypertensive therapy cautiously
Increase oxygen delivery
Increase cardiac output
Transfusion to increase hemoglobin concentration
Supplemental oxygen
Deliberate hypothermia
Mild to moderate systemic hypothermia (32°C to 35°C)
Selective spinal cord hypothermia (epidural cooling, 25°C)
Early detection of spinal cord ischemia
Somatosensory-evoked potentials
Transcranial motor-evoked potentials
Serial neurological examinations
Neuropharmacological protection
Glucocorticoids
Naloxone
Barbiturate or CNS depressants
Magnesium sulfate
Mannitol
Lidocaine
Intrathecal papaverine
Postoperative neurological assessment for early detection of delayed-onset SCI
Serial neurological examinations

Abbreviations: CNS, central nervous system; CSF, cerebrospinal fluid; MAP, mean arterial pressure; SCI, spinal cord ischemia; TEVAR, thoracic endovascular aortic repair.
Reproduced with permission from Ullery BW, Wang GJ, Low D, et al: Neurological complications of thoracic endovascular aortic repair, *Semin Cardiothorac Vasc Anesth.* 2011 Dec;15(4):123-140.

EEG monitoring, jugular venous bulb oxygen saturation ($SjvO_2$), and cerebral oximetry have been suggested as techniques to determine adequacy of cerebral protection during DHCA. Isoelectric EEG indicates that hypothermia has suppressed electrical activity in the brain and hence has significantly reduced oxygen demand. Cerebral oximetry has been used to determine adequacy of cerebral oxygenation during DHCA with saturations below 40% associated with worse neurological outcome. Jugular bulb saturation has similarly been suggested as a guide of the adequacy of cerebral protection (high $SjvO_2$ being associated with cerebral protection and good metabolic suppression with a reduced O_2 demand).

To increase the "safe time" available for surgeons to complete repairs using DHCA, various adjunctive techniques have been employed to deliver oxygenated blood to the brain. Cerebral perfusion supplies oxygenated blood to the brain during DHCA and can be done both antegrade and retrograde. Antegrade cerebral perfusion delivers oxygenated blood during DHCA through a graft attached to the innominate artery or through a graft attached to the right axillary artery.

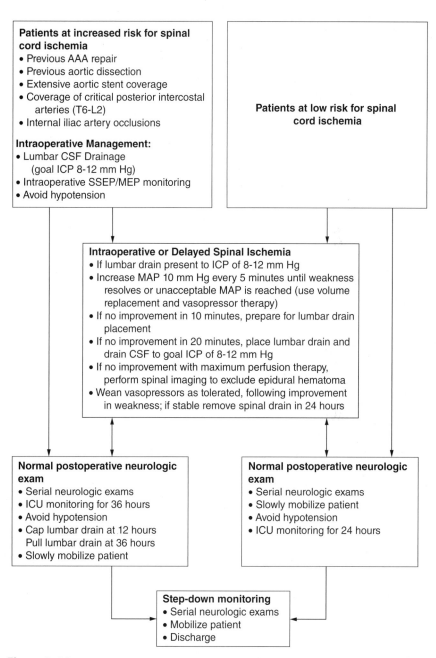

Figure 9–10. Perioperative management strategies to prevent and treat spinal cord ischemia in patients undergoing TEVAR. Abbreviations: AAA, abdominal aortic aneurysm; CSF, cerebrospinal fluid; ICP, intracranial pressure measured through the lumbar cerebrospinal fluid drain; MAP, mean arterial pressure; MEP, motor-evoked potential; SSEP, somatosensory-evoked potential; TEVAR, thoracic endovascular aortic repair. [Reproduced with permission from McGarvey ML, Mullen MT, Woo EY, et al: The treatment of spinal cord ischemia following thoracic endovascular aortic repair, *Neurocrit Care.* 2007;6(1):35-39.]

Unfortunately, cerebral perfusion may be associated with an increased risk of cerebral embolic injury. Nonetheless, a recent meta-analysis demonstrated improved patient survival when selective antegrade cerebral perfusion was used in combination with DHCA.[15] However, this same study did not demonstrate any difference in neurological outcome between DHCA alone and DHCA with selective antegrade cerebral perfusion. Use of antegrade cerebral perfusion with mild to moderate hypothermia has also been suggested as a way to avoid the negative effects of deep hypothermia.[16] However, prolonged arrest under moderately hypothermic conditions may have deleterious effects on the viscera.[17]

Retrograde cerebral perfusion involves delivery of oxygenated blood through the superior vena cava cannula through the venous system to the brain. Retrograde cerebral perfusion may improve cerebral hypothermia and the clearing of emboli from the cerebral vessels but may not deliver significant oxygen to the brain when utilized and may increase the risk of cerebral edema. Still, retrograde cerebral perfusion may be a useful adjunct as studies have demonstrated beneficial mortality and stroke outcomes when employed.[18] Nonetheless, all patients irrespective of whatever protective mechanisms are in place remain at risk for perioperative stroke. Augoustides et al. noted an 8.3% incidence of stroke in patients requiring DHCA.[19] As such, the search to improve neurological outcomes in patients requiring circulatory arrest is likely to continue.

ECHOCARDIOGRAPHY IN THE MANAGEMENT OF THORACIC AORTIC DISEASES

When performing a TEE examination in a patient with aortic pathology, careful consideration should be granted to a few otherwise mundane aspects. The TEE probe should be placed after the patient has been adequately anesthetized to avoid sudden increases in blood pressure, which might aggravate the extent of the dissection or lead to an aneurismal rupture. Given the possibility that a large aortic aneurysm could compress the esophagus, the advancement of the probe in the esophagus should be stopped at the slightest resistance encountered due to the increased risk of aortic rupture.

TEE is routinely employed in the management of patients presenting for emergent and elective thoracic aortic surgery. The aorta is examined for the presence of plaque, which could embolize at the time of aortic cannulation or cross clamping. Epiaortic ultrasonography (EAU) may be employed to complete the evaluation of the ascending aorta as the interposed airway prevents complete TEE examination of the distal ascending aorta and proximal aortic arch.

Patients for elective resection of ascending aneurysms will likely have undergone numerous preoperative echocardiographic examinations. However, a comprehensive TEE evaluation should be performed. As dilatation of the aortic root can lead to profound aortic regurgitation necessitating placement of a composite aortic valve–aortic root graft, the aortic valve is assessed to determine its competency. Following reimplantation of the coronary arteries, TEE can demonstrate coronary blood flow indicating that the flow has been reestablished and not compromised. This information can be particularly useful if new wall motion abnormalities are detected or ventricular function appears reduced compared with prebypass baseline function. In such an instance, presence of flow down the left coronary artery will exclude surgical occlusion of the vessel. The absence of detectable flow, however, may not always indicate vessel occlusion because the coronary arteries are not always clearly visualized by TEE. Coronary artery bypass may be necessary if blood flow via reimplanted native coronary vessels is inadequate following aortic root replacement.

TEE is highly sensitive and specific in diagnosing aortic dissections. Any cardiac surgery patient can develop an aortic dissection secondary to aortic cannulation and aortic manipulation. The appearance of an intimal flap in the ascending and/or descending aorta in multiple views suggests a dissection. Color flow Doppler can be used to detect the entry point as blood passes from the true lumen to the false lumen of the dissected aorta. The aortic valve may be compromised by a dissection resulting in AI, and blood may accumulate in the pericardium.

The true lumen can be discerned from the false lumen by collections of echogenic clot and debris in the false lumen and by the presence of systolic expansion of the true lumen.

Many echo artifacts can be visualized within the aorta and, as such, complicate the intraoperative diagnosis of a new dissection. Examination in multiple examining planes throughout the aorta is necessary. Swan-Ganz catheters in particular can generate echo artifacts that appear as aortic dissection flaps.

CASE SCENARIO

A 77-year-old man presents to the emergency room with severe back pain following syncope. A dissecting aortic aneurysm is reported to extend from just beyond the aortic valve through to the abdominal aorta. What preoperative evaluation is required?

Preoperatively, a brief cardiac history (myocardial ischemia/infarction, stents, medication) is needed. The anesthesia team should note the patient's neurological function and confirm the presence and quality of *all* peripheral pulses. ECG should be examined especially pertaining to chronic or acute myocardial ischemic events. Computed tomography angiography, chest x-ray (CXR), and echocardiography should be reviewed to determine the extent of the dissection and to determine the competency of the aortic valve as well as overall hemodynamics.

What monitors are required and how should induction proceed?

Bilateral radial artery catheters are placed to make sure perfusion is equivalent on both sides of the aortic arch. Also, if right axillary cannulation is considered, the left radial arterial catheter will be used to monitor systemic pressure, while the right radial arterial catheter can be used to monitor cerebral perfusion pressure during anterograde cerebral perfusion and DHCA. Femoral vessels are best left for surgical/perfusion access if possible. Any anesthetic agents may be used assuming the surgeon is not planning on using evoked potentials monitoring. Blood pressure control is essential to prevent further expansion or rupture of the dissecting aortic aneurysm and to avoid organ ischemia.

The surgeon informs you that DHCA is required to repair the aortic arch. How will you proceed?

> After initiation of CPB, the perfusionist cools the patient to a core temperature of less than 15°C and the anesthesia team packs the patient's head in ice. At this point the patient's circulation is suspended. The surgeon repairs the aorta, and the patient is rewarmed.

On separating from bypass the patient has new left ventricular (LV) anterior and lateral wall motion abnormalities. What is the possible differential diagnosis?

> New wall motion abnormalities can occur secondary to myocardial ischemia due to kinking of the coronary arteries if they have been reattached to the aortic graft, air, or particulate emboli entrained though the coronary arteries or inadequate myocardial protection. TEE demonstrates flow in the left coronary artery. Mean arterial pressure is increased through the administration of vasopressin 2 U/h and eventually LV function returns to normal.

The patient is weaned from CPB and protamine is administered slowly; however, the patient continues to bleed profusely from the suture sites. How should you proceed?

> Assuming that the bleeding is not surgical, efforts are undertaken to correct for probable post DHCA and post CPB coagulopathy. Platelets, fresh frozen plasma, cryoprecipitate, and packed red blood cells are given as indicated. If hemorrhage is life threatening, activation of a "mass transfusion" protocol can be helpful to ensure the timely delivery of blood products. Occasionally, to correct the coagulopathy, recombinant factor VII or prothrombin complex concentrate may be administered (Chapter 16).

The coagulopathy is corrected, and the patient is transferred to the ICU. What postoperative issues must be considered?

> Patients following DHCA for aortic surgery may experience stroke, kidney injury, mesenteric ischemia, and myocardial dysfunction secondary to either hypoperfusion or embolic events. If postoperative bleeding due to coagulopathy persists, as will often be the case, blood products will be administered according to the results of laboratory tests such as PT, PTT, thromboelastography, or platelet count.
>
> Discussion of the high risks associated with aortic dissections and other diseases of the thoracic aortic (e.g., stroke and death) and their treatment should be made clear to patients and their families so that expectations are realistic.

REFERENCES

1. DeBakey ME, Henly WS, Cooley DA, et al. Surgical management of dissecting aneurysms of the aorta. *J Thorac Cardiovasc Surg.* 1965;49:130-149.
2. Miller DC, Stinson EB, Oyer PE, et al. Operative treatment of aortic dissections. Experience with 125 patients over a sixteen-year period. *J Thorac Cardiovasc Surg.* 1979;78:365-382.
3. Fattori R, Cao P, De Rango P, et al. Interdisciplinary expert consensus document on management of type B aortic dissection. *J Am Coll Cardiol.* 2013;61:1661-1678.

4. Nienaber C, Kische S, Rousseau H, et al. Endovascular repair of type B aortic dissection: long term results of the randomized investigation of stent grafts in aortic dissection trial. *Circ Cardiovasc Interv.* 2013;6:407-416.

5. Apple J, McQuade K, Hamman B, et al. Initial experience in the treatment of thoracic aortic aneurismal disease with a thoracic aortic endograft at Baylor University Medical Center. *Proc (Bayl Univ Med Center).* 2008;21(2):115-119.

6. Lima B, Nowicki E, Blackstone E, et al. Spinal cord protective strategies during descending and thoracoabdominal aneurysm repair in the modern era: the role of intrathecal papaverine. *J Thorac Cardiovac Surg.* 2012;143:945-952.

7. Safi HJ, Miller C, Huynh T, et al. Distal aortic perfusion and cerebrospinal fluid drainage for thoracoabdominal and descending thoracic aortic repair: ten years of organ protection. *Ann Surg.* 2003;238(3):372-381.

8. Badner N., Nicolaou G, Clarke C, Forbes T. Use of spinal near infrared spectroscopy for monitoring spinal cord perfusion during endovascular thoracic aortic repairs. *J Cardiothorac Vasc Anesth.* 2011;25(2):316-319.

9. Leyvi G, Ramachandran S, Wasnick J, et al. Risk and benefits of cerebrospinal fluid drainage during thoracoabdominal aortic aneurysm surgery. *J Cardiothorac Vasc Anesth.* 2005;19(3):392-399.

10. McGarvey M, Cheung A, Szeto W, et al. Management of complications of thoracic aortic surgery. *J Clin Neurophysiol.* 2007;24(4):336-343.

11. Rizvi A, Sullivan T. Incidence, prevention and management in spinal cord protection during TEVAR. *J Vasc Surg.* 2010;52:86S-90S.

12. Leyvi G, Bello R, Wasnick J, et al. Assessment of cerebral oxygen balance during deep hypothermic circulatory arrest by continuous jugular bulb venous saturation and near-infrared spectroscopy. *J Cardiothorac Vasc Anesth.* 2006;20(6):826-833.

13. Pochettino A, Cheung A. Retrograde cerebral perfusion is useful for deep hypothermic circulatory arrest. *J Cardiothorac Vasc Anesth.* 2003;17(6):764-767.

14. Reich D, Uysal S. Retrograde cerebral perfusion is not an optimal method of neuroprotection in thoracic aortic surgery. *J Cardiothorac Vasc Anesth.* 2003;17(6):768-769.

15. Tian D, Wan B, Bannon P, et al. A meta-analysis of deep hypothermic circulatory arrest alone versus with adjunctive selective antegrade cerebral perfusion. *Ann Cardiothorac Surg.* 2013;2(3):261-270.

16. Urbanski P, Lenos A, Bougioukakis P, et al. Mild to moderate hypothermia in aortic arch surgery using circulatory arrest: a change of paradigm? *Eur J Cardiothorac Surg.* 2012;41:185-191.

17. Khaladj N, Peterss S, Pichlmaier M, et al. The impact of deep and moderate body temperatures on end-organ function during hypothermic circulatory arrest. *Eur J Cardiothorac Surg.* 2011;40:1492-1499.

18. Ueda Y. A reappraisal of retrograde cerebral perfusion. *Ann Cardiothorac Surg.* 2013;2(3):316-325.

19. Augoustides J, Pochettino A, Ochroch A, et al. Clinical predictors for prolonged intensive care unit stay in adults undergoing thoracic aortic surgery requiring deep hypothermic circulatory arrest. *J Cardiothorac Vasc Anesth.* 2006;20(1):8-13.

REVIEWS

Hiratska LF, Bakris GL, Beckman JA, et al. 2010 ACCF/AHA/AATS/ACR/ASA/SCA/SCAI/SIR/STS/SVM guidelines for the diagnosis and management of patients with thoracic aortic disease: executive summary. *Anesth Analg.* 2010:111;279-315.

Ullery BW, Wang GJ, Low D, Cheung AT. Neurological complication of thoracic endovascular aortic repair. *Seminars in Cardiothoracic and Vascular Anesthesia* 2011;15(4):123-140.

Hobbs RD, Ullery BW, Mentzer AR, Cheung AT. Protocol for prevention of spinal cord ischemia after thoracoabdominal aortic surgery. *Vascular.* 2016;24(4):430-434.

Hypertrophic Obstructive Cardiomyopathy and Cardiac Masses

10

Previous chapters discussed how fixed obstructions to blood flowing through the heart can lead to significant morbidity and mortality. Aortic and mitral stenosis are two examples of lesions, which prevent the heart from effectively pumping blood. Hypertrophic obstructive cardiomyopathy (HOCM) represents a specific form of hypertrophic cardiomyopathy (HCM), which also manifests, at rest or with provocation (e.g., elevated heart rate, hypovolemia), with dynamic obstruction of left ventricular outflow tract (LVOT) (Figure 10–1). Dynamic outflow obstruction results in syncope, dyspnea, and, at times, sudden death. Although there is an increased incidence of sudden cardiac death (SCD) in the HCM patient with myocardial wall thickness greater than 30 mm or more, the majority of sudden deaths occur in HCM patients with myocardial wall thicknesses less than 30 mm.[1] Consequently, all HCM patients should undergo SCD risk stratification at initial evaluation. The American College of Cardiology Foundation and the American Heart Association (ACCF/AHA) developed extensive guidelines for the evaluation and management of the HCM.

Although rare, cardiac tumors and other masses at times interfere with valve function, produce emboli, and dynamically obstruct blood flow through the heart. This chapter will examine these different conditions, which are nonetheless linked by their dynamic ability to prevent the heart from properly functioning.

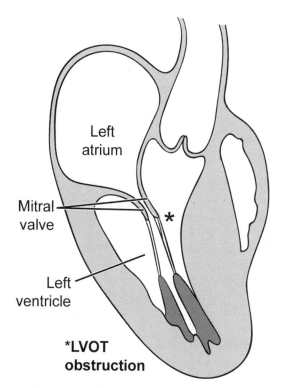

Left atrium

Mitral valve

*

Left ventricle

*LVOT obstruction

Figure 10–1. The midesophageal long-axis view is presented here in outline form. As a consequence of the hypertrophied interventricular septum, flow patterns within the heart are altered such that the anterior leaflet of the mitral valve is drawn during ventricular systole into the LVOT producing obstruction. This is known as systolic anterior motion (SAM) of the mitral valve.

SIGNS, SYMPTOMS, AND DIAGNOSIS OF HCM

HCM is an autosomal dominant trait; roughly one-half of the patients have a blood relative afflicted with HCM.[2,3] The disease can affect both males and females. It is estimated that HCM presents in 1:500 of the general adult population and that these patients are at increased risk for SCD.[4] Certainly, many patients with HCM are not detected and can present with SCD as the first manifestation of their cardiac disease.

Symptoms of HCM include dyspnea, exercise intolerance, palpitations, syncope, chest pain, and SCD. HCM can manifest in both the left and the right heart; however, it is overwhelmingly a disease of the left ventricle. HCM can occur with and without LVOT obstruction.[5] In nonobstructive HCM disease, patients develop a hypertrophied myocardium and diastolic dysfunction without generating high dynamic pressure gradients in the LVOT. As previously discussed in Chapter 2, diastolic dysfunction occurs when the heart is unable to normally accommodate diastolic filling at low pressures. Subsequently, impaired relaxation and ventricular compliance leads to an increased left ventricular end-diastolic pressure (LVEDP), elevated pulmonary arterial pressures (PAPs), increased pulmonary congestion, and decreased coronary perfusion pressure (CPP). Such patients can develop angina, dysrhythmias, systolic heart failure, and sudden death in the absence of any LVOT obstruction. Nonetheless, patients in whom HCM disease produces an obstruction of the LVOT are at a significantly increased risk of death and/or severe heart failure.[5]

Clinically, the diagnosis of HCM with dynamic LVOT obstruction is made by the auscultation of a late systolic murmur. The murmur is heard in late systole as the anterior leaflet of the mitral valve abuts the hypertrophied septum during systole (Videos 10–1 and 10–2). This systolic anterior motion (SAM) of the mitral valve provides the source of dynamic systolic obstruction in these patients (Figure 10–2A and B). Various clinical maneuvers can be employed to increase the murmur by reducing the venous return to the heart (e.g., Valsalva maneuver). By reducing venous return to the heart, the ventricles fill to a lesser degree. In the HCM patient, the fuller the heart, the less likely it is that during systole the mitral valve will be able to obstruct the LVOT. In the underloaded heart, however, the anterior leaflet of the mitral valve can more readily obstruct the ejection of blood.

Not surprisingly, echocardiography is best suited to make the diagnosis of HCM disease.[2] When ventricular wall thickness in diastole is greater than 15 mm, the patient is thought to have HCM disease assuming there are no other conditions that would produce ventricular hypertrophy (e.g., aortic stenosis or systemic hypertension). Symptomatic patients routinely have thickened interventricular septums of 20 to 30 mm.[2]

PATHOLOGY OF HCM

HCM is a genetic disease. Mutations in the genes, which code for the cardiac sarcomeres and their supporting proteins, have been implicated as causes of HCM.[2,3] Mutations in the beta-myosin heavy chain and myosin-binding protein C represent upward of 50% of the genotyped patients.[3] However, other cardiac protein mutations can also be associated with HCM. Additionally, the phenotypic expression of the HCM patient is variable. Thus, even in families with the same mutation, the variations in phenotypic expression can lead to radically different outcomes.[2]

At the cellular level, the myocardium of the HCM patient is a mix of oddly shaped myocytes and fibrotic tissue. The myocytes of the HCM patient lack the neat parallel array of normal ventricular muscle tissue.[2]

This abnormal myocardium can become quite noncompliant leading to diastolic dysfunction. As the LVEDP increases, pressure is transmitted through the left atrium to the pulmonary vasculature resulting in elevated PAPs. The HCM patient can develop dyspnea with minimal exertion. Thus, HCM patients can be symptomatic without having LVOT obstruction. Additionally, the HCM patient can develop associated right ventricular dysfunction and this is correlated to the degree of LV dysfunction and pulmonary hypertension.[6] HCM patients with reduced tricuspid annular plane systolic excursion (TAPSE) (see Chapter 8) have an increased likelihood of death or transplantation.

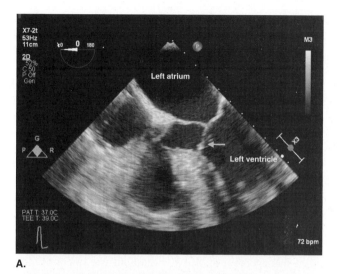

Figure 10–2. (A) Midesophageal four-chamber view showing systolic anterior motion (gray arrow) of the mitral valve abutting the hypertrophied interventricular septum. (B) Midesophageal long-axis view with color flow Doppler showing flow acceleration in the left ventricular outflow tract (gray arrow) and mitral regurgitation posteriorly oriented jet (white arrow).

Systolic function is often initially preserved in the HCM patient. However, over time in a small percentage of patients, the heart's systolic pumping ability fails. In HCM patients especially if LVOT obstruction is present, the increased LV work to overcome elevated pressures will lead to increased wall stress, ischemia, cell death, ventricular fibrosis, and heart failure.[3]

Mitral regurgitation frequently occurs in HCM during obstruction of the LVOT. Mechanisms for development of mitral regurgitation include elevated intraventricular pressures, SAM of the mitral leaflet, abnormally positioned papillary muscles, and redundant mitral leaflets. Mitral regurgitation may result in left atrial dilatation, atrial fibrillation, decreased stroke volume, and further impairment of the ventricular function.

SCD is one of the most dreaded complications of HCM.[7] Consequently, many patients with this condition are provided with an implantable cardioverter defibrillator (ICD) after a risk stratification and selection process. In particular, a history of ventricular fibrillation, sustained ventricular tachycardia, unexplained syncope, and a family history of SCD should be investigated in the HCM patient. ACCF/AHA recommendations suggest ICD placement in patients with a past history of cardiac arrest, ventricular fibrillation, or sustained ventricular tachycardia. They recommend as a class IIa guideline that it is reasonable to place an ICD in patients with myocardial wall thickness greater than 30 mm. ICD placement is not indicated for routine management of HCM without an assessment of increased risk or to facilitate participation in competitive athletics

MEDICAL THERAPY FOR HCM

The majority of patients with HCM are managed medically when symptoms warrant.[2] Asymptomatic patients are routinely managed expectantly; however, ICD placement may be considered in those with a strong family history of SCD. Medical therapy is centered primarily upon determining the nature of HCM encountered. The nonobstructive HCM patient presents with signs and symptoms of diastolic dysfunction.[2] Both beta-blockers and calcium antagonists have been used in this setting with variable results. It is possible that these agents improve symptoms by reducing the incidence of myocardial ischemia. Patients presenting with signs of heart failure in the nonobstructive HCM patient can be treated with judicious administration of diuretics to relieve symptoms of pulmonary congestion. However, reduced ventricular volumes could prove problematic as the noncompliant, dysfunctional ventricle requires an adequate SV to generate an acceptable cardiac output. Rhythm disturbances such as atrial fibrillation should also be corrected to permit adequate LV filling during diastole.

Patients with obstructive HCM can develop intraventricular pressure gradients during systole. Gradients across the LVOT of over 100 mm Hg can be detected between different regions of the LV cavity (Video 10–3). Indeed, the presence of obstruction with gradients as low as 30 mm Hg is predictive of worse outcomes and increased mortality in the HCM patient population.[5] Therapy is aimed at reducing myocardial contractility to reduce the LVOT gradient during systole. Beta-blockers, verapamil, and disopyramide are employed to this end. These agents have negative inotropic effects and reduce the systolic gradient. Likewise, efforts are made to maintain a large, well-filled left ventricle. Any situation leading to a reduction in the size of the left ventricle (e.g., hypovolemia, increased myocardial contractility, and decreased systemic vascular resistance) will increase the likelihood or severity of dynamic obstruction during ventricular systole.

DYNAMIC OBSTRUCTION OF THE LVOT

HCM patients can be symptomatic whether they have the obstructive form or the nonobstructive form of cardiomyopathy. It is important to realize that both presentations can lead to perioperative complications resulting from arrhythmia, hypotension, and even SCD. Although the cardiac anesthesiologist is likely to encounter that subset of obstructive HCM patients not amenable to medical therapy, it is critical to understand that the HCM patient may undergo a variety of procedures and have varying anesthetic requirements.

What differentiates the obstructive form of HCM from the nonobstructive form is the dynamic development of a pressure gradient across the LVOT.

The LVOT provides the pathway for oxygenated blood as it leaves the LV cavity and is ejected out through the aortic valve. The SAM of the mitral valve in the LVOT is the most common cause of dynamic obstruction generating significant pressure gradients (> 50 mm Hg) across the LVOT. The hypertrophied bulge of the intraventricular septum at the level of the LVOT may direct the flow in the heart in such a way that it drags the anterior leaflet into the LVOT producing obstruction.[8] The development of increased LV intracavitary pressure can soon lead to mitral valve incompetence and worsening symptoms of systolic and diastolic heart failure.

ANESTHETIC MANAGEMENT OF THE HCM PATIENT FOR NONCARDIAC SURGERY

Only certain HCM patients are brought to surgery for myectomy and/or mitral valve replacement. Many patients will nonetheless require anesthesia at some point for noncardiac surgery. Management is directed at minimizing the degree of outflow obstruction, lessening the impact of diastolic dysfunction, and controlling arrhythmias. Both general and neuraxial anesthesia techniques can produce wide swings in hemodynamics. As mentioned, during anesthesia induction in the patient with a fixed obstruction to systolic ejection, such as aortic stenosis, it often becomes necessary to administer fluids and vasoconstrictors to prevent hemodynamic instability. In the patient with dynamic obstruction, the greater the decrease in venous return, the worse the degree of obstruction. Agents, which decrease sympathetic tone and peripheral vascular resistance, likewise can increase the degree of dynamic obstruction, as the left ventricle is free to contract against less resistance. An increase in heart rate associated with laryngoscopy, intubation, and surgical stimulation should be avoided, as this will decrease the time for LV diastolic filling resulting in worsening of the degree of dynamic obstruction and hypotension. Consequently, these patients are frequently managed with fluid and vasopressor administration at the time of induction and intraoperative arterial and transesophageal echocardiography

(TEE) monitoring. Short-acting beta-blockers such as esmolol can be used to reduce myocardial contractility, decrease the heart rate, and counteract the effects of increased catecholamine release during intubation, emergence, and other periods associated with surgical stress.

Neuraxial anesthesia approaches can be employed in these patients and have also been used in the patient with HCM for labor analgesia.[4] The decrease in sympathetic tone with its associated reduction in venous return and decrease in peripheral vascular resistance makes the use of neuraxial techniques potentially deleterious. Careful titration of local anesthetic to obtain the appropriate level of anesthesia is clearly important if these approaches are to be safely employed. Likewise, invasive monitoring may prove helpful in this setting to detect acute deteriorations. Regional techniques that leave sympathetic tone relatively unaffected (e.g., peripheral nerve blocks) are of use when indicated in the HCM patient.

HCM patients frequently have undergone the placement of an ICD. The perioperative management of these devices is discussed in Chapter 15.

Anesthetic management may be further complicated by diastolic dysfunction. Additionally, patients often have some degree of mitral regurgitation, which further increases left atrial pressure, pulmonary venous pressure, and pulmonary congestion. Treatment is aimed at reducing the degree of dynamic obstruction, favoring adequate systolic ejection and thereby, reducing MR and pulmonary congestion. Although diuresis to unload the heart might be desirable in the patient with a high grade of diastolic dysfunction, care must be taken not to reduce ventricular volume such that the obstruction across the LVOT is increased.

ANESTHETIC MANAGEMENT FOR SURGICAL REPAIR OF HCM

For those patients who do not benefit from medical management, there are surgical approaches to relieve dynamic obstruction and restore adequate mitral valve function. Anesthetic management remains centered upon minimizing the degree of LVOT obstruction during the hemodynamic shifts associated with general anesthesia. Monitoring is similar to that employed in any cardiac surgical case requiring cardiopulmonary bypass (CPB). The utility of the PA catheter in this setting is unproven. However, TEE is essential to the performance of the operation. In this procedure, TEE is not merely a monitor of ventricular function or an additional surveillance tool—it is essential for the surgical management of the patient.[8,9] There is close interaction between the anesthesiologist and the surgeon during the surgery.

A variety of induction and maintenance agents can be employed in these patients. More important than the drug choice for anesthesia induction is directing therapy toward maintaining an adequate preload and high afterload and on avoiding elevation in heart rate. Catecholamine release associated with inadequate anesthetic depth can increase obstruction secondary to tachycardia and augmented myocardial contractility.

As mentioned in the previous section, hemodynamic derangements such as hypotension or tachycardia at the time of induction should be treated promptly

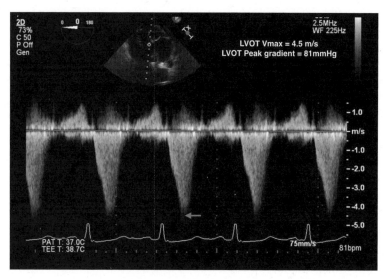

Figure 10–3. Continuous wave Doppler across the left ventricular outflow tract (LVOT) shows a characteristic late peaking "dagger-shape" spectral Doppler envelope. LVOT peak velocity (V_{max}) is 4.5 m/s and the LVOT peak gradient is 81 mm Hg.

using vasoconstrictors, fluids, or short-acting beta-blockers. Antiarrhythmics and beta-blockers should be continued perioperatively. Intraoperative therapeutic interventions may be monitored using TEE guidance to demonstrate relief of obstruction and reduced/absent dynamic pressure gradient.

Video 10–3 demonstrates the LVOT being obstructed by the anterior leaflet of the mitral valve abutting the bulging septum. The deep gastric view is employed, and as such there is a good alignment between the LVOT and the Doppler beam. Using continuous wave Doppler (CWD), it is possible to determine the velocity of flow across the obstruction. Video 10–3 displays the velocity-time integral of a patient with a severe dynamic gradient. Using Bernoulli's equation, it is possible to calculate the peak pressure gradient present across the LVOT:

$$\text{Pressure gradient} = 4V^2$$

where V is the peak blood flow velocity. As can be seen, the gradient can be rather significant (Figure 10–3).

Patients with severe gradients can quickly deteriorate perioperatively developing profound hypotension. Additionally, these patients have a significantly elevated LVEDP. Recalling the formula for coronary perfusion pressure:

$$\text{CPP} = \text{DBP} - \text{LVEDP}$$

The combination of profound systemic hypotension and elevated LVEDP will result in a reduced CPP in patients with HCM leading to a downward spiral of ischemia, hypotension, arrhythmias, and eventually cardiac arrest.

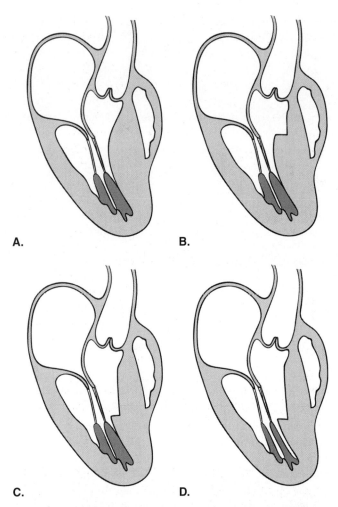

A.   **B.**

C.   **D.**

Figure 10–4. (A) Schematic of the long-axis view of the hypertrophic obstructive cardio-myopathy patient. Flow dynamics associated with the enlarged ventricular septum push the anterior leaflet of the mitral valve into the outflow track. (B) A subaortic myectomy may not be enough to redirect flow so that it does not intercept the tips of the mitral valve, so systolic anterior motion may still persist. In panels (C) and (D) an extensive myectomy is performed and the papillary muscles are partially excised to direct the flow of blood more anteriorly toward the LVOT rather than posteriorly. The coaptation point of the mitral valve leaflets is thus more posterior in the ventricle away from the anteriorly placed left ventricular outflow tract. [Adapted with permission from Sherrid MV, Chaudhry FA, Swistel DG, et al: Obstructive hypertrophic cardiomyopathy: echocardiography, pathophysiology, and the continuing evolution of surgery for obstruction, *Ann Thorac Surg*. 2003 Feb;75(2):620-632.]

THE SURGICAL APPROACH TO HCM REPAIR

Surgery is directed at reducing the muscle mass of the intraventricular septum in the region where it contacts the anterior leaflet of the mitral valve (Figure 10–4).[8,9] After institution of CPB and heart arrest by administration of cardioplegia, the aorta is opened and the surgeon carefully retracts the leaflets of the aortic valve. Looking down the LVOT, the surgeon is able to identify the muscle mass and reduce its size. Measurements obtained by TEE in the operating room assist the surgeon in guiding the repair. The echocardiographer determines the thickness of the septum and the distance from the aortic valve to the point where the mitral valve leaflet makes contact with the septum during systole. Additionally, TEE is used to determine the competency of the mitral valve. Should the mitral valve be deformed or incompetent, it may have to be repaired or replaced. Primarily, however, surgery is directed at removing the bulge in the ventricular septum.[8] By removing the septal bulge, the drag forces, which push the anterior leaflet of the mitral valve into the LVOT, are removed and the coaptation point of the mitral valve moves more posteriorly in relationship to the LVOT. Consequently, the SAM of the mitral valve is relieved and the gradient across the LVOT reduced (Figure 10–5). Figure 10–4D demonstrates the broad area of septum removed to reduce drag force on the mitral valve and thereby relieve SAM.

Once the surgical repair is completed, the aorta is closed, and the patient weaned from CPB in the usual fashion, TEE is again employed to make sure the surgeon has not created a ventricular septal defect (VSD) during the repair by cutting out too much of the intraventricular septum. Additionally, the mitral and aortic valves are examined by TEE to be sure that any mitral repair is competent and that the aortic leaflets have not been damaged during retraction to expose the LVOT.

Often a dobutamine challenge is performed to determine the adequacy of the repair. In this setting, dobutamine (5-10 µg/kg/min) is administered to the patient. This will cause increases in heart rate and contractility and a decrease is afterload, conditions that can increase the likelihood of LVOT obstruction, as well

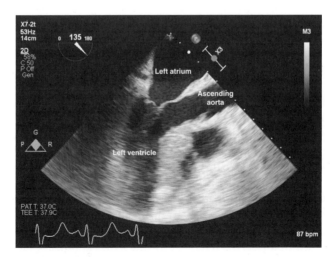

Figure 10–5. Midesophageal long-axis view in a patient with hypertrophic obstructive cardiomyopathy after septal myectomy. The systolic anterior motion of the mitral valve has disappeared, and the left ventricular outflow tract appears free of obstruction.

as a decrease in peripheral vascular resistance. The LVOT is examined for signs of dynamic obstruction and any residual gradients measured. In addition to creation of VSD, heart block requiring pacemaker insertion can develop in upward of 10% of these patients.[8]

Alcohol septal ablation (ASA) is also employed to reduce the size of the septal bulge. In this catheter-based technique, the left anterior descending artery (LAD) is entered and a septal branch located. The area of distribution of flow from the branch is determined, and if confined to the septum, absolute alcohol is injected producing a controlled myocardial infarction. Risks include spread of the alcohol outside of the septum, ventricular arrhythmias, and heart block. The infarcted septum gradually reduces in size upon healing and changes the flow patterns in the ventricle reducing drag on the anterior leaflet of the mitral valve and relieving obstruction.

The 2011 ACCF/AHA guidelines suggest as a class IIa recommendation that surgical septal myectomy be the first consideration for the majority of eligible patients with HCM with severe drug refractory symptoms and LVOT obstruction. They suggest as a class IIb recommendation that ASA is an alternative for patients following a balanced and thorough discussion. They note that the effectiveness of ASA is uncertain in patients with HCM with > 30 mm septal hypertrophy and discourage the procedure in that patient population. Sorajja et al. in a 2012 retrospective study demonstrated favorable and similar outcomes in patients treated with ASA compared with surgical myectomy.[10] Ball et al. in a study of 403 invasively treated HCM patients failed to detect a difference in 5-year survival in patients undergoing either myectomy or septal alcohol ablation.[11] Ideally, myectomy and/or ASA should be performed by experienced centers in the treatment of HCM.[12]

CARDIAC MASSES

Cardiac tumors are rare[13,14] but have the potential to create dynamic obstruction in their own right. Cardiac tumors may be primary or secondary, malignant or benign. Primary cardiac tumors are frequently histologically benign. Myxomas (Figure 10–6) are the most frequent cardiac tumors; (Video 10–4) other benign tumors include lipomas, fibromas, papillary fibroelastomas, and rhabdomyomas. The most frequent malignant primary cardiac tumors are angiosarcomas; other malignant tumors include rhabdomyosarcoma, liposarcoma, fibrosarcoma, and malignant lymphoma.

Metastatic tumors to the heart are far more common than primary tumors, tend not to be intracavitary lesions, and have a grim prognosis. Intraventricular thrombi can develop following myocardial infarction and can be confused with cardiac masses. The incidence of postinfarction thrombi formation has decreased with the routine use of anticoagulating agents peri-infarction. Nonetheless, intraventricular thrombi can occur and be the source of embolic phenomenon. They are surgically resected if operative therapy is indicated for the patient's primary cardiac disease and if they have become symptomatic. Video 10–5 demonstrates the appearance on echocardiography of intraventricular thrombi.

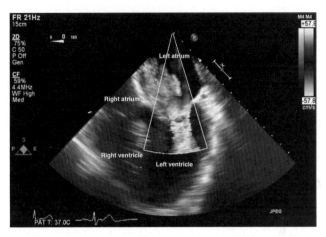

Figure 10–6. Midesophageal four-chamber view showing a myxoma (arrow) in the left atrium attached to the interatrial septum. Flow acceleration across the mitral valve occurs due to partial obstruction of flow by the myxoma.

The clinical presentations, which herald the presence of intracardiac masses, include stroke, dyspnea, and chest pain. Cardiac masses may result in embolization, obstruction, and impairment in ventricular filling or disruption in valvular integrity. Cardiac masses are diagnosed through the use of echocardiography and cardiac magnetic resonance imaging.

Where indicated, surgical management focuses upon removal of the mass and repair or replacement of any valvular structure damaged as a consequence of the lesion.

Anesthetic management of these cases centers upon the primary impact of the lesion on the flow of blood through the heart. Patients, whose venous return to the heart is blocked by the mass, will behave similarly to patients with tamponade. These patients are likely to collapse hemodynamically at induction due to vasodilatation and positive pressure ventilation. Patients with obstructing left-sided lesions may develop pressure gradients in the LVOT in a manner similar to that described for the HCM patient. Volume loading and maintenance of vascular tone at the time of induction will help to minimize hemodynamic instability at the time of induction. In certain patients, smaller masses may result in valvular insufficiency. Therefore, should a small mass produce aortic or mitral regurgitation, anesthesia is administered to lower systemic resistance and promote forward blood flow. Should the mass produce a restriction to blood flow through the valve, the patient would be managed in a manner similar to that for stenotic valvular lesions.

When cardiac masses are present, there is the ever-present risk of embolization. Embolization to the bowel, extremities, renal arteries, viscera, and brain can occur. Should right-sided lesions be present in addition to tricuspid and pulmonic valvular insufficiency, these patients are at risk for pulmonary arterial embolization. PA line placement in the presence of right-sided cardiac masses could dislodge vegetation, clot, or other mass leading to perioperative pulmonary embolism.

CASE SCENARIO: 22-YEAR-OLD MAN WITH SUDDEN CARDIAC DEATH

A 22-year-old man suffers ventricular fibrillation while playing college football. At the scene, cardiopulmonary resuscitation (CPR) is commenced. He is successfully defibrillated and transported to the emergency room.

What is the differential diagnosis of sudden ventricular fibrillation?

Differential diagnosis includes coronary artery disease, pulmonary embolism, tension pneumothorax, cerebral hemorrhage, and primary dysrhythmias.

In the emergency room, his vital signs are BP 60/40 mm Hg, HR 120 bpm, sinus rhythm, mechanical ventilation, and SaO_2 100%. What therapy and evaluation are required?

Physical examination, ECG, and chest x-ray are obtained. Breath sounds are bilateral and chest x-ray is unremarkable. Rhythm appears sinus. Two large-bore IVs are started, and an arterial line placed.

A TEE is performed emergently showing the findings in the TEE (**Video 10–1**). What is the diagnosis?

HCM.

What medical therapy is required at this time?

Medical therapy should include beta-blockers to reduce heart rate and myocardial contractility, volume administration, and vasoconstrictors to augment vascular tone.

The patient is scheduled for surgery for myectomy and mitral valve repair. What are the anesthetic concerns for this patient?

This patient requires maintenance of preload and heart rate, preservation of vascular tone, and reduction of myocardial contractility.

REFERENCES

1. Ross R, Sherrid M, Casey M, et al. Does surgical relief of obstruction improve prognosis for hypertrophic cardiomyopathy? *Prog Cardiovasc Dis.* 2012;54:529-534.
2. Sherrid M. Pathophysiology and treatment of hypertrophic cardiomyopathy. *Prog Cardiovasc Dis.* 2006;49(2):123-151.
3. Gersh B, Maron B, Bonow R, et al. 2011 ACCF/AHA guideline for the diagnosis and treatment of hypertrophic cardiomyopathy: a report of the American College of Cardiology Foundation/American Heart Association Task Force on Practice Guidelines. *J Am Coll Cardiol.* 2011;58:e212-260.
4. Poliac L, Barron M, Maron B. Hypertrophic cardiomyopathy. *Anesthesiology.* 2006;104(1):183-192.
5. Maron M, Olivotto I, Betocchi S, et al. Effect of left ventricular outflow tract obstruction on clinical outcome in hypertrophic cardiomyopathy. *NEJM.* 2003;348(4):295-303.
6. Finocchiaro G, Knowles J, Pavlovic A, et al. Prevalence and clinical correlates of right ventricular dysfunction in patients with hypertrophic cardiomyopathy. *Am J Cardiol.* 2014;113:361-367.
7. Maron B, Spirito P, Shen W, et al. Implantable cardioverter-defibrillators and prevention of sudden cardiac death in hypertrophic cardiomyopathy. *JAMA.* 2007;298(4):405-412.
8. Sherrid M, Chaudhry F, Swistel D. Obstructive hypertrophic cardiomyopathy: echocardiography, pathophysiology, and continuing evolution of surgery for obstruction. *Ann Thorac Surg.* 2003;75:620-632.

9. Balaram S, Sherrid M, DeRose J, Hillel Z, Winson G, Swistel D. Beyond extended myectomy for hypertrophic cardiomyopathy: the resection-plication-release (RPR) repair. *Ann Thorac Surg.* 2005;80:217-223.

10. Sorajja P, Ommen S, Holmes D, et al. Survival after alcohol septal ablation for obstructive hypertrophic cardiomyopathy. *Circulation.* 2012;126:2374-2380.

11. Ball W, Ivanov J, Rakowski H, et al. Long-term survival in patients with resting obstructive hypertrophic cardiomyopathy. *J Am Coll Cardiol.* 2011; 58:2313-2321.

12. Olivotto I, Ommen S, Maron M, Cecchi F, Maron B. Surgical myectomy versus alcohol septal ablation for obstructive hypertrophic cardiomyopathy: will there ever be a randomized trial? *JACC.* 2007;50(9):831-834.

13. Elbardissi A, Dearani J, Daly R, et al. Survival after resection of primary cardiac tumors: a 48-year experience. *Circulation.* 2008;118:s7-s15.

14. Buyukates M, Aktunc E. Giant left atrial myxoma causing mitral valve obstruction and pulmonary hypertension. *Can J Surg.* 2008;51(4):E97-E98.

Ventricular Assist Devices and Heart Transplantation

11

TOPICS

Adult heart surgery patients are increasingly older with varying degrees of preoperative ventricular failure. Patients routinely present with both systolic and diastolic ventricular dysfunction, ventricular remodeling, fluid retention, and pulmonary congestion. Additionally, even those patients with well-preserved preoperative ventricular function can deteriorate intraoperatively secondary to inadequate myocardial preservation, embolism, myocardial ischemia, protamine reactions, and other "catastrophic" events (e.g., anaphylaxis and aortic dissection). Of course, the overwhelming majority of patients experiencing intra-operative right or left ventricular failure can be treated with a combination of inotropes and/or inhaled pulmonary vasodilators. However, others lack sufficient ventricular function to provide adequate delivery of oxygenated blood to the tissues. Such patients readily develop kidney dysfunction, acidosis, and cardiogenic shock unless provided mechanical assistance to support or replace the heart's pump function. This chapter reviews the anesthetic management of patients in need of intra-aortic balloon counterpulsation (IABP), ventricular assist devices (VADs), and heart transplantation (HT).

INTRA-AORTIC BALLOON COUNTERPULSATION AND THE HEART SURGERY PATIENT

IABP counterpulsation is employed to assist the failing heart (Video 11–1). It is not a substitute for a beating ventricle and as such does not replace the function of the ventricle it is assisting. IABPs are generally introduced via the femoral artery into the thoracic aorta and positioned distal to the takeoff of the left subclavian artery. The IABP inflates with helium during diastole and deflates during systole. Thus, it creates a counterpulsation to the pulsation generated by the native heart. By inflating during diastole at the point of aortic valve closure, the IABP augments diastolic blood pressure and thus improves coronary artery perfusion pressure.

Recall,

$$CPP = \text{Diastolic blood pressure (DBP)} - \text{Left ventricular end-diastolic pressure (LVEDP)}$$

During systole, the IABP deflates reducing the afterload against which the heart must eject, thereby potentially improving forward blood flow.

The cardiac anesthesiologist is likely to encounter the IABP in several situations:

1. Many patients presenting with myocardial ischemia refractory to medical or percutaneous interventions are provided an IABP in the cardiac catheterization laboratory to relieve ischemic chest pain. By increasing DBP and lowering LVEDP, the IABP improves the balance of LV myocardial oxygen supply and demand. In a 1997 review of 4,756 IAPB uses in a single institution over a period of 30 years, Torchiana et al. suggested that preoperative placement of an IABP in those with medically refractory ischemia can improve patient outcome.[1] Guidelines continue to evolve in parallel with new evidence regarding the utility of the IABP in patients with ST-segment elevation myocardial infarction (STEMI) and cardiogenic shock to affect clinical outcomes (e.g., mortality). MacKay et al. recently reviewed the role of IABP use in cardiovascular practice and report that various guidelines have downgraded the strength of the recommendation for IABP use in the setting of STEMI. However, recent meta-analyses have demonstrated a mortality benefit in high-risk coronary artery bypass surgery patients when an IABP is placed preoperatively.

2. In patients with cardiogenic shock, the IABP is placed to augment cardiac output in the immediate preoperative period should emergent heart surgery be warranted. Of note, the IABP is contraindicated in patients with aortic dissections, aortic aneurysms, severe aortic insufficiency, and severe atherosclerotic disease in the descending aorta. The relatively recent development and availability of percutaneous left ventricular assist devices (LVAD) has raised the question that these devices might offer improved survival compared to IABP placement in cardiogenic shock patients. Cheng et al. in a meta-analysis concluded that although hemodynamic indices (e.g., cardiac index, mean arterial pressure, and pulmonary wedge pressure) were better improved with percutaneous LVAD support compared to IABP, there was no impact upon 30-day mortality irrespective of the circulatory support device employed.[2] The PROTECT II trial examined preprocedural placement of either an IABP or a percutaneous LVAD (Impella 2.5) in high-risk patients before percutaneous coronary interventions (PCI). MacKay et al. in their review of the trial determined that although no statistical difference was seen at 30 or 90 days following the procedure in major

adverse events there was a nonsignificant statistical trend that favored the use of the Impella device over the IABP.

3. IABPs are placed in the operating room in those patients whose poor ventricular function prevents separation from cardiopulmonary bypass (CPB) in spite of maximal inotropic and vasopressor support. Temporary LVAD and extracorporeal membrane oxygenation (ECMO) are also used to support patients should they fail to adequately separate from CPB.

4. In patients with a sudden-onset ventricular septal defect (VSD) or papillary muscle/chordal rupture secondary to acute myocardial infarction, the IABP is placed to reduce afterload, and hence decrease left-to-right shunt or MR, respectively.

Several parameters are important for the adequate operation of the IABP, and these are set at the IABP console. Synchronization of the IABP with the cardiac rhythm and timing of the balloon inflation and deflation can be done using either the ECG tracing or the arterial pressure tracing. Balloon inflation occurs at the dicrotic notch of the arterial pressure waveform, which indicates the closure of the aortic valve and the beginning of diastole. Timing of the inflation and deflation of the IABP is critical to achieve maximal diastolic augmentation of the blood pressure and maximal afterload reduction. Another parameter that can be set is the ratio of IABP counterpulsations to ventricular pulsations. The IABP can cycle with every beat (1 to 1 assist), every other beat, or every third beat of the heart. In this way the degree of assist can be regulated when the patient is to be weaned from IABP support. The volume of gas used to inflate the balloon and the time required for inflation and deflation can also be adjusted.

Complications of IABP use include femoral artery injuries, aortic dissections, thromboembolism, and balloon rupture with subsequent gas embolism. At times IABP complications require exploration and repair of the femoral artery and arterial embolectomy.

VENTRICULAR ASSIST DEVICES: DESIGNS AND INDICATIONS

Unlike IABPs that require a left ventricle capable of producing some cardiac output to be effective, ventricular assist devices (VADs) can function in lieu of a completely dysfunctional left or right ventricle. VADs are often placed when medical therapy has been exhausted in efforts to improve end-organ perfusion. Because deteriorations in ventricular function occur both acutely and chronically, VAD placement can be completed either emergently or electively depending upon the patient's condition.

The decision to place a VAD and the type of device to be employed is dependent upon both the patient's associated illnesses and the estimated time that VAD therapy will be required. VADs can be placed to provide short-term ventricular support in those cases where recovery of cardiac function or heart transplantation (HT) is expected. Both percutaneous and implantable devices have been used in this setting. At other times, recovery of heart function is not considered likely and VADs are placed to support organ perfusion in patients awaiting heart transplantation. Still, other patients are thought not to be suitable candidates for the limited number of hearts available for transplantation and are provided a VAD as "destination" therapy. In other words, it is hoped that the VAD will provide patients crippled by heart failure both longer and better-quality lives. The decision to commit an individual to long-term VAD support is not lightly undertaken and should be considered in situations when kidney, liver, pulmonary, and neurologic dysfunction are not so advanced that patient survival is not thought possible even with improved cardiac output. Usually, the patient's cardiologist together with a cardiothoracic surgeon will determine whether a VAD as "destination" therapy, a VAD as a bridge to HT, or immediate HT (if a heart is available) is warranted. Proposed short-term emergent VAD placement following failure to separate from cardiopulmonary bypass (CPB) should occur only after the surgeon and the anesthesiologist discuss the immediate patient management plan.

VADs are used to support the function of the left, right, or both ventricles. They can be classified according to how blood flows when they are employed. Flow through a VAD can be either continuous or pulsatile. Continuous flow VADs include most currently used devices placed percutaneously for temporary support of ventricular function (e.g., Impella) and devices implanted (e.g., HeartMate II, HeartMate III, and HeartWare). Pulsatile VADs, included extracorporeal devices (e.g., Abiomed BVS) for short-term support and those previously used for support of longer duration (e.g., HeartMate I).[3] ECMO circuits are also used for transient hemodynamic support as well as to support pulmonary function.

SHORT-TERM VAD PLACEMENT

VADs can be placed emergently whenever ventricular function is severely compromised. Often candidates for emergent VAD placement are in cardiogenic shock requiring multiple vasoactive medications and possible IABP counterpulsation. VAD placement may prevent the development of multiorgan system failure giving time for the heart to recover function or may provide a "bridge to decision" during which the patient, healthcare providers, and family members can discern the best course of therapy.

The type of VAD to be placed and whether one or both of the ventricles will be supported depends upon the clinical conditions. A left ventricular assist device (LVAD) is placed in the setting of cardiogenic shock and poor left ventricular systolic function (Videos 11–2A and 11–2B). A right ventricular assist device (RVAD) is placed when the right heart fails such as during a right ventricular infarction, or right ventricular dysfunction after left VAD placement or HT. In this setting the LV is often underloaded as the RV does not deliver sufficient blood to the LV to eject into the systemic circulation resulting in cardiogenic shock. At times, both ventricles require mechanical support.

Emergent short-term VADs include both percutaneously and surgically placed devices. Percutaneous devices can be placed in the cardiac catheterization laboratory and thus can provide mechanical assistance without the need for surgical interventions. The TandemHeart[4-6] device provides left atrial-to-femoral artery blood flow. TandemHeart is a continuous flow centrifugal device using an extracorporeal pump.

The inflow cannula is inserted via the femoral vein through the interatrial septum into the left atrium. Oxygenated blood is then pumped from the left atrium and returned to the systemic circulation via a cannula placed in a femoral artery providing retrograde flow to most of the body. Because the lungs continue to oxygenate blood flowing into the left atrium, TandemHeart can be employed during high-risk percutaneous coronary interventions (PCIs) to provide circulatory support without requiring extracorporeal oxygenation (Figure 11–1). Although

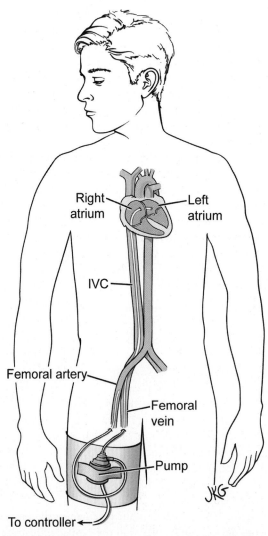

Figure 11–1. The tandem heart device provides circulatory support but not extracorporeal oxygenation. Blood is drawn from the left atrium and returned to the arterial system via the femoral artery.

TandemHeart was found capable of improving hemodynamics in a randomized trial of patients with cardiogenic shock following acute myocardial infarction compared to those treated with IABP support, the 30-day mortality was similar between the groups.[5]

Devices in the Impella family are used to support left ventricular function.[7] The device generally is placed via a peripheral artery (e.g., femoral or axillary) and threaded across the aortic valve into the left ventricle. Patients with postoperative LV failure treated with an Impella device were found to have a similar mortality to that of patients supported with an IABP.[7] Ouweneel et al. in a recent study demonstrated that mortality was unaffected through the use of a percutaneous mechanical support device (Impella CP) versus an IABP in patients following acute myocardial infarction complicated with cardiogenic shock (Figure 11–2). However, the 2015 Society of Cardiovascular Angiography and Interventions/American College of Cardiology/Heart Failure Society of America/Society of Thoracic Surgeons consensus statement on the use of percutaneous mechanical circulatory support devices in cardiovascular care suggests that in the "setting of profound cardiogenic shock, IABP is less likely to provide benefit than continuous flow pumps including the Impella CP and TandemHeart."

Pressure-volume loops illustrate the effects of mechanical circulatory support on cardiac work.[8] Figure 11–3 demonstrates the reduction of stroke volume and the increase in left ventricular end-diastolic pressure and volume in cardiogenic shock following acute myocardial infarction. Figure 11–4 displays the effects on cardiac function with the introduction of IABP, percutaneous LVADs such as Impella and TandemHeart, and extracorporeal membrane oxygenation. Percutaneous ventricular assist devices significantly lower left ventricular volume, pressure, and stroke volume (SV), therefore reducing cardiac work. The IABP increases SV while lowering end-diastolic pressure. Veno-arterial (VA) ECMO without adequate unloading of the left ventricle (either by LV venting or maintaining some degree of contractility) may increase LV systolic and diastolic pressure and may increase myocardial oxygen demand secondary to an increase in afterload.

Both the Impella device and TandemHeart require anticoagulation. Sufficient right heart function is necessary to deliver adequate oxygenated blood volume to the left heart to then be drained from the left atrium in the case of TandemHeart or the left ventricle in the case of Impella. Temporary support of right heart function can also be provided by continuous flow devices that drain the right heart and eject blood into the pulmonary artery. Both TandemHeart and Impella provide continuous blood flow, and both have their limitations. TandemHeart requires a transatrial septal puncture to drain blood from the left atrium. The Impella devices cross the aortic valve and thus are contraindicated in patients with severe aortic valvular disease or mechanical prosthetic aortic valve. Left ventricular thrombus is also a contraindication to Impella placement.

Short-term VAD support can be employed by surgical (through a median sternotomy) placement of extracorporeal, centrifugal pumps. For LVAD support, a drainage cannula is placed in the left atrium or the left ventricle apex and blood is drained into the pump to be returned to the patient through a synthetic graft

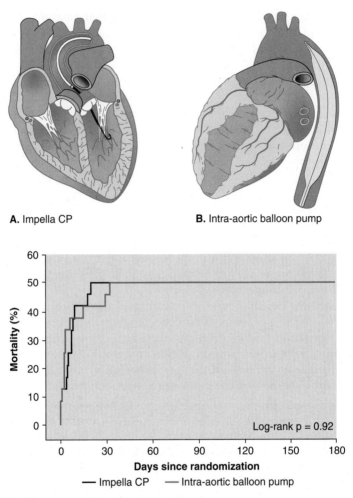

A. Impella CP   **B.** Intra-aortic balloon pump

C. All-cause mortality, ≤ 6 months

Figure 11–2. Schematic drawings of the heart and aorta showing the two mechanical support devices used in the study: (A) Impella CP (Abiomed, Danvers, Massachusetts). (B) The intra-aortic balloon pump (IABP). (C) Time-to-event Kaplan-Meier curves up to 6 months after randomization for all-cause mortality. LV, left ventricular. [Reproduced with permission from Ouweneel DM, Eriksen E, Sjauw KD, et al: Percutaneous Mechanical Circulatory Support Versus Intra-Aortic Balloon Pump in Cardiogenic Shock After Acute Myocardial Infarction, *J Am Coll Cardiol.* 2017 Jan 24;69(3):278-287.]

attached to the aorta. Similarly, cannulas are placed in the right atrium and the pulmonary artery to assist right heart function.

Conditions that impede the delivery of blood to the left atrium (e.g., right heart failure, clot, hypovolemia) can reduce LVAD output. Many patients with long-standing LV failure have significant pulmonary hypertension and RV failure. If RV function is inadequate, the VAD will be underfilled because blood will not be

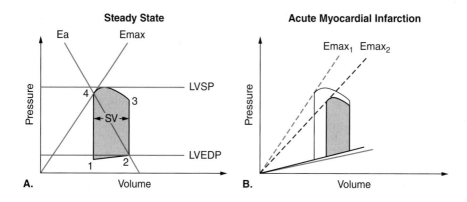

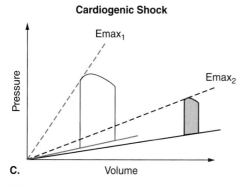

Figure 11–3. Normal and abnormal pressure-volume loops. Each pressure-volume (PV) loop represents one cardiac cycle (A). Beginning at the end of isovolumic relaxation (point 1), LV volume increases during diastole (phase 1 to 2). At end-diastole (point 2), LV volume is maximal and isovolumic contraction (phase 2 to 3) begins. At the peak of isovolume contraction, LV pressure exceeds aortic pressure and blood begins to eject from the LV into the aorta (point 3). During this systolic ejection phase, LV volume decreases until aortic pressure exceeds LV pressure and the aortic valve closes, which is known as the end-systolic pressure-volume point (ESPV) (point 4). Stroke volume (SV) is represented by the width of the PV loop as the volume difference between end-systolic and end-diastolic volumes (points 1 and 2). The shaded area within the loop represents stroke work. Load-independent LV contractility also known as Emax, is defined as the maximal slope of the ESPV point under various loading conditions, known as the ESPV relationship (ESPVR). Effective arterial elastance (Ea) is a component of LV afterload and is defined as the ratio of end-systolic pressure and stroke volume. Under steady-state conditions, optimal LV pump efficiency occurs when the ratio of Ea:Emax approaches 1. (B) Representative PV loop in AMI. LV contractility (Emax) is reduced; LV pressure, SV, and LV stroke work may be unchanged or reduced; and LVEDP is increased. (C) Representative PV loop in cardiogenic shock. Emax is severely reduced; LVEDV and LVEDP are increased; and SV is reduced. [Reproduced with permission from Rihal CS, Naidu SS, Givertz MM, et al: 2015 SCAI/ACC/HFSA/STS Clinical Expert Consensus Statement on the Use of Percutaneous Mechanical Circulatory Support Devices in Cardiovascular Care (Endorsed by the American Heart Association, the Cardiological Society of India, and Sociedad Latino Americana de Cardiologia Intervencion; Affirmation of Value by the Canadian Association of Interventional Cardiology-Association Canadienne de Cardiologie d'intervention), *J Card Fail.* 2015 Jun;21(6):499-518.]

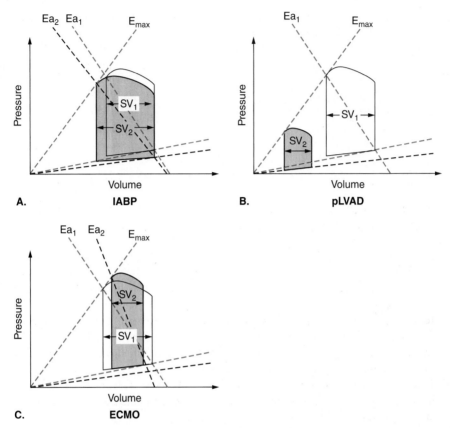

Figure 11–4. Cardiac effects of mechanical support. Illustrations of PV loops after activation of device therapy (gray loops). (A) Intra-aortic balloon pump (IABP) counter-pulsation reduces both peak LV systolic and diastolic pressures and increases LV stroke volume. The net effect is a reduced slope of arterial elastance (Ea_2). (B) Percutaneous LV assist devices (pLVAD: Impella and TandemHeart) significantly reduce LV pressures, LV volumes, and LV stroke volume. The net effect is a significant reduction in cardiac work-load. (C) Veno-arterial extra-corporeal membrane oxygenation (VA-ECMO) without a LV venting strategy increases LV systolic and diastolic pressure, while reducing LV stroke volume. The net effect is an increase in arterial elastance (Ea). [Reproduced with permission from Rihal CS, Naidu SS, Givertz MM, et al: 2015 SCAI/ACC/HFSA/STS Clinical Expert Consensus Statement on the Use of Percutaneous Mechanical Circulatory Support Devices in Cardiovascular Care (Endorsed by the American Heart Association, the Cardiological Society of India, and Sociedad Latino Americana de Cardiologia Intervencion; Affirmation of Value by the Canadian Association of Interventional Cardiology-Association Canadienne de Cardiologie d'intervention), *J Card Fail.* 2015 Jun;21(6):499-518.]

pushed across the pulmonary vasculature to return to the LA for drainage into the LVAD pump. Likewise, should a patent foramen ovale (PFO) be present, systemic hypoxemia might occur as deoxygenated blood will flow across the inter-atrial septum from the right atrium into the left atrium. By draining blood from the left atrium, the VAD will lower the pressure in this chamber; therefore, deoxygenated blood will follow the pressure gradient and will enter the systemic circulation through a PFO or other septal defect leading to a right-to-left shunt. Consequently, transesophageal echocardiography (TEE) examination prior to VAD placement must rule out the presence of any septal defects.

Veno-arterial ECMO is similar to a cardiopulmonary bypass system where venous blood is drained from the venous circulation and returned to the arterial system (see Chapter 17). Several VA ECMO configurations exist: (1) peripheral VA ECMO cannulas are usually placed in the descending aorta through the femoral artery and right atrium through the femoral vein and inferior vena cava, and (2) central VA ECMO cannulas are placed directly in the ascending aorta and the right atrium, respectively. Venous blood that is drained into the ECMO circuit will be fully oxygenated and carbon dioxide swept away. However, if the patient's lung function is impaired, any blood that passes through the pulmonary artery will be oxygenated only to the extent that the lungs are able to do so. Consequently, in this circumstance, blood ejected from the heart will be of lower oxygen saturation than blood that enters the arterial system through the ECMO circuit. This can lead to different oxygen tension in arterial blood depending upon where the blood sample is obtained. For example, oxygen saturation from the femoral artery catheter returning blood to the patient from the ECMO circuit will be 100% saturated. However, blood sampled from a right radial artery catheter may reflect lower oxygen saturation if large volumes of blood passed through the pulmonary circulation and were inadequately oxygenated and then ejected by the heart into the system circulation. Effective drainage from the right heart reduces the amount of blood that passes through the pulmonary vasculature and thus decreases the potential for pulmonary flow to affect oxygen saturation.

Patients occasionally present to the OR for placement of an Impella device using surgical access. Anesthetic management is similar to that described below for the routine anesthetic care of long-term VAD devices. Patients are routinely supported with inotropes (e.g., epinephrine, milrinone, dopamine) and may or may not have already had an IABP placed. Preservation of right heart function is critical to permit adequate delivery of blood to the left ventricle. Pulmonary hypertension is routinely treated with inhaled nitric oxide or other pulmonary vasodilators. As patients presenting for temporary VAD support generally manifest signs of cardiogenic shock, they frequently present from the ICU with full arterial line monitoring and central venous access. Perioperative echocardiography is used to guide device placement, assess left and right ventricular function, evaluate valvular function (especially the aortic valve in the case of placement of an Impella LVAD), and rule out any abnormal connections between the right and left heart (e.g., patent foramen ovale, atrial septal defect, ventricular septal defect).

LONG-TERM VAD PLACEMENT

Pulsatile flow, axial (non-pulsatile) flow, and centrifugal (non-pulsatile) flow type devices have been designed to provide long-term VAD support either as a "bridge to transplantation" or as "destination" therapy.

Blood is drained from the apex of the LV and returned through a graft sutured in the ascending aorta. As with short-term LVAD therapy, TEE is essential in the perioperative management of these devices. Patients with septal defects could shunt blood from right to left leading to hypoxemia following drainage of blood from a cannula placed in the apex of the LV. Aortic insufficiency would likewise complicate LVAD flow as well. A leaking aortic valve will merely drain blood back into the LV following delivery of the blood flow through the graft sutured to the ascending aorta. At times, surgeons will suture closed a leaky aortic valve or replace it with a bioprosthetic valve if necessary, to prevent creating a flow loop between the ascending aorta and LV cavity.

First-generation implantable pulsatile VADs (e.g., HeartMate I) were shown to decrease the death rate in patients awaiting heart transplantation and to improve survival after these patients undergo heart transplantation.[9] These initial implanted devices were somewhat large and placed in the abdominal cavity.

The REMATCH (randomized evaluation of mechanical assistance for the treatment of congestive heart failure) trial demonstrated that VADs could be employed in patients who were not candidates for heart transplantation with improved quality of life and survival.[10]

Variations in VAD design have been attempted to improve patient survival, mobility, and quality of life while reducing the incidence of complications such as bleeding, stroke, and infection. Non-pulsatile, continuous flow assist devices are currently employed and continually under development (Figure 11–5)[11,12] (Videos 11–3A and 11–3B). Although pulsatile devices provided excellent support, they were both noisy and subject to failure as they included a number of moving parts to displace and eject blood into the aorta. Pulsatile devices are no longer employed. Conversely, continuous flow devices are smaller and have fewer parts permitting them to be implanted in small patients for whom the old pulsatile devices were too large. Additionally, devices such as HeartWare or HeartMate III can be implanted entirely in the pericardial cavity.

Continuous flow devices direct blood flow either in an axial or centrifugal manner. The rotating impeller propels blood from the left ventricle into the aorta. Increasing the speed of the device increases the flow assuming the left ventricle has been adequately volume loaded. Delivery of sufficient volume to the left ventricle is necessary for the pump to be adequately loaded. Inadequate preload secondary to hypovolemia or right ventricular failure can lead to the walls of the left ventricle being "sucked down" impeding LVAD outflow. Likewise, LVAD flow is impaired if the device must work against increased afterload. The pulsatility index reflects the contribution to flow from contraction of the LV as well as the loading conditions of the heart.

ANESTHETIC MANAGEMENT OF VADs

The anesthetic management of the patient for VAD placement is largely dependent upon the circumstances in which VAD placement is being undertaken. The patient with heart failure presenting for elective VAD placement as "bridge to transplantation" presents challenges both similar and different from the patient undergoing temporary VAD placement for salvage following cardiac surgery.

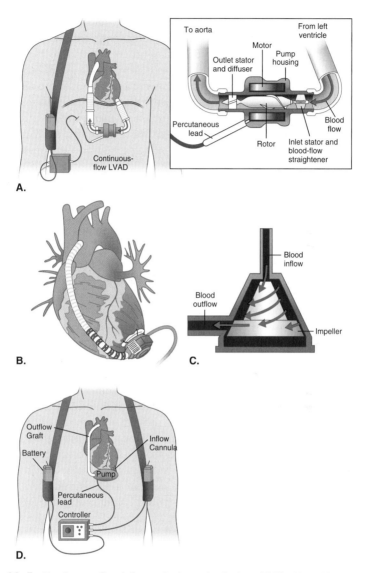

Figure 11–5. Continuous-flow left ventricular assist devices. (A) The HeartMate II, an axial-flow CF LVAD, propels blood parallel to the axis of rotation of the rotor. (B) The HeartWare ventricular assist device is smaller than the HeartMate II and attaches directly to the left ventricular apex. It provides centrifugal flow in which inflowing blood is propelled forward in a perpendicular direction, shown in (C). (D) Various components of an implantable LVAD, including the inflow cannula and outflow graft, percutaneous lead, system controller, and batteries. CF LVAD, continuous flow left ventricular assist device; LVAD, left ventricular assist device. [Image (A) reproduced with permission from Slaughter MS, Rogers JG, Milano CA, et al: Advanced heart failure treated with continuous-flow left ventricular assist device, *N Engl J Med*. 2009 Dec 3;361(23):2241-2251. Images (C) and (D) reproduced with permission from Mancini D, Colombo PC: Left Ventricular Assist Devices: A Rapidly Evolving Alternative to Transplant, *J Am Coll Cardiol*. 2015 Jun 16;65(23):2542-2555.]

Patients presenting for elective placement of an implantable VAD secondary to systolic heart failure are approached in a manner similar to any patient for cardiac surgery with severely compromised ventricular function. Hemodynamic collapse at the time of anesthetic induction should be anticipated irrespective of anesthetic agents employed. Inotropic agents are often necessary until CPB can be initiated. The exact choice of narcotics, inhalational agents, and muscle relaxants is less important than tailoring the anesthetic management to the goal of hemodynamic stability, preservation of blood pressure, and tissue perfusion. Many patients present with right heart failure producing hepatic congestion and subsequent coagulopathy. Patients with pulmonary hypertension and right ventricular dysfunction might not adequately deliver sufficient volume to an LVAD once placed, and the anesthesiologist must be prepared to both augment right heart function and decrease pulmonary artery pressures. Although elective VAD placement is preferred before the onset of significant organ impairment, kidney injury may likewise complicate perioperative management. Patients at high risk of hemodynamic collapse upon anesthesia induction may be supported with an IABP or percutaneous device. Some patients may have had a previous sternotomy making surgical exposure difficult. In this instance, femoral cardiopulmonary bypass can be initiated should hemodynamic collapse ensue or to support the patient during difficult surgical exposure (see Chapter 17). Assuming correction of other cardiac lesions (tricuspid regurgitation, aortic insufficiency, mitral stenosis) is not needed, LVADs can be placed with the patient on CPB without the need to arrest the heart with cardioplegia.

Following placement of the device, the surgical team will carefully de-air the VAD prior to initiation of pumping function. Once an LVAD is placed, its loading will be dependent upon right heart function, preload, and afterload. Unfortunately, many patients with long-standing severe heart failure have developed pulmonary hypertension. Consequently, high PA pressures and RV failure may prevent maximal loading of the new LVAD leading to inadequate flow. Inhaled nitric oxide or other pulmonary vasodilators are used to decrease pulmonary arterial resistance along with agents such as levosimendan or milrinone to support RV function. Should these maneuvers fail in improving RV function, temporary mechanical support of the right ventricle will be necessary.

LVAD flow is begun, and the patient is weaned from CPB. TEE is used to adjust VAD speed. Mean blood pressure > 70 mm Hg is maintained with preload and afterload adjusted based upon TEE assessment and pulsatility index. Hypovolemia and RV failure can lead to inadequate delivery of blood to the left ventricle resulting in a "suction event." In this situation, LVAD speed is temporarily reduced, allowing the ventricle to refill, and volume status (in the setting of hypovolemia) or RV function (in the setting of RV dysfunction) is optimized.

Following reversal of heparin, other blood products may be administered to achieve hemostasis (see Chapter 16). Anticoagulation with heparin, warfarin, and/or antiplatelet therapy are begun by the ICU team once postsurgical bleeding is corrected. Bleeding is a complication in patients managed with implantable LVADs. In addition to the effects of anticoagulation, LVAD patients develop type 2A von Willebrand disease secondary to sheer stress effects on the von Willebrand factor.

The postoperative management of the LVAD patient is discussed in Chapter 14.

Patients who are already in surgery may require a temporary VAD should separation from CPB not be possible only with inotropic and IABP support. A percutaneous or surgically placed device (Impella) can be employed to provide short-term support of the left ventricle with the hope that LV function will recover in the postoperative period. Anesthetic management is centered upon preservation of right ventricular function should only an LVAD be placed. Coagulopathy is corrected and intravascular volume maintained to adequately load left, right, or biventricular devices. Vascular tone can be preserved with the use of norepinephrine or vasopressin infusions as would be routinely employed in any patient with post CPB vasoplegia syndrome. Pulmonary vasodilation may unload the right ventricle and can be achieved by administration of inhaled pulmonary vasodilators (see Chapter 9) and inodilators.

With the VAD delivering a suitable cardiac output, bleeding is controlled, the surgical procedure completed, and the patient transported to the intensive care unit. Antithrombotic medications are administered based upon the requirements of the particular device.

At times, patients recover ventricular function such that mechanical support can be discontinued. In such instances the heart is weaned from VAD support, and the device explanted.

TEE AND VADs

TEE is critical in the perioperative management of the patient receiving a VAD.[13] Prior to placement of a VAD, a comprehensive TEE examination is mandatory. TEE is essential in diagnosing: (1) intracardiac shunts such as PFO and atrial or ventricular septal defects, (2) intracavitary thrombi especially in the left atrial appendage and left ventricle apex, (3) mitral valve stenosis which may restrict LVAD inflow, (4) aortic valve insufficiency which would hinder forward flow of the LVAD outflow into the systemic circulation, (5) aortic stenosis which would prevent intermittent opening of the aortic valve in left ventricles supported with continuous flow devices, (6) ascending aorta aneurysms or atheroma, and (7) right ventricle function and tricuspid valve regurgitation. Table 11–1 identifies abnormal echocardiographic findings and appropriate interventions.

After placement of the LVAD, TEE is critical to determine correct position and adequate flow through the VAD's inflow cannula.[14] The apical inflow continuous flow LVAD cannula should be angled toward the mitral valve and aligned with the LV inflow tract.[15] Color flow and continuous wave Doppler should demonstrate continuous, unidirectional flow with slight pulsatility. High-velocity flows suggest partial obstruction of the inflow cannula (> 1.5 m/s). Similarly, high outflow velocity (> 2 m/s) may indicate outflow graft obstruction or kinking (Figure 11–6). When continuous flow devices are employed, increasing VAD flow can compromise inflow if the ventricle walls are "sucked down" preventing adequate loading

Table 11-1. Management of Pre-Operative Echocardiographic Abnormalities in LVAD Candidates

Abnormality	Intervention
Aortic insufficiency	Repair, replace, or oversew
Tricuspid regurgitation	Controversial; consider repair or annuloplasty if moderate to severe
Mitral stenosis	Valvotomy
Mitral regurgitation	Usually none if not organic
Patent foramen ovale or atrial septal defect	Repair
Aortic root dilation or atheroma	Consider alteration in outflow cannula placement
Intracardiac thrombus	Consider surgical thrombectomy
Severe right ventricular dysfunction	Consider short-term RVAD or durable BiVAD

Abbreviations: BiVAD, biventricular assist device; LVAD, left ventricular assist device; RVAD, right ventricular assist device.
Reproduced with permission from Cohen DG, Thomas JD, Freed BH: Echocardiography and Continuous-Flow Left Ventricular Assist Devices: Evidence and Limitations, *JACC Heart Fail.* 2015 Jul;3(7):554-564.

of the VAD. RV function should be reevaluated after placement of the LVAD. Drainage of the LV can alter the relationship between the right ventricle and the interventricular septum leading to ineffective RV function. TEE is also employed perioperatively to ensure effective de-airing of the ventricle following VAD placement. Air entrainment in the right coronary artery can lead to transient right ventricular dysfunction. Lastly, TEE is used in VAD patients along with other modalities of hemodynamic monitoring (e.g., PA catheters) to discern the causes of hemodynamic instability and to assess response to therapy. The American Society of Echocardiography provides extensive recommendations on the use of echocardiography in the management of the LVAD patient. Table 11–2 presents the postoperative complications that can be detected by echocardiography. Moreover, they provide comprehensive guidance on the echo evaluation of the LVAD patient (see Table 11–3).

Figure 11–7 demonstrates fluoroscopic and echocardiographic images of an Impella device crossing the aortic valve.

HEART TRANSPLANTATION

The increasing number of patients with heart failure has been a major driving force behind the development of ventricular assist devices. Heart transplantation (HT) offers the heart failure patient the opportunity to live free from mechanical assistance. Unfortunately, the number of hearts available for transplantation is relatively small and as such the number of operations performed in the United States in any particular year is in the thousands. Because most of these operations are concentrated in a few heart transplant centers, the average cardiac anesthesiologist is not likely to be involved in their care. As with the VAD patients, anesthetic management is focused on maintaining hemodynamic stability in spite of greatly impaired systolic and diastolic function up until CPB can be initiated. Following

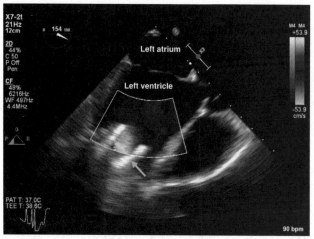

A.

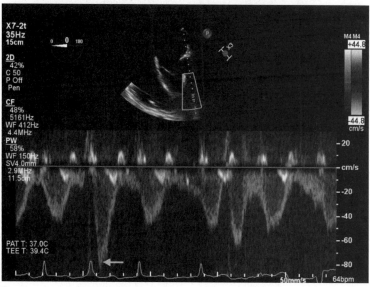

B.

Figure 11-6. (A) Mid-esophageal long-axis view with color flow Doppler demonstrating left ventricular assist device (LVAD) inflow cannula (arrow) at the left ventricular apex in adequate position with laminar flow. (B) Pulsed wave Doppler of blood flow through the LVAD inflow cannula demonstrating adequate peak velocities (arrow). (C) Ascending aorta in long-axis showing position of the LVAD outflow cannula (arrow). (D) Continuous wave Doppler of flow through the LVAD outflow cannula demonstrating adequate peak velocities (arrow).

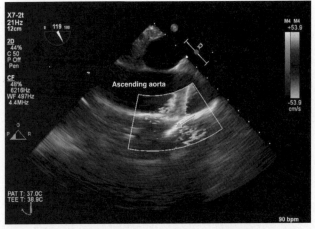

C.

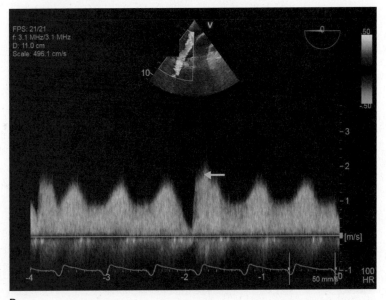

D.

Figure 11–6. (Continued)

placement of arterial and central venous access, anesthesia induction is undertaken using a variety of techniques depending upon patient's comorbidities and individual preference of the anesthesiologist. Inotropes and vasoconstrictors are employed to maintain blood pressure until CPB can be initiated. Should sternotomy not be readily accomplished, femoral-femoral bypass should be considered if the patient's hemodynamics deteriorate and access to the heart and great vessels is delayed. Sterile techniques as with all cardiac surgery patients must be scrupulous. Pulmonary

Table 11–2. Continuous-Flow LVAD Postimplant Complications and Device Dysfunction Detected by Echocardiography

---

Pericardial effusion
With or without cardiac tamponade including RV compression. *Tamponade*: respirophasic flow changes; poor RVOT SV.

LV failure secondary to partial LV unloading
(by serial exam comparison)
a. 2D/3D: increasing LV size by linear or volume measurements; increased AV opening duration, increased left atrial volume.
b. Doppler: increased mitral inflow peak E-wave diastolic velocity, increased E/A and E/e′ ratio, decreased deceleration time of mitral E velocity, worsening functional MR, and elevated pulmonary artery systolic pressure.

RV failure
a. 2D: increased RV size, decreased RV systolic function, high RAP (dilated IVC/leftward atrial septal shift), leftward deviation of ventricular septum.
b. Doppler: increased TR severity, reduced RVOT SV, reduced LVAD inflow cannula and/or outflow-graft velocities (i.e., < 0.5 m/s with severe failure); inflow-cannula high velocities if associated with a suction event. Note: a "too-high" LVAD pump speed may contribute to RV failure by increasing TR (septal shift) and/or by increasing RV preload.

Inadequate LV filling or excessive LV unloading
Small LV dimensions (typically < 3 cm and/or marked deviation of interventricular septum towards LV). Note: May be due to RV failure and/or pump speed too high for loading conditions.

LVAD suction with induced ventricular ectopy
Underfilled LV and mechanical impact of inflow cannula with LV endocardium, typically septum, resolves with speed turndown.

LVAD-related continuous aortic insufficiency
Clinically significant—at least moderate and possibly severe—characterized by an AR proximal jet-to-LVOT height ratio > 46%, or AR vena contracta ≥ 3 mm; increased LV size and relatively decreased RVOT SV despite normal/increased inflow cannula and/or outflow graft flows.

LVAD-related mitral regurgitation
a. Primary: inflow cannula interference with mitral apparatus.
b. Secondary: MR-functional, related to partial LV unloading/persistent heart failure.
Note: Elements of both a and b may be present.

Intracardiac thrombus
Including right and left atrial, LV apical, and aortic root thrombus

Inflow-cannula abnormality
a. 2D/3D: small or crowded inflow zone with or without evidence of localized obstructive muscle trabeculation, adjacent MV apparatus or thrombus; malpositioned inflow cannula.
b. *High-velocity* color or spectral Doppler at inflow orifice. Results from malposition, suction event/other inflow obstruction: aliased color-flow Doppler, CW Doppler velocity > 1.5 m/s.
c. *Low-velocity* inflow (markedly reduced peak systolic and nadir diastolic velocities) may indicate internal inflow-cannula thrombosis or more distal obstruction within the system. Doppler flow velocity profile may appear relatively "continuous" (decreased phasic/pulsatile pattern).

Outflow-graft abnormality
Typically due to obstruction/pump cessation.
a. 2D/3D imaging: visible kink or thrombus (infrequently seen).
b. Doppler: peak outflow-graft velocity ≥ 2 m/s* if near obstruction site; however, diminished or absent spectral Doppler signal if sample volume is remote from obstruction location, combined with lack of RVOT SV change and/or expected LV-dimension change with pump-speed changes.

(Continued)

Table 11–2. Continuous-Flow LVAD Postimplant Complications and Device Dysfunction Detected by Echocardiography (*Continued*)

Hypertensive emergency
New reduced/minimal AV opening relative to baseline exam at normal BP, especially if associated with new/worsened LV dilatation and worsening MR. Note: hypertension may follow an increase in pump speed.

Pump malfunction/pump arrest:
a. Reduced inflow-cannula or outflow-graft flow velocities on color and spectral Doppler or, with pump arrest, shows diastolic flow reversal.
b. Signs of worsening HF: including dilated LV, worsening MR, worsened TR, and/or increased TR velocity; attenuated speed-change responses: decrease or absence of expected changes in LV linear dimension, AV opening duration, and RVOT SV with increased or decreased pump speeds; for HVAD, loss of inflow-cannula Doppler artifact.

2D, Two-dimensional; 3D, three-dimensional; A, mitral valve late peak diastolic velocity; AR, aortic regurgitation; AV, aortic valve; BP, blood pressure; CW, continuous-wave; E, mitral valve early peak diastolic velocity; e′, mitral annular velocity; HVAD, HeartWare ventricular assist device; IVC, inferior vena cava; LV, left ventricular; LVAD, left ventricular assist device; LVOT, left ventricular outflow tract; MR, mitral regurgitation; MV, mitral valve; RAP, right atrial pressure; RV, right ventricular; RVOT, right ventricular outflow tract; SV, stroke volume; TR, tricuspid regurgitation.
*Note: based on observational data. The "normal" outflow graft peak velocities are not well defined. Because the HVAD outflow graft diameter is smaller than that of the HM II device. Therefore, the normal Doppler-derived HVAD outflow velocities may be somewhat higher on average than those observed for the HM II LVAD.
Adapted with permission from Estep JD, Chang SM, Bhimaraj A, et al: Imaging for ventricular function and myocardial recovery on nonpulsatile ventricular assist devices, *Circulation.* 2012 May 8;125(18):2265-2277.

Table 11–3. Perioperative TEE Protocol/Checklist

Two-Part Exam
1. Preimplantation Perioperative TEE Exam
Goals: confirm previous echocardiography (TTE or TEE) findings; detect unexpected abnormal findings before and after LVAD implantation
Blood pressure: via arterial line; for hypotension, consider vasopressor agent to assess AR severity
LV: size, systolic function, assess for thrombus
LA: size, assess for LA appendage/LA thrombus
RV: size, systolic function, catheters/leads
RA: size, assess for thrombus, catheters/leads
Interatrial septum: detailed 2D, color Doppler, IV saline contrast; *red flag:* PFO/ASD
Systemic veins: assess SVC, IVC
Pulmonary veins
Aortic valve: *red flags:* > mild AR, prosthetic valve
Mitral valve: *red flags:* ≥ moderate mitral stenosis, prosthetic mitral valve
Pulmonary valve: *red flags:* > mild PS, ≥ moderate PR, if RVAD planned; prosthetic valve
Pulmonary trunk: *red flags:* congenital anomaly (PDA, pulmonary atresia or aneurysm)
Tricuspid valve: TR, systolic PA pressure by TR velocity; *red flags:* ≥ moderate TR, > mild TS, prosthetic valve
Pericardium: screen for effusion; consider constrictive physiology
Aorta: root, ascending, transverse, and descending thoracic aorta; screen for aneurysm, congenital anomaly, dissection, or complex atheroma at each level

(*Continued*)

Table 11–3. Perioperative TEE Protocol/Checklist *(Continued)*

2. Postimplantation Perioperative TEE Exam
Goals: monitor for intracardiac air; rule out shunt; confirm device and native heart function
Pump type:
Pump speed:
Blood pressure: via arterial line; for hypotension (MAP of < 60 mmHg), consider vasopressor agent before assessing AR severity and other hemodynamic variables
Intracardiac air: left-sided chambers and aortic root during removal from CPB
LV: size, inflow-cannula position and flow velocities, septal position; *red flags:* small LV (over-pumping or RV failure), right-to-left septal shift; large LV (obstructed or inadequate pump flows)
Inflow-cannula position: 2D/3D, assess for possible malposition
Inflow-cannula flow: spectral and color Doppler (*red flag:* abnormal flow pattern/high/low velocities, especially after sternal closure)
LA: Assess LA appendage
RV: size, systolic function; *red flags:* signs of RV dysfunction
RA: size, assess for thrombus, catheters/leads
Interatrial septum: repeat IV saline test and color Doppler evaluation of IAS (*red flags:* PFO/ASD)
Systemic veins: (SVC, IVC)
Pulmonary veins: inspect
Aortic valve: degree of AV opening and degree of AR (*red flags:* > mild AR)
Mitral valve: exclude inflow-cannula interference with submitral apparatus; assess MR
Pulmonary valve: assess PR, measure RVOT SV if able
Pulmonary trunk: (if applicable, demonstrate RVAD outflow by color Doppler); assess PR
Tricuspid valve: assess TR (*red flags:* ≥ moderate TR); systolic PA pressure by TR velocity (if not severe TR)
Pericardium: screen for effusion/hematoma
Aorta: exclude iatrogenic dissection
Outflow graft: identify conduit path adjacent to RV/RA with color and spectral Doppler (when able)
Outflow graft-to-aorta anastomosis: assess patency/flow by color and spectral Doppler (when able) *red flags:* kinked appearance/turbulent flow/velocity > 2 m/s, particularly after sternal closure

2D, Two-dimensional; *3D*, three-dimensional; *AR*, aortic regurgitation; *ASD*, atrial septal defect; *AV*, aortic valve; *CPB*, cardiopulmonary bypass; *IAS*, interatrial septum; *IV*, intravenous; *IVC*, inferior vena cava; *LA*, left atrium; *LV*, left ventricle; *LVAD*, left ventricular assist device; *LVOT*, left ventricular outflow tract; *MAP*, mean arterial pressure; *MR*, mitral regurgitation; *PA*, pulmonary artery; *PFO*, patent foramen ovale; *PDA*, patent ductus arteriosus; *PR*, pulmonary regurgitation; *PS*, pulmonary stenosis; *RA*, right atrium; *RV*, ventricle; *RVAD*, right ventricular assist device; *RVOT*, right ventricular outflow tract; *SV*, stroke volume; *SVC*, superior vena cava; *TEE*, transesophageal echocardiography; *TR*, tricuspid regurgitation; *TS*, tricuspid stenosis; *TTE*, transthoracic echocardiography. Reproduced with permission from Stainback RF, Estep JD, Agler DA: Echocardiography in the Management of Patients with Left Ventricular Assist Devices: Recommendations from the American Society of Echocardiography, *J Am Soc Echocardiogr.* 2015 Aug;28(8):853-909.

arterial catheters are usually not placed, as the native heart will be excised; however, if desired, a PA catheter can be placed in a sterile sheath for advancement into the grafted heart to assist in separation from cardiopulmonary bypass. Close communication between the anesthesia team, the surgical team, and the organ procurement team is critical to coordinate timely delivery of the heart to be transplanted to minimize the ischemic time prior to implantation.

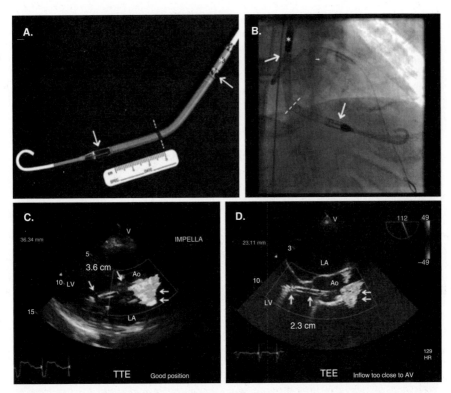

Figure 11–7. (A) Photograph of the Impella CP Percutaneous LVAD, showing the pump impeller housing (*), blood-inflow zone (downward arrow) and blood-outflow zone (upward arrow) zones, with the distal pigtail catheter component. (B) Fluoroscopic X-ray image of the Impella CP device in situ. Blood-inflow zone (downward arrow), blood-outflow zone (upward arrow), impeller housing (*). The radiopaque marker (immediately below dotted line) indicates the desired aortic annulus level, which is 3.5 cm from the middle of the inflow zone. (C) TTE parasternal long-axis view. The Impella device crosses the AV. The distance from the blood inflow area (left single arrow) to the aortic annulus (right single arrow) is approximately 3.6 cm. (D) On TEE, the distance from the inflow area (left single arrow) to the aortic annulus (right single arrow) is 2.3 cm; this is not far enough into the left ventricle to provide a safety margin, although the device is functioning normally). In views (C) and (D), the double arrows indicate a typical pump-impeller aliased color-Doppler artifact. [Reproduced with permission from Stainback RF, Estep JD, Agler DA: Echocardiography in the Management of Patients with Left Ventricular Assist Devices: Recommendations from the American Society of Echocardiography, *J Am Soc Echocardiogr.* 2015 Aug;28(8):853-909.]

HT begins with the identification of a suitable donor. Once a donor is identified, multiple procurement teams begin the collection of various organs for transplantation. Prior to procuring the heart, cardioplegia solution is administered and the heart is removed from the chest and prepared for transport. Once the procurement team is satisfied with the condition of the graft and surgeons give the "go" order, the recipient is prepared for general anesthesia. The patient's last intake by mouth is confirmed and the anesthetic induction managed accordingly (e.g., cricoid pressure, rapid sequence induction). Induction and maintenance are determined by the individual preferences of the anesthesia team involved. As HT patients generally have severely limited left ventricular function, the sympathectomy and reduction of vascular tone that often accompany anesthetic induction can result in profound hypotension. Vasopressin can readily restore vascular tone and support the blood pressure. Inotropes are administered to improve ventricular function. Many patients will be supported by home milrinone therapy. Should the heart fail and severe hemodynamic instability ensue while awaiting the graft, CPB is initiated to preserve organ perfusion. Often the HT patient will be supported with a previously placed continuous flow LVAD that will be explanted with their native heart following institution of CPB.

Following surgical anastomosis of the graft, the patient is weaned from CPB in the usual manner. The surgical team will request the perioperative administration of various immunosuppressive agents (e.g., methylprednisolone, cyclosporine, simulect) It is important to confirm with the surgical team exactly what agents are desired and the exact timing for their delivery before the start of the case. Direct-acting inotropes are used since the grafted heart is denervated from the native sympathetic and parasympathetic nervous systems. TEE is extensively employed to assess right and left graft heart function. The right ventricle of the transplanted heart may not be accustomed to the elevated pulmonary artery pressures present in many heart failure patients. Interventions to prevent right heart failure include avoidance of hypercarbia and hypoxemia, the use of inhaled pulmonary vasodilators (e.g., inhaled nitric oxide) and inotropic support (e.g., epinephrine, milrinone). Temporary mechanical support of the right ventricle is occasionally necessary. Separation from bypass is undertaken in the usual fashion; protamine is administered, and blood products are given as indicated. Over-administration of fluids and blood products can produce right heart overload. Echocardiography is essential in the assessment of right ventricular function and loading.

In patients with severe pulmonary hypertension and biventricular failure, combined heart lung transplants are undertaken. The total artificial heart has been a work in progress since 1982 with the first implantation in Dr. Barney Clark.[16] Pulsatile devices such as the CardioWest have been used as a bridge to transplant. Pneumatic drive lines displace blood from the chambers of the artificial heart generating the stroke volume. Blood pressure is dependent upon supporting the vascular tone and the stroke volume generated by the device. Continuous flow total artificial hearts are under investigation.

CASE SCENARIO

A 42-year-old man presents for coronary artery bypass surgery following anterior myocardial infarction. The estimated ejection fraction is 20% preoperatively.

Following completion of three bypass grafts, the anesthesiologist weans the patient from CPB. BP is 60/40 mm Hg, and PA pressure is 60/40 mm Hg.

TEE demonstrates biventricular failure. What actions might the anesthesiologist now attempt?

The anesthesiologist starts milrinone, epinephrine, and vasopressin infusions.

The BP increases to 65/45 mm Hg, and the PA pressures increase to 65/46 mm Hg. The patient develops ventricular fibrillation. What should be the next response of the anesthesiologist?

The bypass cannulas are still in place, and the patient is returned promptly to CPB. (No protamine had been given.) The surgeon defibrillates the heart using internal paddles. The patency of the grafts and adequacy of surgical revascularization is confirmed. The epinephrine infusion is increased and an IABP is placed at 1:1 support permitting the patient to be successfully separated from CPB. Norepinephrine infusion may be added to ensure adequate systemic perfusion pressure.

Had the IABP not been effective, what other options would the surgery team have?

Failure to wean from CPB could result in intraoperative death. Additionally, after assessment of left and right ventricular function, a ventricular assist device could be placed. If a VAD is to be placed, a comprehensive TEE examination should evaluate for mechanical factors that might hinder adequate function of the VAD (intracardiac shunts, mitral valve stenosis, aortic valve insufficiency, etc.). After placement of the VAD, TEE should evaluate proper VAD function including cannula position, inflow, and outflow. If biventricular failure is placed, both left and right heart mechanical support can be performed.

REFERENCES

1. Torchiana DF, Hirsch G, Buckley M. Intraaortic balloon pumping for cardiac support: trends in practice and outcome, 1968 to 1995. *J Thorac Cardiovasc Surg.* 1997;113(4):758-769.
2. Cheng J, den Uil C, Hoeks S, et al. Percutaneous left ventricular assist devices vs. intra-aortic balloon pump counterpulsation for treatment of cardiogenic shock: a meta-analysis. *Eur Heart J.* 2009;30:2101-2108.
3. Mather P, Konstam M. Newer mechanical devices in the management of acute heart failure. *Heart Fail Rev.* 2007;12:167-172.
4. Aragon J, Lee M, Kar S, Makkar R, et al. Percutaneous left ventricular assist device: "Tandem Heart" for high-risk coronary surgery. *Catheter Cardiovasc Interv.* 2005;65:346-352.
5. Thiele H, Sick P, Boudriot E, et al. Randomized comparison of intra-aortic balloon support with a percutaneous left ventricular assist device in patients with revascularized acute myocardial infarction complicated by cardiogenic shock. *E Heart J.* 2005;26:1276-1283.
6. Burkoff D, O'Neill W, Brunckhorst C, et al. Feasibility study of the use of the TandemHeart percutaneous ventricular assist device for treatment of cardiogenic shock. *Catheter Cardiovasc Interv.* 2006;68:211-217.
7. Ouweneel D, Eriksen E, Sjauw K, et al. Percutaneous mechanical circulatory support versus intra-aortic balloon pump in cardiogenic shock after acute myocardial infarction. *JACC.* 2017;69(3):278-287.
8. Rihal C, Naidu S, Givertz M, et al. 2015 SCAI/ACC/HFSA/STS Clinical expert consensus statement on the use of percutaneous mechanical circulatory support devices in cardiovascular care (endorsed by the American Heart Association, The Cardiological Society of India, and Sociedad Latino Americana de Cardiologia Intervencion; Affirmation of value by the Canadian Association of Interventional Cardiology-Association Canadienne de Cardiologie d'intervention). *J Card Fail.* 2015;21(6):499-518.

9. Frazier O, Rose E, McCarthy P, et al. Improved mortality and rehabilitation of transplant candidates treated with a long-term implantable left ventricular assist system. *Ann Surg.* 1995;22(3):327-338.

10. Rose E, Gelijns A, Moskowitz A, et al. Long term use of a left ventricular assist device for end-stage heart failure. *NEJM.* 2001;345(20):1435-1443.

11. Slaughter M, Pagani F, Rogers J, et al. Clinical management of continuous flow left ventricular assist devices in advanced heart failure. *J Heart Lung Transplant.* 2010;29:S1-S39.

12. Miller L, Pagani F, Russell S, et al. Use of a continuous flow device in patients awaiting heart transplantation. *NEJM.* 2007;357:885-896.

13. Chumnanvej S, Wood M, McGillivray T, Vidal Melo M. Perioperative echocardiographic examination for ventricular assist device implantation. *Anesth Analg.* 2007;105:583-601.

14. Castillo J, Anyanwu A, Adams D, et al. Real time 3-dimensional echocardiographic assessment of current continuous flow rotary left ventricular assist devices. *J Cardiothorac Vasc Anesth.* 2009;23(5):702-710.

15. Catena E, Tasca G. Role of echocardiography in the perioperative management of mechanical circulatory assistance. *Best Pract Res Clin Anaesthesiol.* 2012;26:199-216.

16. Sale S, Smedira N. Total artificial heart. *Best Pract Res Clin Anaesthesiol.* 2012;26:147-165.

REVIEWS

Stainback R, Estep J, Agler D, et al. Echocardiography in the management of patients with left ventricular assist devices: recommendations from the American Society of Echocardiography. *J Am Soc Echocardiogr.* 2015;28:853-909.

Cohen D, Thomas J, Greed B, et al. Echocardiography and continuous flow left ventricular assist devices. *JACC Heart Fail.* 2015;3(7):554-564.

Chung M. Perioperative management of the patient with a left ventricular assist device for non cardiac surgery. *Anesth Analg.* 2018;126(6):1839-1850.

Meng M, Spellman J. Anesthetic management of the patient with a ventricular assist device. *Best Pract Res Clin Anaesthesiol.* 2017;31:215-226.

MacKay E, Patel P, Gutsch J, et al. Contemporary clinical niche for intra-aortic balloon counterpulsation in perioperative cardiovascular practice: an evidence based review for the cardiovascular anesthesiologist. *J Cardiothorac Vasc Anesth.* 2017;31:309-320.

Rihal C, Naidu S, Givertz M, et al. 2016 SCAI/ACC/HFSA/STS clinical expert consensus statement on the use of percutaneous mechanical circulatory support devices in cardiovascular care. *J Card Fail.* 2015;21(6):499-518.

Dangas G, Kini A, Sharma S, et al. Impact of hemodynamic support with Impella 2.5 versus intra aortic balloon pump on prognostically important clinical outcomes in patients undergoing high risk percutaneous coronary intervention (from the PROTECT II trial). *Am J Cardiol.* 2014;113:222-228.

Nguyen L, Banks D. Anesthetic management of the patient undergoing heart transplantation. *Best Pract Res Clin Anaesthesiol.* 2017;31:189-200.

Ramsingh D, Harvey R, Runyon A, Benggon M. Anesthesia for heart transplantation. *Anesthesiology Clin.* 2017;35:453-471.

Anesthesia for Patients With Congenital Heart Disease

12

TOPICS

The incidence of congenital heart defects is approximately 8 in 1000 births.[1] Over the course of the past decades survival of children with congenital heart disease (CHD) has improved. Today, adults frequently present for routine general surgery and obstetric care after having had various congenital cardiac surgical repairs in childhood. Unfortunately, the frequently multistaged surgical repairs necessary to improve survival in children often result in complex cardiac physiology in adulthood. Knowledge of the anatomy of the original structural defect and the repairs undertaken is essential in the choice of appropriate monitoring and anesthetic techniques for otherwise routine procedures. Moreover, CHD patients may require additional heart surgery and/or cardiac transplantation later in life. For children with CHD identification of those patients at highest risk for anesthesia complications is critical. Such children include those with a functional single ventricle, children with suprasystemic pulmonary hypertension, children with left ventricular outflow tract obstruction, and lastly patients with dilated cardiomyopathy.[2] This chapter highlights the anatomy, physiology, and correction of common congenital heart defects. In general, surgical repairs are directed at ensuring the delivery of oxygenated blood to the systemic tissues and eliminating communications between the right and left heart. Of course, for some CHD patients the distinction of which is the right heart and which is the left heart may not be entirely clear. Consequently, when considering the CHD patient, tracing the flow of blood through the chambers of the heart into the circulation and back again provides the basis toward acquiring an understanding of CHD.

ATRIAL SEPTAL DEFECTS

Atrial septal defects (ASDs) are abnormal communications between the left atrium (LA) and right atrium (RA). A patent foramen ovale (PFO) may be present in up to 25% of the population and produces a small interatrial communication as a consequence of failure of the septum primum and septum secundum to fuse. ASDs account for 6% to 10% of the CHD population and present in a variety of ways.[3] Eighty percent of ASDs are of the ostium secundum type (Figure 12–1 and **Videos 12–1A and 12–1B**) located in the middle of the interatrial septum. Defects located lower in the atrial septum [toward the atrial-ventricular (AV) valves] are

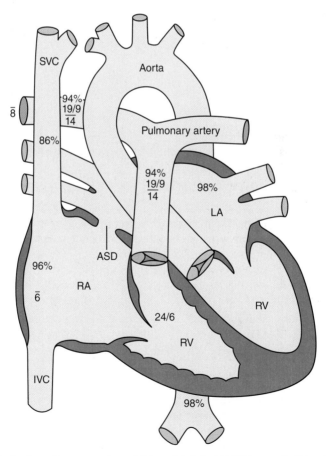

Figure 12–1. An ostium secundum atrial septal defect (ASD) is seen in this schematic. Pressures and oxygen saturations in the various parts of the heart are displayed.

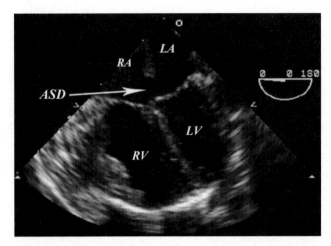

Figure 12–2. An ostium primum atrial septal defect (ASD) in a midesophageal four-chamber view. LA = left atrium; LV = left ventricle; RA = right atrium; RV = right ventricle. [Reproduced with permission from Burch TM, Mizuguchi KA, DiNardo JA: Echocardiographic assessment of atrial septal defects, *Anesth Analg.* 2012 Oct;115(4):772-775.]

ostium primum ASDs and are at times associated with a ventricular septal defect (VSD) (Figure 12–2). Sinus venosus ASDs occur close to the junctions of the superior vena cava (SVC) or inferior vena cava (IVC) with the RA (Figure 12–3). Sinus venosus ASDs are often associated with pulmonary vein anomalies and anomalous return of oxygenated pulmonary vein blood to the right atrium.

ASDs generally produce a left-to-right shunt of blood across the defect. Thus, oxygenated blood is delivered into the right heart circulation to be returned to the lungs through the pulmonary artery. The oxygen saturation of the RA is increased, and RA and right ventricular (RV) volume is increased. The amount of blood, which flows between the chambers, is dependent upon both the size of the defect and the pressure gradient between the chambers. A ratio of the pulmonary blood flow (Qp) to the systemic blood flow (Qs) of less than 1.5 is often adequately tolerated; however, when the Qp/Qs ratio exceeds 3, symptoms secondary to overload of the pulmonary circulation appear.[4] Over time, pulmonary artery hypertension can develop resulting in RV hypertrophy and failure. Eventually, right-sided pressures can exceed those of the left heart resulting in an Eisenmenger syndrome where deoxygenated venous blood flows in a right-to-left direction producing hypoxemia.

Over time many small defects of < 3 mm will close spontaneously; however, defects greater than 8 mm generally will not resolve spontaneously.[4-6] Approximately 20% of ASDs will close during the first year of life and many go undetected even into adulthood. However, patients with ASDs are at risk for bacterial endocarditis and paradoxical right-to-left embolism and stroke. Larger ASDs often become manifest in the patient's third decade heralded by complaints of dyspnea, arrhythmias, and congestive heart failure (CHF).[4]

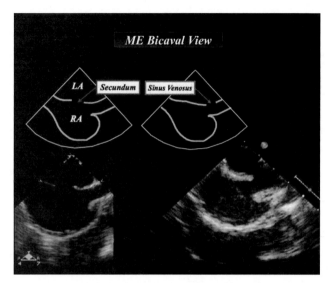

Figure 12–3. A comparison of an ostium secundum atrial septal defect (ASD) and a superior sinus venosus ASD seen in a bicaval view. LA = left atrium; ME = midesophageal; RA = right atrium. [Reproduced with permission from Burch TM, Mizuguchi KA, DiNardo JA: Echocardiographic assessment of atrial septal defects, *Anesth Analg.* 2012 Oct;115(4):772-775.]

The indications for surgical or catheter-mediated repair of an ASD include:

- RV volume overload
- Qp/Qs > 2

Although some ASDs will close spontaneously, sinus venosus and ostium primum ASDs will not close without intervention.

Surgical closure of ASDs requires the use of cardiopulmonary bypass (CPB). Depending upon the size of the defect being repaired, surgeons can perform either a primary suture closure of the defect or use a pericardial or synthetic patch.

Children taken to surgery for ASD repair are premedicated with oral or intravenous midazolam. Invasive arterial pressure monitoring is employed. Anesthesia induction can be through the use of inhalational agents or intravenous agents. Maintenance of anesthesia in the pediatric population is with a combination of opioids, inhalational agents, and muscle relaxants. Prior to cannulation for the initiation of CPB, heparin is administered as in the adult population. Often CPB times are relatively brief and the patients are generally separated from CPB with little need for inotropic support. Following repair of the ASD, pressure within the LA will increase and right atrial pressure (CVP) will decrease secondary to elimination of left-to-right flow into the RA. The surgeon can place a left atrial pressure line to discern left ventricular preload.[4] Surgical mortality is low, and the hospital length of stay is generally less than 4 days.

Many ASDs can be closed with devices delivered by a cardiac catheter. These procedures are performed under fluoroscopic and echocardiographic guidance and eliminate the need for sternotomy and CPB. Patient selection is essential to identify those most amenable to catheter-mediated repairs. Ostium primum and sinus venosus ASDs generally are not correctable by catheter-based approaches due to the location of the defect and associated pathologies. The Amplatzer septal occluder system (AGA Medical Corporation, Golden Valley, Minnesota) consists of two attached circular discs. The larger of the two discs faces the LA, while the smaller disc faces the RA (Figure 12–4). The device straddles the defect in the atrial septum after being introduced via a catheter placed in a femoral vein. Endothelialization occurs over roughly 6 months following device placement. The procedure is usually performed under general anesthesia. Complications are rare but include air embolization, device dislodgement into the left atrium, and device impingement onto the tricuspid and mitral valve. An antithrombotic regimen is required for 6 months

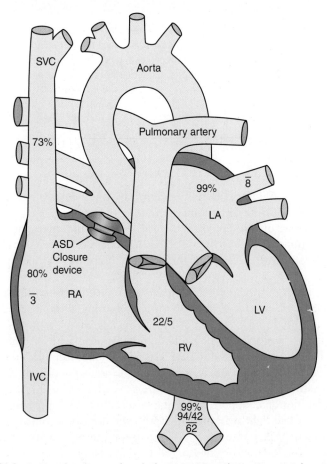

Figure 12–4. An Amplatzer septal occluder is positioned across an atrial septal defect.

or longer to prevent clot formation on the surface of the device. Additionally, antibiotic prophylaxis is indicated for dental procedures following device placement.

VENTRICULAR SEPTAL DEFECTS

Ventricular septal defects (VSDs) are abnormal communications between the left and the right heart through the ventricular septum (Videos 12–2 and 12–3). VSDs represent 20% of congenital heart defects.[7] VSDs are classified by their location along the ventricular septum:[8]

- Type I: 5% to 7% of VSDs are Type I or subarterial VSDs. They are also known as supracristal, outlet, subpulmonary, infundibular, conal, and doubly committed. They are present near the aortic and pulmonic valves (Figure 12–5). They can cause herniation of the right coronary cusp of the aortic valve into the VSD resulting in aortic insufficiency.

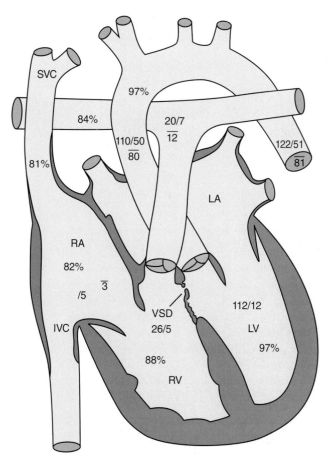

Figure 12–5. Type I, supracristal VSD.

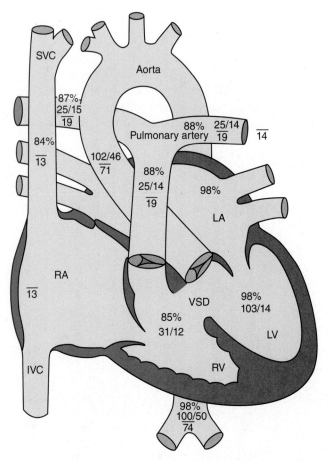

Figure 12–6. Type II, perimembranous VSD.

- Type II: Approximately 80% of VSDs are perimembranous VSDs. They are also known as infracristal, paramembranous, and conoventricular VSDs. The defect is in the membranous portion of the interventricular septum (Figure 12–6). This defect is associated with septal malalignment, overriding aorta, subaortic stenosis, and tricuspid valve leaflet herniation into the septal defect.
- Type III: 5% to 8% of VSDs are inlet VSDs. These are also known as canal-type VSDs or endocardial cushion defects. They are located inferior to the atrioventricular (AV) valve.
- Type IV: 5% to 20% of VSDs are muscular VSDs and are found in the muscular part of the interventricular septum (Figure 12–7).

Many VSDs are small and will close spontaneously. Spontaneous closure occurs most frequently during the first year of life. Some small, restrictive VSDs result in a minimal trans-septal blood flow and limited risk.[9] Others result in free communications between the ventricles, and the degree to which blood is shunted across the

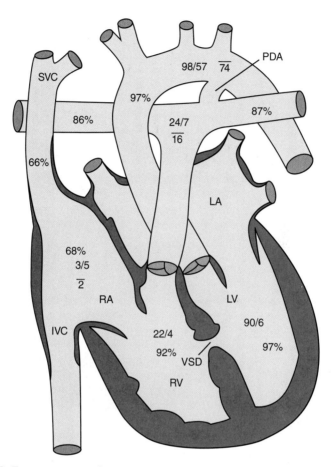

Figure 12–7. Type IV, muscular VSD.

septum is dependent upon the ratio of systemic to pulmonary vascular resistance. When pulmonary vascular resistance is low, flow from the left heart into the right is increased. The result is volume overload and CHF. Over time, pulmonary vascular resistance increases secondary to development of pulmonary vascular occlusive disease leading to reversal of the shunt (flow becomes right-to-left), so-called Eisenmenger syndrome.[8] Approximately 10% of patients with an uncorrected VSD will develop Eisenmenger syndrome, which carries a high incidence of early death.

Prevention of overcirculation in the pulmonary vasculature is essential to avoid pulmonary hypertension, right ventricular failure, and Eisenmenger syndrome. Initial anesthetic management for surgical closure of VSDs is similar to that described for ASD repair. However, nitric oxide (NO) along with infusions of the inotropic medications may be required to effectively separate from CPB in the setting of ventricular failure and pulmonary hypertension. Conduction defects secondary to manipulation of the interventricular septum may occur necessitating temporary and at times permanent pacing following repair.

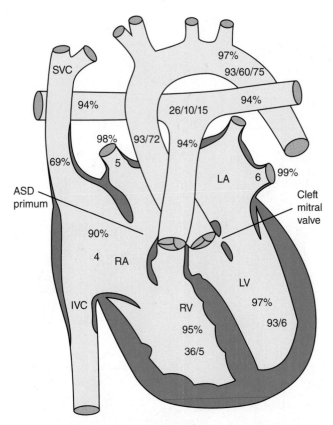

Figure 12–8. A partial AV canal with cleft mitral valve and ostium primum ASD.

Defects in the atrioventricular canal or endocardial cushion can result in an ostium primum ASD, a cleft anterior leaflet of the mitral valve, and an inlet VSD. They represent approximately 2.9% of CHD patients. AV canal defects can be associated with Down syndrome. Figure 12–8 demonstrates a so-called "partial" AV canal defect consisting of a primum ASD and a cleft mitral valve. Figure 12–9 reveals a complete AV canal defect with the addition of an inlet VSD. Patients develop an initial left-to-right shunt with associated CHF. If left untreated, pulmonary hypertension develops leading to flow reversal from right to left. Surgical therapy often consists of not only closure of the atrial and ventricular septal defects but also correction of any abnormalities found in the patient's atrioventricular valves. Inotropic support, inhaled pulmonary vasodilator therapy, and temporary pacing are often necessary to successfully separate the AV canal patient from CPB.

VSDs can occur acutely in the adult population following myocardial infarction or secondary to iatrogenic mishap (e.g., excessive myectomy resected hypertrophic cardiomyopathy surgery). Patients are often quite unstable and are taken to surgery for attempts at salvage.

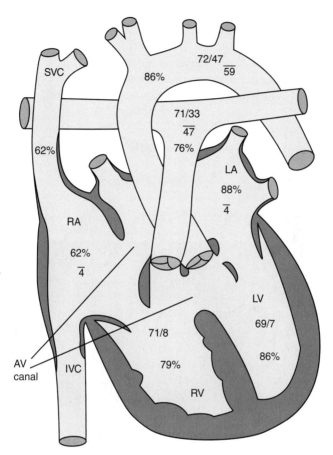

Figure 12–9. Complete AV canal.

TETRALOGY OF FALLOT

Tetralogy of Fallot (TOF) is the most common cyanotic heart disease representing 10% of all CHD patients (**Video 12–4**). TOF consists of four anatomic abnormalities:

1. Right ventricular outflow tract (RVOT) obstruction
2. RV hypertrophy
3. A large, unrestricted VSD
4. An aorta that overrides both the left and right ventricle receiving flow from both chambers (Figure 12–10).

Additionally, coronary artery abnormalities may present (5%–12%) with the left anterior descending coronary artery (LAD) branching from the right coronary artery (RCA). Other associated anomalies include pulmonary valve atresia, ASD, persistent left SVC, anomalous pulmonary vein connections, and dextrocardia.

The presentation of the TOF patient is dependent upon the degree of RVOT obstruction. Patients with significant RVOT obstruction will have a right-to-left

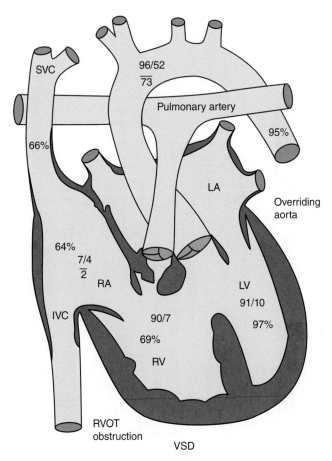

Figure 12–10. Tetralogy of Fallot: VSD, overriding aorta, RV hypertrophy, and right ventricular outflow obstruction.

shunt resulting in severe hypoxemia and cyanosis with saturations ranging from 70% to 80%. On the other hand, those with minimal obstruction "pink tet" will have VSD physiology with a left-to-right shunt. Often RVOT obstruction has a dynamic component leading to acute increases of obstruction and exacerbation of right-to-left shunting. Such episodes, referred to as "tet spells," may produce transient cerebral ischemia and loss of consciousness. These may occur secondary to infundibular spasm secondary to increased activity in the sympathetic nervous system as might occur with crying.[10]

Induction of anesthesia can produce a fall in systemic vascular resistance (SVR) leading to a worsening right-to-left shunt and hypoxemia. Should tet spells present in the perioperative period, they can be relieved by:

- Hyperventilation with 100% FiO_2
- Volume administration
- Phenylephrine

- Knee-chest position
- Increasing anesthetic depth to reduce infundibular spasm secondary to inadequate anesthetic depth

Ultimately, therapy is directed at increasing systemic vascular resistance, relieving infundibular spasm, and decreasing pulmonary vascular resistance.

The presence of chronic cyanosis can lead to polycythemia and the potential for embolic stroke across the VSD. Infectious vegetations are also a source of systemic emboli in TOF and other CHD patients at increased risk for endocarditis.

The majority of TOF patients are repaired in infancy except those whose pulmonary arteries are too underdeveloped.[10,11] A palliative Blalock-Taussig-Thomas (BTT) shunt can be performed, whereby the subclavian artery is anastomosed to the ipsilateral branch of the pulmonary artery (Figure 12–11). The BTT shunt provides additional blood flow to the pulmonary vasculature to relieve cyanosis until a

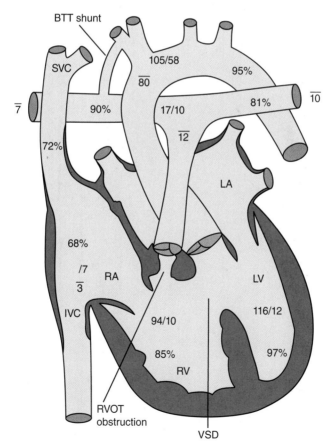

Figure 12–11. A BTT shunt has been placed to increase pulmonary blood flow in this schematic of a patient with tetralogy of Fallot (TOF).

definitive repair can be completed. In those patients thought to be candidates for a complete surgical repair, TOF surgery consists of:

- Ligation of any previous BT shunt
- Relief of RVOT obstruction through resection of excess muscle mass (Figure 12–12)
- Closure of the VSD
- Patch to enlarge subannular or transannular area of RVOT
- RV to PA conduit if pulmonary atresia is present

Perioperative anesthetic management of the TOF patient is centered upon promoting pulmonary blood flow and avoiding cyanosis. Dehydration should be avoided preoperatively. Oral midazolam can be given with the child appropriately monitored to reduce perioperative anxiety, crying, and potentially the incidence of tet spells. An inhalational induction with sevoflurane is acceptable if intravenous access is not available. Nonetheless, limited pulmonary blood flow may slow an inhalational induction. The myocardial depressant effects of inhalational agents

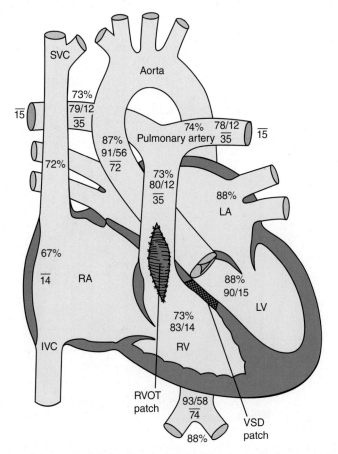

Figure 12–12. Repair of TOF includes closure of VSD and enlargement of the RVOT.

may be useful in limiting any infundibular spasm, RVOT obstruction, and right-to-left shunting across the VSD. On the other hand, systemic vasodilation and tachycardia caused by inhalational agents may increase right-to-left shunting and hypoxemia. If an intravenous line is readily available, etomidate, ketamine, and fentanyl used in combination with muscle relaxants and vasopressors can be employed. The presence of a right-to-left shunt may decrease the time for anesthetic effect following intravenous induction with some drug bypassing the lungs. Obviously, in any patient with right-to-left shunts all intravenous lines must be purged of air to prevent systemic air emboli perioperatively.

Systemic vascular resistance is maintained perioperatively with the use of phenylephrine and the patient's volume augmented with fluid boluses. Inotropes generally are not used in the peri-induction period as they might worsen infundibular spasm and promote right-to-left shunting. Should infundibular spasm be suspected, small doses of esmolol could be given.

A radial artery catheter is placed opposite to that of any BT shunt because the shunt can "steal" blood from the patient's upper extremity. Central venous access is obtained to deliver fluids and other medications perioperatively.

Maintenance of anesthesia is achieved with combinations of narcotics, muscle relaxants, and inhalational agents. High airway pressures are avoided to minimize the impact of mechanical ventilation upon PVR.

Separation from CPB following surgical repair may require high right-sided filling pressures secondary to a generally poorly compliant RV in the TOF patient.[12] RV dysfunction is common following TOF repair. Adequate preload, inotropic support, and afterload reduction are mainstays of therapy for weaning from CPB. Complete heart block and right bundle branch block are common perioperatively, and temporary pacing is often necessary. Pressure-controlled ventilation with 100% oxygen and the lowest airway pressure to maintain a $PaCO_2$ of 25 to 33 mm Hg is employed. As such, PVR is minimized to the degree possible. The majority of patients are extubated within 12 hours and require 1 to 2 days of ICU care.

Unfortunately, many patients following TOF repair are at risk for a variety of long-term complications, which can complicate anesthetic management of these patients for noncardiac surgery. Residual VSD and pulmonic valvular incompetence are most unwelcome surgical sequelae. Those patients with hemodynamically significant VSD are at risk for developing pulmonary hypertension and should be reoperated to correct this defect.[13] RV dysfunction can also complicate long-term management. Ventricular dysrhythmias are common and can emanate from various foci including the area of infundibular resection and areas near the VSD patch.[14] Although isolated PVCs may be well-tolerated, potentially lethal ventricular rhythms can develop with the overall incidence of sudden death of 0.3% per patient a year after surgical repair.[15] Anesthesiologists may be called upon to care for the patient following TOF repair undergoing electrophysiologic studies and placement of antiarrhythmia implantable devices. All patients with TOF whether repaired or not require endocarditis prophylaxis.[16]

Anesthetic management of the TOF patient requiring noncardiac surgery is similar to that described for cardiac surgical repair. Interventions are directed toward the maintenance of pulmonary blood flow and the avoidance of right-to-left shunting. Appropriate antibiotic prophylaxis *must* be administered, and the patient monitored as described above for any major surgical intervention.

TRANSPOSITION OF THE GREAT ARTERIES

Transposition of the great arteries (TGA) essentially means ventricular arterial discordance. These lesions represent 5% to 7% of all CHD and have a high mortality within the first year of life.[17] Complete transposition describes a patient with atrioventricular concordance but ventriculo-arterial discordance. As such, the right atrium is connected to the right ventricle via the tricuspid valve but the right ventricle is connected to the systemic artery, the aorta (Figure 12–13). The left atrium is likewise connected via the mitral valve to the left ventricle, which in turn is connected incorrectly to the pulmonary artery. The coronary arteries emerge from the aorta. Consequently, without other defects in the heart, deoxygenated blood would only be delivered to systemic circulation as blood flow is in parallel and

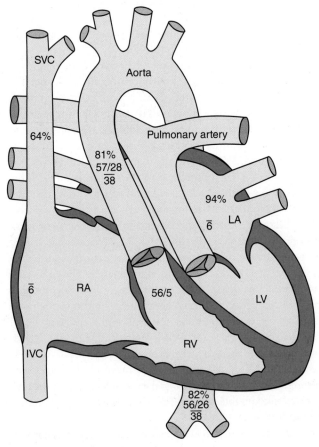

Figure 12–13. Transposition of the great vessels.

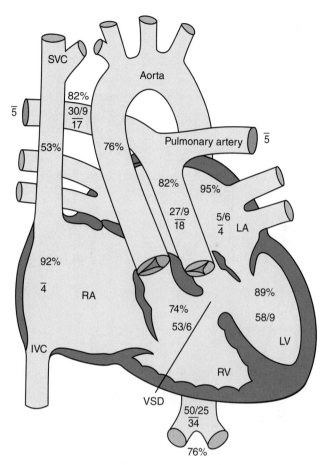

Figure 12–14. Associated abnormalities permit intermixing of blood in TGA patients as seen in this schematic.

not in series. However, this condition is associated with other defects including a patent ductus arteriosus (PDA), PFO, and VSD (Figure 12–14). Consequently, oxygenated and deoxygenated blood intermix permitting transient survival until surgical repair can be undertaken. Without mixing of blood secondary to other structural defects, life would not be possible. In patients with TGA and a VSD mixing occurs in the ventricle. In those patients born with an intact interventricular septum, blood mixing is dependent upon a PFO, ASD, or PDA. Prostaglandin E_1 infusions are at times needed to preserve PDA blood flow. Likewise, balloon atrial septostomy in the catheterization laboratory can be performed to increase the connection between the systemic and pulmonary circulations at the atrial level (Figure 12–15). Other patients may be provided a BTT shunt to improve pulmonary blood flow (Figure 12–16).

Definitive surgical repair is the arterial switch or Jatene operation. Both the ascending aorta and pulmonary artery are transected above their respective valves.

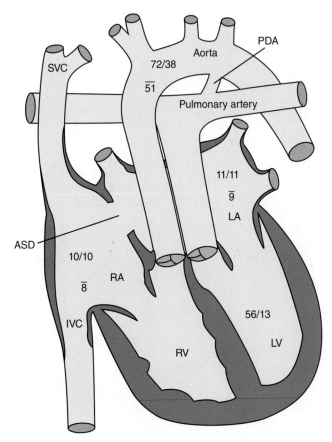

Figure 12–15. The ASD and PDA in this schematic permit the intermixing of oxygenated and deoxygenated blood in this TGA patient.

The pulmonary artery is attached to the right ventricular outflow tract (RVOT) and the aorta to the left ventricular outflow tract (LVOT) (Figure 12–17). The coronary arteries that follow the aorta during development must be explanted from the region of the RVOT and reimplanted into the aorta. Twisting of the coronary arteries during performance of the Jatene procedure can lead to myocardial ischemia and ventricular dysfunction. The Rastelli (Figure 12–18) and Damus-Kaye-Stansel procedures are employed when an arterial switch is not possible. Following these procedures, oxygenated blood is directed into the systemic circulation while deoxygenated venous blood enters the lungs. The direction of oxygenated and deoxygenated blood can also be changed at the atrial level.[18] Atrial switch procedures (Mustard and Senning) create an intra-atrial baffle and thus direct systemic venous blood to the mitral valve (MV), LV, and pulmonary artery. Conversely, pulmonary venous return is directed to the tricuspid valve (TV), RV, and aorta (Figure 12–19). The RV remains the systemic pumping chamber, TV faces systemic pressure, and over time TV regurgitation and

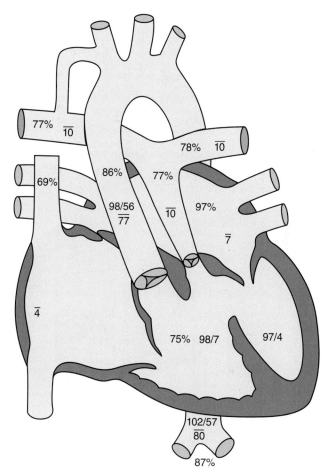

Figure 12–16. A BT shunt has been created in this TGA patient to improve the delivery of blood to the lungs for oxygenation.

RV failure may occur. Likewise, many patients experience varying degrees of arrhythmias.

In rare cases of TGA so-called congenitally corrected TGA can occur. In this arrangement the right atrium is connected to the mitral valve and the left ventricle, which in turn pumps blood into the pulmonary artery. The left atrium is connected to the tricuspid valve and the right ventricle, which in turn is connected to the systemic artery, the aorta. Consequently, in congenitally corrected TGA a morphological right ventricle becomes the systemic pumping chamber of the heart; however, because of the serial connections in the circulation, deoxygenated blood reaches the lungs and oxygenated blood is pumped into the systemic circulation. This TGA variant can remain asymptomatic for some time (third-fifth decade) until the RV fails as the systemic pumping chamber of the heart, tricuspid regurgitation develops, or conduction abnormalities ensue.[19]

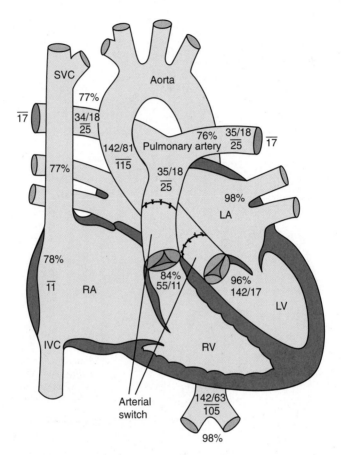

Figure 12–17. An arterial switch procedure.

Anesthetic management of patients undergoing TGA surgeries is complicated and requires a thorough knowledge of the patient's circulation. Inotropes and vasodilators might be needed following arterial switch when the low-pressure left ventricle assumes its proper role as the systemic pumping chamber of the heart. Signs of myocardial ischemia secondary to occlusion of coronary arteries after their reimplantation have to be sought. Patients whose right ventricle must serve as the systemic ventricles are potentially subject to ventricular failure and tricuspid valve regurgitation. All patients are prone to develop various dysrhythmias.

SINGLE VENTRICLE PATIENTS

There are many pathologic conditions that give rise to single ventricle (SV) physiology. In one subset of patients, such as the majority of those with tricuspid atresia (Figure 12–20), pulmonary blood flow is inadequate and oxygenation of the blood becomes possible only through flow via the PDA. Such patients often present with

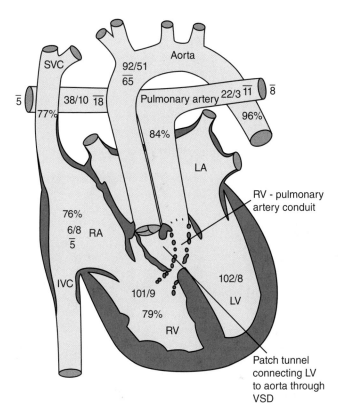

Figure 12–18. The Rastelli procedure directs oxygenated blood to the systemic circulation and deoxygenated blood to the pulmonary circulation.

cyanosis. Other patients [e.g., those with hypoplastic left heart syndrome (HLHS)] have an undeveloped left (systemic) ventricle and ascending aorta. They suffer from inadequate systemic perfusion. Systemic circulation is provided by flow through a PDA into the aorta (Figure 12–21). Consequently, HLHS patients have systemic hypoperfusion but pulmonary hyperperfusion. Depending upon the anatomic variant, SV patients can have either too much or too little pulmonary blood flow. If there is too much blood flow, the patient will manifest signs of pulmonary congestion and systemic hypoperfusion. If there is too little pulmonary blood flow, the patient can become cyanotic. The initial management of the SV patient is centered upon the resuscitation of the affected newborn. The goal of management is to bring into balance the patient's Qs and Qp, which should approach a ratio of 1.[20] Prostaglandin E_1 infusion is used to maintain ductal patency.

Irrespective of the anatomic lesions, palliation of the SV patient is usually accomplished over two to three stages during infancy and early childhood. The goals are to dedicate the SV to the systemic circulation and direct systemic venous return to the pulmonary arteries. In patients with decreased pulmonary blood flow a systemic artery to pulmonary artery shunt (BTT shunt) is performed to relieve

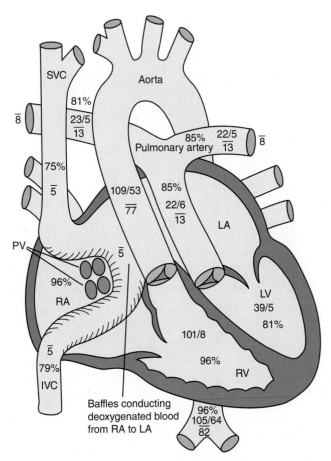

Figure 12–19. Redirection of oxygenated and deoxygenated blood at the atrial level.

cyanosis (Figure 12–22). In those patients with pulmonary hyperperfusion and systemic hypoperfusion, initial management may include the placement of a pulmonary artery (PA) band to prevent excessive pulmonary blood flow.

The anesthetic management of patients for initial SV palliation depends upon the degree of pulmonary hypo- or hyperperfusion encountered. The patient with pulmonary hyperperfusion for PA banding requires maintenance of pulmonary vascular resistance to prevent further "stealing" of blood from the systemic to the pulmonary circulation. Inotropic support is often needed secondary to SV volume overload. Patients requiring BTT shunts for pulmonary hypoperfusion require high-inspired oxygen concentrations and controlled hyperventilation to reduce PVR. Both BTT shunt and PA banding procedures can be performed without the use of CPB.

Patients with HLHS are treated by the Norwood procedure (Figure 12–23). A new aorta is created from the hypoplastic aorta and the main pulmonary artery. The RV becomes the systemic pumping chamber and pulmonary blood flow is

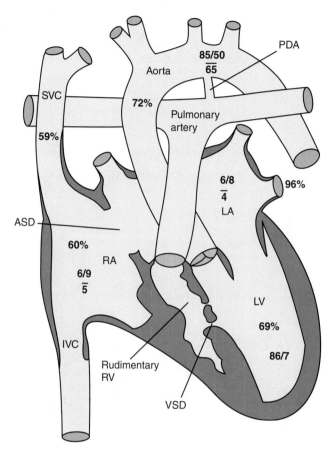

Figure 12–20. Single ventricle with tricuspid atresia and an ASD. [Reproduced with permission from Leyvi G, Wasnick JD: Single-ventricle patient: pathophysiology and anesthetic management, *J Cardiothorac Vasc Anesth.* 2010 Feb;24(1):121-130.]

provided by a BTT shunt or Sano shunt (RV to PA).[21] A combination of pulmonary artery banding and radiologically guided stenting of the PDA can also be performed for newborns with HLHS[22] (Figure 12–24). In this hybrid approach, the pulmonary arteries are banded to reduce pulmonary hyperperfusion and the PDA is stented to provide systemic perfusion from the SV into the aorta.

The second stage of palliative procedures for the SV patient generally involves creation of a Glenn shunt. In the Glenn procedure, venous return from the SVC is directed into the pulmonary artery (Figure 12–25). Cyanosis is not corrected by the Glenn procedure because IVC flow still returns to the SV and is ejected into the systemic circulation. As patients grow, flow from the IVC increases gradually decreasing the patient's arterial saturation. The bidirectional Glenn shunt (BDG) delivers SVC flow to both the right and left lungs. However, IVC flow is not delivered to the lungs resulting in the potential for developing pulmonary arteriovenous

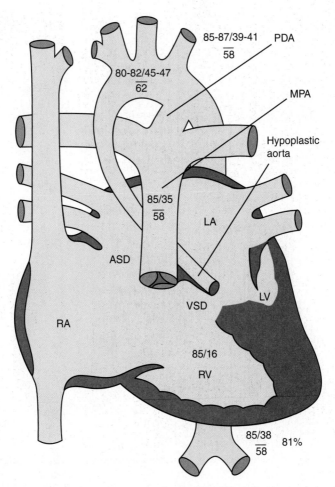

Figure 12–21. Hypoplastic left heart syndrome. [Reproduced with permission from Leyvi G, Wasnick JD: Single-ventricle patient: pathophysiology and anesthetic management, *J Cardiothorac Vasc Anesth.* 2010 Feb;24(1):121-130.]

malformations (AVMs). It is believed to be secondary to the absence of hepatic venous factor delivered directly to the lungs.[23]

The third stage of palliation for the SV patient is the Fontan procedure.[24] The Fontan procedure completes the process by which the SV is dedicated exclusively to the systemic circulation. The goal of the procedure is to direct all SVC and IVC venous return to the pulmonary vasculature, bypass the function of the right ventricle, and establish the single ventricle as the systemic pumping chamber of the heart. The Fontan procedure today creates a total cavopulmonary connection (TCPC) as a lateral tunnel (Figure 12–26) or extracardiac conduit (Figure 12–27).

Anesthetic management of the second and third stages of SV palliation can be quite challenging. The SV, which was exposed to volume overload at the time of

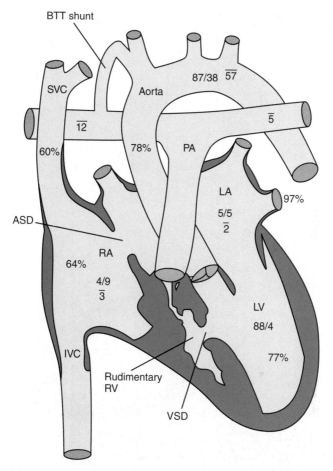

Figure 12–22. A BTT shunt has been placed to increase pulmonary blood flow in this cyanotic patient. [Reproduced with permission from Leyvi G, Wasnick JD: Single-ventricle patient: pathophysiology and anesthetic management, *J Cardiothorac Vasc Anesth.* 2010 Feb;24(1):121-130.]

systemic to pulmonary artery shunt or other circumstances of parallel circulation, is prone to ventricular failure. Pulmonary vascular resistance should be low in Fontan candidates but can be underestimated resulting in the impedance of blood flow through the lungs. Anesthetic induction can be achieved with inhalational or intravenous agents. Direct arterial pressure monitoring is obtained as well as adequate venous access for resuscitation in children who most likely have already had one to two prior sternotomies. At times surgeons will cannulate both the femoral artery and femoral vein to establish femoral-femoral CPB in the event of cardiac or vascular injury upon sternal opening. Anesthetic maintenance is with combinations of narcotics, inhalational agents, muscle relaxants, and neuraxial narcotics for postoperative pain control to facilitate early extubation.[25] Fontan repair can be completed

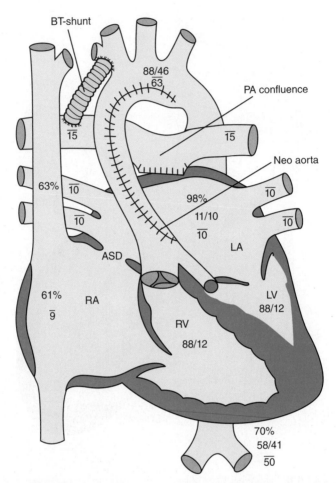

Figure 12–23. The Norwood procedure for HLHS. The RV becomes the heart chamber which pumps systemically. Pulmonary blood flow is provided by a shunt. [Reproduced with permission from Leyvi G, Wasnick JD: Single-ventricle patient: pathophysiology and anesthetic management, *J Cardiothorac Vasc Anesth*. 2010 Feb;24(1):121-130.]

with or without the use of CPB.[26] A 2012 review of early outcomes comparing Fontan procedures with and without the use of CPB did not demonstrate a significant difference in early outcomes in children undergoing the procedure.[27]

Following surgical repair, anesthetic management is directed at reducing PVR and promoting passive pulmonary blood flow. Patients are maintained on high-inspired FiO_2 and ventilated to produce a moderate hypocarbia with low inspiratory pressures. Nitric oxide or inhaled prostacyclin may be needed to decrease PVR and improve pulmonary blood flow. Monitoring of both venous pressure and atrial pressure are helpful in perioperative management. The central venous pressure measures pressure within the venous system delivering deoxygenated blood to the

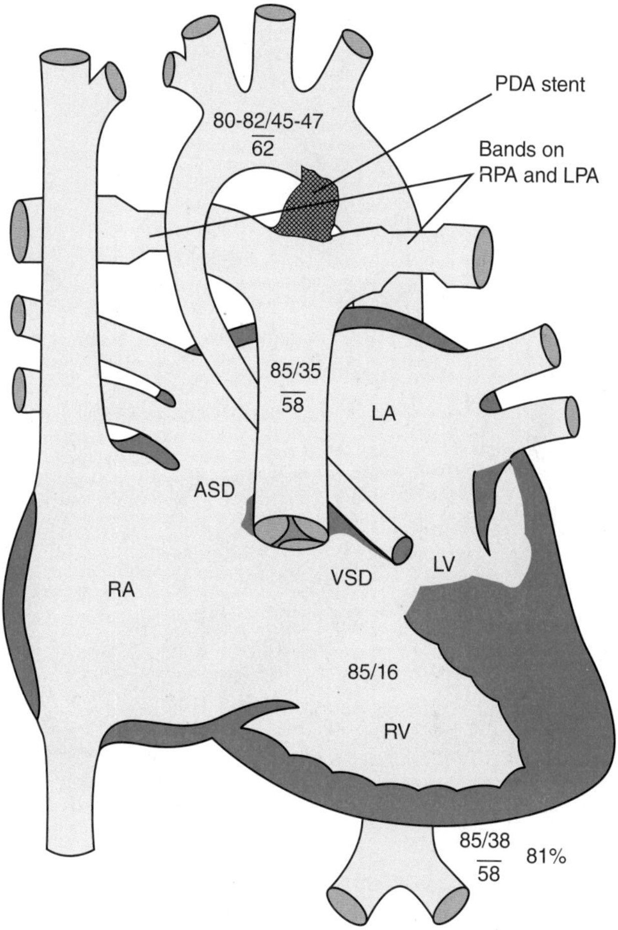

Figure 12–24. A hybrid approach to HLHS palliation restricts pulmonary blood flow through the placement of pulmonary artery bands. Systemic flow is through a stented patent ductus arteriosus. [Reproduced with permission from Leyvi G, Wasnick JD: Single-ventricle patient: pathophysiology and anesthetic management, *J Cardiothorac Vasc Anesth.* 2010 Feb;24(1):121-130.]

pulmonary arteries bypassing the heart. The atrial pressure reflects the pressure in the single atrium receiving oxygenated blood via the pulmonary veins to be ejected into the systemic circulation by the SV. Ideally, the CVP is 15 mm Hg with an atrial pressure of 8 mm Hg. If the atrial pressure measured by a surgically placed transthoracic atrial line is elevated, dysfunction of the single ventricle or AV valve regurgitation should be suspected. SV dysfunction can be treated by inotropes and afterload reduction. However, if the atrial pressure is normal and the central venous pressure increased, then increased PVR is suggested and nitric oxide therapy is initiated. Positive pressure ventilation decreases pulmonary blood flow. Pulmonary flow

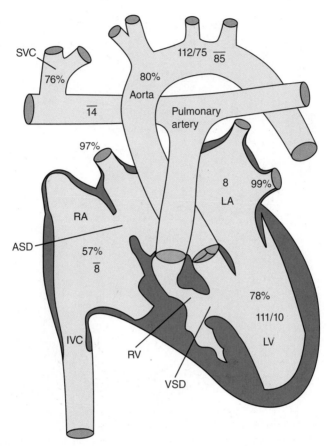

Figure 12–25. The bidirectional Glenn procedure directs superior vena cava flow to the pulmonary arteries. [Reproduced with permission from Leyvi G, Wasnick JD: Single-ventricle patient: pathophysiology and anesthetic management, *J Cardiothorac Vasc Anesth.* 2010 Feb;24(1):121-130.]

in the positive pressure ventilated Fontan patient is improved by adjusting ventilatory parameters to achieve the lowest possible mean airway pressure consistent with ventilatory goals. The benefits of positive end-expiratory pressure (PEEP) in promoting alveolar recruitment must be balanced against the potential to increase intrathoracic pressure and decrease pulmonary blood flow. Early extubation and spontaneous ventilation are encouraged when tolerated, because negative transthoracic pressure augments pulmonary blood flow and increases cardiac output.

Adult patients following Fontan palliation should be managed in a manner similar to that for the child undergoing Fontan creation. Spontaneous ventilation is encouraged as is the use of anesthetic techniques with minimal negative inotropic effects. Sufficient intravascular volume is necessary to perfuse the pulmonary vasculature and preserve the cardiac output.

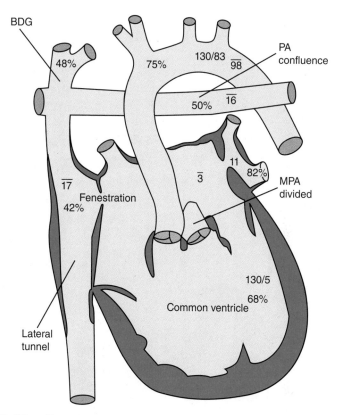

Figure 12–26. Palliation of the single ventricle by the Fontan procedure using a lateral tunnel to direct venous flow to the pulmonary artery. [Reproduced with permission from Leyvi G, Wasnick JD: Single-ventricle patient: pathophysiology and anesthetic management, *J Cardiothorac Vasc Anesth.* 2010 Feb;24(1):121-130.]

ANESTHESIA FOR NONCARDIAC SURGERY IN ADULTS WITH CONGENITAL HEART DISEASE

Specific anesthetic techniques must be designed for each individual patient following review of the patient's records and discussion with the patient's primary physicians. The degree to which a patient's underlying defect has or has not been corrected needs to be discerned. Generally, management is directed toward:

- Avoiding air or other emboli in patients with shunts present
- Avoiding myocardial depression
- Reducing airway pressure
- Balancing pulmonary and systemic flow ratio

Even the most straightforward simple congenital lesions can be associated with a number of long-term complications including:

- Pulmonary hypertension
- Ventricular dysfunction

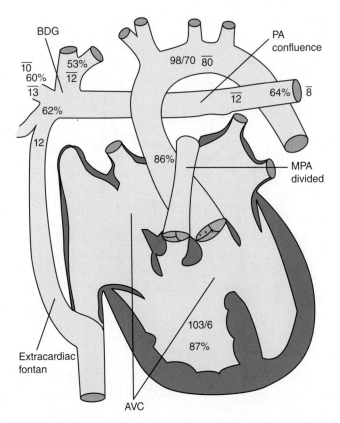

Figure 12–27. Fontan palliation using an extracardiac conduit. AVC = atrioventricular canal; BDG = bidirectional Glenn shunt; MPA = main pulmonary artery. [Reproduced with permission from Leyvi G, Wasnick JD: Single-ventricle patient: pathophysiology and anesthetic management, *J Cardiothorac Vasc Anesth.* 2010 Feb;24(1):121-130.]

- Dysrhythmias
- Conduction defects
- Residual shunts
- Valvular lesions
- Arteriovenous malformations and vascular lesions

Pulmonary hypertension can be present in patients secondary to long-standing large, nonrestrictive defects resulting in an initial left-to-right shunt and pulmonary hyperperfusion when Qp>>>Qs. Congenital mitral valvular disease and ventricular failure can also lead to increases in pulmonary artery pressures. Eisenmenger syndrome occurs with less frequency today due to early surgical interventions. Elective surgery should be carefully considered in patients with Eisenmenger syndrome. In patients with pulmonary hypertension, increases in PVR are avoided by:

- Minimizing sympathetic stimulation
- Preventing hypoxia and hypercarbia

- Maintaining normal airway pressures if possible
- Employing pulmonary vasodilators (e.g., NO) when necessary

Sudden increases in PVR may precipitate right heart failure, oxygen desaturation, and reduced systemic cardiac output. Regional techniques can be employed where indicated.

Cyanosis following CHD repairs usually reflects residual right-to-left shunting. Long-standing cyanosis results in a compensatory erythrocytosis yielding an increase in blood viscosity and the propensity for thrombosis. Iron deficiency may accompany erythrocytosis making red cells less deformable further promoting clot formation. Perioperatively patients should be adequately hydrated when fasted.

CHD patients whether corrected or not are at risk for varying degrees of both systolic and diastolic right and left heart failure. Regimens used to treat left and right heart failure are applied in the CHD patient as they are in the general population. Similarly, many patients with CHD have various atrial and ventricular arrhythmias. Anesthesiologists can from time to time encounter CHD patients in electrophysiology laboratories when they present for ablative therapy.

CHD patients are at risk for endocarditis. The American Heart Association (AHA) provides guidelines to assist physicians in determining when prophylaxis is needed.[16] As many patients following repair of CHD lesions have various shunts, baffles, and conduits, the potential for infection should never be discounted. As these guidelines often change, practitioners should frequently review the AHA's recommendations. The American College of Cardiology/ American Heart Association has developed guidelines for the management of adult patients with CHD. In particular, they note the importance of regional adult CHD centers in coordinating the care of these patients.

CARDIAC SURGERY AND PREGNANCY

With CHD patients evermore surviving into adulthood, an increasing number of pregnancies can be expected among women with repaired CHD.[28] Moreover, acquired valvular or ischemic heart disease can necessitate surgical or catheter-mediated interventions in the pregnant patient. The European Society of Cardiology (ESC) has provided extensive guidelines to assist in the management of the 0.2% to 4% of women whose pregnancy is complicated by cardiovascular disease.[29] In addition to CHD patients becoming pregnant, the increasing age of first pregnancy in the western world and the increased prevalence of conditions leading to cardiovascular disease (e.g., diabetes, hypertension, and obesity) have combined to make heart disease the major cause of maternal death during pregnancy. Peripartum cardiomyopathy is a potentially lethal complication of pregnancy developing between the final month of pregnancy and the fifth postpartum month.[30] The U.S. incidence is 1/3000 live births with 50% of women affected fully recovering. The remaining patients are at risk for significant morbidity and mortality. Consequently, the anesthesiologist is increasingly likely to encounter the pregnant patient with CHD or newly acquired heart disease.

The physiologic changes associated with normal pregnancy include:

- Decreased systemic vascular resistance
- Increased cardiac output
- Decreased pulmonary vascular resistance
- Decreased systolic and diastolic blood pressure
- Increased oxygen consumption
- Anemia
- Decreased functional residual capacity
- Airway edema and potential for difficult intubation

Patients with impaired ventricular or valvular function may be unable to adapt to the normal physiology of pregnancy, leading to hemodynamic collapse. In particular, patients with pulmonary hypertension are at increased risk for heart failure during pregnancy as are patients with prepregnancy cardiomyopathy.[31]

Patients with repaired CHD may be candidates for vaginal or cesarean delivery depending upon their medical conditions. Ventricular function should be assessed during the prenatal period and the history of previous repairs reviewed. Limited ventricular reserve, as might be seen in patients with Fontan circulation, may prevent the patient from responding to the hemodynamic challenges of delivery. Additionally, many CHD and mechanical valve patients are taking warfarin. Warfarin use during the first trimester is associated with embryopathy. Heparin does not cross the placenta and is frequently employed during this period in patients who require anticoagulation. Anesthesiologists should be aware of the anticoagulation regimen employed. Cesarean section is generally not mandated unless indicated for obstetrical purposes. The volume shifts associated with labor analgesia and delivery may not be tolerated by the CHD patient with impaired ventricular function leading to hemodynamic collapse and heart failure. Invasive monitoring may be employed on an individual basis as indicated.

From time to time, anesthesiologists may be called upon to care for the pregnant patient who must undergo heart surgery requiring the use of CPB. Although cardiac surgery can be safely performed for the mother, there are numerous perioperative risks affecting fetal survival.[32] Fetal heart rate monitoring can be employed after 22 weeks' gestational age. Fetal bradycardia is associated with hemodilution, sustained uterine contraction, hypotension, and medications. High flows (> 2.4 L/min/m^2), CPB pressures of > 70 mm Hg, and normothermia have been suggested to improve fetal viability. Expeditious surgical times and avoidance of hyperkalemia secondary to repeated doses of cardioplegia solution are also recommended. Heparin and protamine do not cross the placenta. Because coagulation is enhanced during pregnancy, anti-fibrinolytic agents are avoided in the pregnant patient requiring CPB. Left uterine displacement should be done by placing a wedge under the right hip to avoid aorto-caval compression. A maternal hematocrit $> 28\%$ is likewise suggested during CPB. Anesthetic agents cross the placenta as do opioids; however, muscle relaxants do not cross the placenta.

Peripartum cardiomyopathy is an idiopathic cardiomyopathy presenting as LV systolic failure at the end of pregnancy or in the immediate months postpartum.

The etiology is unclear but may result from an oxidative stress response resulting in the proteolytic cleavage of prolactin into a fragment that promotes apoptosis and anti-angiogensis which damage the myocardium.[33] Management of peripartum heart failure is similar to that of other heart failure with added consideration for placental transfer of drugs and their safety during lactation. Review of the European Society of Cardiology guidelines is helpful in regard to those medications to be employed in the perioperative management of cardiac disease in the pregnant patient.

Patients with peripartum cardiomyopathy may present for ventricular assist device placement or cardiac transplantation.

TEE AND CHD

Review of TEE examinations of patients with CHD both before and after surgical repair can be challenging for adult echocardiographers at all levels. The basic echocardiographer should be able to recognize the abnormal structure of the CHD patient's heart. Basic echocardiographers should seek the assistance of individuals with specific experience with the CHD patient when bringing these patients to surgery. Kamra et al. provide a useful review of the role of transesophageal echocardiography in the management of pediatric patients with CHD.[34]

REFERENCES

1. Perloff JK, Warnes CA. Challenges posed by adults with repaired congenital heart disease. *Circulation.* 2001;103:2637-2643.

2. Gottlieb E, Andropoulos D. Anesthesia for the patient with congenital heart disease presenting for noncardiac surgery. *Curr Opin Anesthesiol.* 2013;26(3):318-326.

3. Samanek M, Slavik Z, Zborilova B, et al. Prevalence, treatment and outcome of heart disease in live-born children: a prospective analysis of 91,823 live born children. *Pediatr Cardiol.* 1989;10:205-211.

4. Cooper JR, Jr, Goldstein MT. Septal and endocardial cushing defect and double outlet right ventricle perioperative management. In: Lake CL (ed). *Pediatric Cardiac Anesthesia.* 3rd ed. Stamford, CT: Appleton & Lange; 1998:285-302.

5. Hudson JK, Deshpande JK. Septal and endocardial cushion defects. In: Lake CL, Booker PD (eds). *Pediatric Cardiac Anesthesia.* 4th ed. Philadelphia, PA: Lippincott Williams & Wilkins; 2005:329-343.

6. Radzik D, Davignon A, van Doesburg N, et al. Predictive factors for spontaneous closure of atrial septal defect diagnosed in the first three months of life. *J Am Coll Cardiol.* 1993;22:851-853.

7. Mavroudis C, Backer CL, Jacobs JP. Ventricular septal defect. In: Mavroudis C, Backer CL (eds). *Pediatric Cardiac Surgery.* Philadelphia, PA: Mosby; 2003:298-338.

8. Neumayer U, Stone S, Somerville J, et al. Small ventricular septal defects in adults. *Eur Heart J.* 1998;19:1573-1582.

9. Feldt RH, Edwards WD, Coburn JP, et al. Atrioventricular septal defects. In: Allen HD, Gutgesell HP, Clark EB, et al. (eds). *Moss and Adams, Heart Disease in Infants, Children and Adolescents.* Philadelphia, PA: Lippincott Williams & Wilkins; 2001:618-635.

10. Morgan BC, Guntheroth WG, Bloom RS, et al. Clinical profile of paroxysmal hyperpnea in cyanotic congenital heart disease. *Circulation.* 1965;31:66-69.

11. Van Arsdell GS, Maharaj GS, Tom J, et al. What is the optimal age for repair of tetralogy of Fallot? *Circulation.* 2000;102 (suppl III):123-129.

12. Chaturvedi RR, Shore DF, Lincoln C, et al. Acute right ventricular restrictive physiology after repair of tetralogy of Fallot: association with myocardial injury and oxidative stress. *Circulation.* 1999;100:1540-1547.

13. Ruzyllo W, Nihill MR, Mullins CE, et al. Hemodynamic evaluation of 221 patients after intracardiac repair of tetralogy of Fallot. *Am J Cardiol.* 1974;34:565-576.

14. Gatzoulis MA, Balaji S, Webber SA, et al. Risk factors for arrhythmia and sudden cardiac death late after repair of tetralogy of Fallot: a multicentre study. *Lancet.* 2000;356:975-981.

15. Cullen S, Celemajer DS, Franklin RC, et al. Prognostic significance of ventricular arrhythmia after repair of tetralogy of Fallot: a multicentre study. *Am J Cardiol.* 1994;23:1151-1155.

16. Wilson W, Taubert KA, Gewitz M, et al. Prevention of infective endocarditis: guideline from the American Heart Association: a guideline from the American Heart Association Rheumatic Fever, Endocarditis, and Kawasaki Disease Committee, Council on Cardiovascular Disease in the Young, and the Council on Clinical Cardiology, Council on Cardiovascular Surgery and Anesthesia, and the Quality of Care and Outcomes Research Interdisciplinary Working Group. *Circulation.* 2007;116:1736-1754.

17. Liebman J, Cullum L, Belloc NB, et al. Natural history of transposition of the great arteries. Anatomy at birth and death characteristics. *Circulation.* 1969;40:237-262.

18. Losay J, Touchot A, Serraf A, et al. Late outcome after atrial switch operation for transposition of the great arteries. *Circulation.* 2001;104:I121-I126.

19. Graham TP, Bernard YD, Mellen BG, et al. Long-term outcome in congenitally corrected transposition of the great arteries. *J Am Coll Cardiol.* 2000;36:255-261.

20. Hoffman G, Stuth EAE. Hypoplastic left heart syndrome. In: Lake CL, Booker PD (eds). *Pediatric Cardiac Anesthesia.* Philadelphia, PA: Lippincott Williams & Wilkins; 2005:445-466.

21. Sano S, Ishino K, Kado H, et al. Outcome of right ventricle-to-pulmonary artery shunt in first-stage palliation of hypoplastic left heart syndrome: a multi-institutional study. *Ann Thorac Surg.* 2004;78:1951-1957.

22. Bacha EA, Daves S, Hardin J, et al. Single ventricle palliation for high-risk neonates: the emergence of an alternative hybrid strategy. *J Thorac Cardiovasc Surg.* 2006;131:163-171.

23. Shah MJ, Rychik J, Fogel MA, et al. Pulmonary AV malformations after superior cavopulmonary connection: resolution after inclusion of hepatic veins in the pulmonary circulation. *Ann Thorac Surg.* 1997;63:960-963.

24. Fontan F, Mounicot FB, Baudet E, et al. "Correction" of tricuspid atresia. 2 cases "corrected" using a new surgical technic. *Ann Chir Thorac Cardiovasc.* 1971;10:39-47.

25. Leyvi G, Bennett HL, Wasnick JD. Pulmonary artery flow patterns after Fontan procedure are predictive of postoperative complications. *J Cardiothorac Vasc Anesth.* 2009;23:54-61.

26. Tam V, Miller BE, Murphy K. Modified Fontan without use of cardiopulmonary bypass. *Ann Thorac Surg.* 1999;68:1698-1703.

27. McCammond A, Kuo K, Parikh V, et al. Early outcomes after extracardiac conduit Fontan operation without cardiopulmonary bypass. *Pediatr Cardiol.* 2012;33(7):1078-1085.

28. Arendt K, Abel M. The pregnant patient and cardiopulmonary bypass. In: Cohen NH (ed). *Medically challenging patients undergoing cardiothoracic surgery. A Society of Cardiovascular Anesthesiologists monograph,* 2009:215-244.

29. Regitz-Zagrosek V, Lundqvist C, Borghi C, et al. ESC guidelines on the management of cardiovascular disease during pregnancy. *Eur Heart J.* 2011;32:3147-3197.

30. Nickens M, Long R, Geraci S. Cardiovascular disease in pregnancy. *South Med J.* 2013;106(11):624-630.

31. Ruys T, Roos-Hesselink J, Hall R, et al. Heart failure in pregnant women with cardiac disease: data from the ROPAC. *Heart* 2014;100:231-238.

32. Mahli A, Izdes S, Coskun D. Cardiac operations during pregnancy: review of factors influencing fetal outcome. *Ann Thorac Surg.* 2000;69:1622-1626.

33. Bhattacharyya A, Basra S, Kar B. Peripartum cardiomyopathy. *Tex Heart Inst J.* 2012;39(1):8-16.

34. Kamra K, Russell I, Miller-Hance W. Role of transesophageal echocardiography in the management of pediatric patients with congenital heart disease. *Pediatr Anesth.* 2011;21:479-493.

REVIEWS

Chandrasekhar S, Cook C, Collard C. Cardiac surgery in the parturient. *Anesth Analg.* 2009;108:777-785.

Burch TM, Mizuguchi K, DiNardo J. Echocardiographic assessment of atrial septal defects. *Anesth Analg.* 2012;115(4):772-775.

Jooste E, Haft W, Ames W, et al. Anesthetic care of parturients with single ventricle physiology. *JCA.* 2013;25:417-423.

Jolley M, Colan S, Rhodes J, DiNardo J. Fontan physiology revisited. *Anesth Analg.* 2015;121(1):172-182.

Warnes C, Williams R, Bashore T, et al. ACC/AHA guidelines for the management of adults with congenital heart disease: executive summary; a report of the American College of Cardiology/American Heart Association Task Force on Practice Guidelines (Writing Committee to Develop Guidelines of the Management of Adults with Congenital Heart Disease). *Circulation.* 2008;118:2395-2451.

Bhatt A, Foster E, Kuehl K, et al. Congenital heart disease in the older adult: a scientific statement from the American Heart Association. *Circulation.* 2015;131:1884-1931.

Rouine Rapp K, Russell I, Foster E. Congenital heart disease in the adult. *Int Anesthesiol Clin.* 2012;50(2):16-39.

Off-Pump, Robotic, and Minimally Invasive Heart Surgery

TOPICS

During the 1990s, cardiologists and surgeons began a quest to identify new, less invasive methods of treating heart disease. Angioplasty and stents were developed. Surgeons began to perform coronary artery bypass through keyhole-sized incisions assisted by thoracoscopic techniques.[1,2] Subsequently, robotic surgery was introduced into the cardiac surgery operating room to further reduce surgical incision size. Some surgeons attributed most of the difficulties associated with cardiac surgery to the use of cardiopulmonary bypass (CPB). As such, they continued to operate on patients using a full sternotomy but completed their bypass grafts without the use of CPB operating off-pump on the beating heart.

All minimally invasive surgical approaches present different potential challenges for anesthesiologists. During cardiac surgery with CPB, the surgical manipulations of the heart do not generally affect the patient's hemodynamics—after all, the patient is on bypass. In the course of off-pump procedures, the heart must continue to beat and to supply blood to the tissues even when handled in the chest and potentially rendered ischemic during the sewing of vascular anastomoses. Consequently, the off-pump patient can deteriorate acutely requiring resuscitative measures and emergent institution of CPB. Anesthesiologists should never consider off-pump or minimally invasive procedures to be less demanding than those performed on-pump.

MINIMALLY INVASIVE SURGICAL APPROACHES

There are a variety of surgical approaches that are designated as being "minimally invasive." Many off-pump procedures are done through a fully invasive median sternotomy. So, minimally invasive and off pump are not the same although minimally invasive procedures can be completed off pump. Likewise, minimally invasive procedures (e.g., mitral valve replacement) are performed on CPB with robotic assistance. Consequently, surgeons can perform minimally invasive procedures using CPB, or a procedure can be performed off pump but nonetheless require a full sternotomy incision.

For this discussion, "minimally invasive" implies that the surgeon is using something other than a full sternotomy to access the heart. The heart can be approached using various ministernotomies, thoracotomies, and robotic and/or thoracoscopic assistance. Many of these minimally invasive approaches present different challenges to the anesthesiologist.

Off-pump revascularization of the coronary arteries can be completed using minimally invasive approaches or via a full sternotomy.

Off-Pump Coronary Artery Bypass Via Full Sternotomy

When a full sternotomy incision is used for off-pump coronary artery bypass surgery (OPCAB), the beating heart is stabilized using various support devices to permit the completion of multiple coronary bypass grafts. During off-pump bypass surgery, the surgeon occludes blood flow to the vessel being bypassed both proximally and distally using silastic snares and other occlusive devices. The surgical field is occasionally flooded with carbon dioxide to minimize entrainment of air into the coronary artery during surgical manipulation. Because the beating heart, when operated upon, presents the surgeon with a moving target, there are various stabilization devices (Figure 13–1) commercially available, which relatively

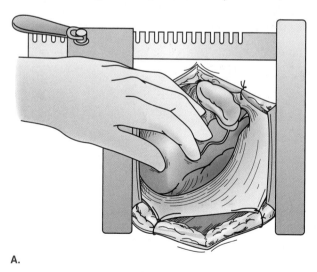

A.

Figure 13–1. (A) During OPCAB surgery using a full sternotomy, the heart is frequently lifted by the surgeon to gain exposure to the vessel to be bypassed. (B) Using stabilization devices, the heart is positioned to optimize surgical exposure and to provide a relatively still target for bypass graft placement. (C) With the heart positioned, the coronary artery to be bypassed is stabilized.

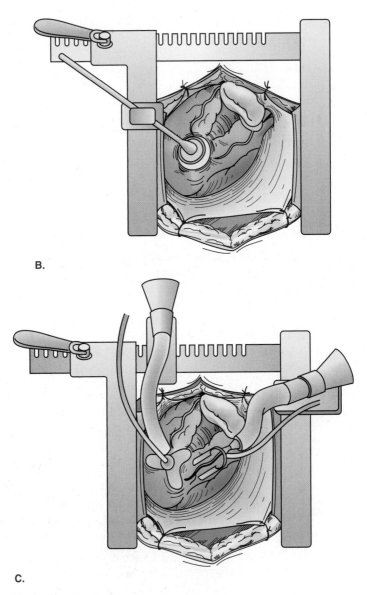

B.

C.

Figure 13–1. (Continued)

immobilize that region of the myocardium where the surgeon plans to create the bypass anastomoses. The surgeon must position the heart in such a manner that surgical access is suitable to complete the surgical repair. During positioning of the heart, venous return can be impaired leading to hemodynamic instability and hypotension. Often, however, once the heart is positioned in such a way that the graft can be placed, venous return becomes adequate and the heart pumps a suitable cardiac output to maintain perfusion even when the heart is lifted and retracted in the thorax. Frequently, the surgeon will occlude the coronary artery to be bypassed for a brief period to determine the patient's response to vessel occlusion and to possibly provide ischemic preconditioning. Following this trial, the surgeon reperfuses the vessel in the hope that through ischemia preconditioning the myocardium supplied by that vessel will be more resilient to future episodes of myocardial ischemia. The vessel is reoccluded and the anastomosis completed. During this period, the coronary artery being bypassed is snared, and, thus, the myocardium dependent on that vessel's flow distribution may become ischemic. Of course, since the vessel requires bypass in the first place, there may have been little flow from it to the myocardium, thereby minimizing the effect of vessel occlusion. However, if that vessel provides sufficient flow to an area of viable heart muscle not supplied by collaterals, the heart may become rapidly ischemic during surgical repair. The surgeon can place a shunt in the coronary artery being bypassed to provide arterial flow while the bypass graft is being sutured into position. Systemic heparin (a dose of 100-300 units/kg) is administered before vessel occlusion to a target of activated clotting time of 250 to 300 seconds. There is considerable variability in the anticoagulation regimen for off-pump bypass surgery from hospital to hospital.[3] Should efforts to support the circulation be inadequate during off-pump bypass, the surgical team should be prepared for full heparinization and institution of CPB.

Robotic, Minimally Invasive, and Hybrid Procedures

Single bypass of the left anterior descending artery (LAD) with the left internal mammary artery (LIMA) can be completed using a variety of minimally invasive robotic and thoracoscopically assisted approaches. The LIMA to LAD graft improves survival of patients treated for coronary artery disease. Hybrid coronary revascularization (HCR) employs a robotically performed minimally invasive LIMA to LAD graft in concert with percutaneous coronary interventions (PCI) of other occluded coronary arteries. HCR procedures reduce surgical trespass and may decrease but not eliminate the inflammatory response associated with on-pump coronary artery bypass surgery.[4,5]

Surgeons also use minimally invasive and robotic surgical techniques for valvular surgery. Minimally invasive aortic valve surgery can be done through a ministernotomy or a right anterior thoracotomy. Mitral valve surgery can be performed through a right anterolateral thoracotomy. Venous drainage is generally accomplished through a cannula placed in the right atrium via the femoral vein and inferior vena cava. Arterial (aortic) cannulation can be performed directly into the ascending aorta or through the right axillary or femoral artery. At times surgeons may request the anesthesiologist to aid with placement of a coronary sinus catheter from the internal jugular vein for the administration of retrograde cardioplegia and/or to place a vent in the pulmonary artery to decompress the left ventricle during CPB. TEE is employed to assist in positioning these catheters (Figures 13–2 and 13–3 and **Video 13–1**). The surgeon applies a transthoracic aortic cross clamp with subsequent cardioplegia delivery. Endo-aortic balloon clamps are also used with TEE guidance to occlude the aorta (Figure 13–3 and **Video 13–2**).

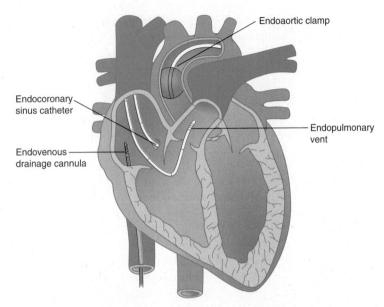

Figure 13–2. Endocoronary sinus catheter, endoaortic clamp, endopulmonary vent, and endovenous drainage cannula used for robotic cardiac surgery. [Reproduced with permission from Wang G, Gao C: Robotic cardiac surgery: an anaesthetic challenge, *Postgrad Med J.* 2014 Aug;90(1066):467-474.]

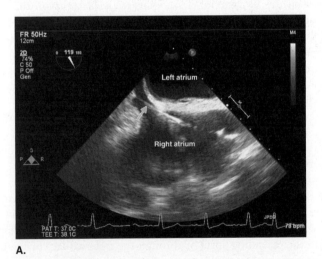

A.

Figure 13–3. (A) Mid-esophageal bicaval view showing the coronary sinus catheter (gray arrow) for delivery of retrograde cardioplegia engaging the coronary sinus ostium. (B) Mid-esophageal bicaval view showing the coronary sinus catheter (gray arrow) in the coronary sinus and the venous cannula (white arrow) engaging the superior vena cava. (C) Mid-esophageal aortic valve long-axis showing the ascending aorta in long axis and the endoclamp catheter (gray arrow) with the endoclamp balloon not yet inflated. (D) Same view as panel (C). The endoclamp balloon has been inflated (gray arrow) and cardioplegia (white arrow) is being delivered in the aortic root.

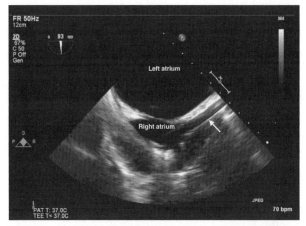

B.

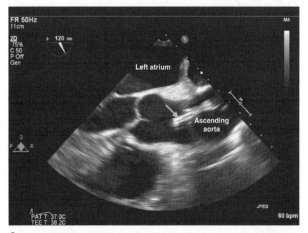

C.

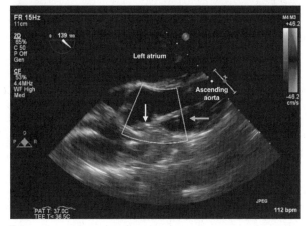

D.

Figure 13–3. (Continued)

ANESTHETIC CHALLENGES FOR OFF-PUMP AND MINIMALLY INVASIVE SURGERY

Prior to establishing invasive arterial monitoring and central venous access, the anesthesiologist and the surgeon should discuss the surgical plan especially regarding which vessels will be cannulated for initiating CPB if this is planned and if the placement of a retrograde coronary sinus catheter through the internal jugular vein is necessary. If the case involves a ministernotomy with CPB cannulas placed in the chest, the procedure will unfold similarly to other procedures requiring a full sternotomy. Because neither a ministernotomy nor a robotic approach permits full access to the heart, external defibrillation/pacemaker pads must be placed if internal paddles are unable to properly make contact with the epicardium.

If the procedure is to be performed through a thoracotomy incision or with thoracic port access (e.g., robotic mitral valve repair or replacement), the ability to provide one-lung ventilation is required (Figure 13–4). Double-lumen endotracheal tubes or bronchial blockers are used depending upon patient characteristics, anesthesiologist's preference, and need for postoperative mechanical ventilation. Carbon dioxide may be insufflated into the hemithorax to improve thoracoscopic or robotic access. Hypoxemia and hemodynamic instability may accompany one lung ventilation and CO_2 insufflation.

Choice of anesthetic agent for minimally invasive surgery parallels that of conventional cardiac surgery. Anesthetics should be designed to provide fast-track emergence and extubation as patient parameters permit. Combinations of opioids (short-acting or carefully titrated longer acting), inhalational agents, and propofol have all been used in these cases successfully. Paravertebral blocks and other regional techniques are used to facilitate fast track management (see Chapter 18). As with all cardiac anesthesia practice, careful management of the patient's hemodynamics is far more important than the particular anesthetic method chosen. Monitoring of patients during minimally invasive procedures is similar to that employed in fully

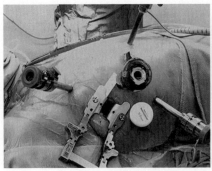
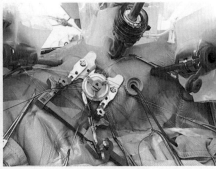

A.   B.

Figure 13–4. External view. (A) A setup for robotic mitral valve replacement including robort ports and rib retractor for working port. (B) Mitral prosthesis deployment through a rib retractor. [Reproduced with permission from Kuo CC, Chang HH, Hsing CH, et al: Robotic mitral valve replacements with bioprosthetic valves in 52 patients: experience from a tertiary referral hospital, *Eur J Cardiothorac Surg.* 2018 Nov 1;54(5):853-859.]

invasive cardiac surgery. In procedures performed through small incisions, the anesthesiologist often cannot see the beating heart, which can otherwise be a reasonable monitor of cardiac function. Therefore, TEE monitoring of heart function during minimally invasive procedures becomes ever more important. However, when the heart is lifted from the chest to facilitate placement of a bypass graft during full sternotomy off-pump surgery, TEE imaging becomes difficult and may not always be useful in detecting perioperative ischemia. When TEE images are available, the appearance of new wall motion abnormalities during coronary artery occlusion can signal the development of myocardial ischemia. Release of coronary arterial snares and the restoration of blood flow will usually resolve ischemia. Hypotension, increased pulmonary arterial pressures, new ST-segment changes, and arrhythmias can complicate off-pump surgical procedures. Surgical use of coronary artery shunts may at times relieve ischemia and facilitate off-pump bypass grafting. Often vasopressors are necessary to support the blood pressure when the heart is lifted out of the chest or rendered ischemic by snare ligatures. Conversely, when the heart is returned to its normal position and/or myocardial ischemia is relieved, the patient's cardiac output will improve, potentially increasing blood pressure to the point of the patient developing unexpected hypertension.

As mentioned above, the surgical and anesthesia teams should be prepared at all times to convert the procedure from an off-pump minimally invasive procedure to a full sternotomy, on-pump procedure should hemodynamic instability ensue and should efforts to restore blood pressure and relieve surgically induced coronary ischemia falter.

During robotic or minimally invasive on-pump procedures, surgeons employ various transthoracic and intra-aortic cross clamps to isolate the heart from the systemic circulation to permit surgical repair.[6] TEE is used in these situations to ensure that the intra-aortic balloon clamps do not become malpositioned in the aorta potentially occluding flow to the innominate artery. Aortic dissections can also occur, and TEE examination should include an assessment of the aorta.

During robotic cardiac surgery muscle paralysis is essential, as the robotic arms are fixed and may cause trauma should the patient move or cough during surgery.

Postoperatively, patients undergoing minimally invasive surgery are ideal candidates for early extubation in the operating room. Particular attention should be paid to adequate control of bleeding, correction of any existing coagulopathy, adequate control of pain, and maintenance of normothermia. The patient must be actively warmed throughout surgery and room temperature controlled. The usual blood gases and routine lab values should be monitored and corrected as with any cardiac surgery patient. Because of concern regarding the above-mentioned factors (bleeding, pain, hemodynamic instability), anesthesiologists may elect to keep the patient intubated and sedated for a short period of observation prior to extubation in the ICU following minimally invasive surgery.

IS OFF-PUMP SURGERY BETTER THAN ON-PUMP SURGERY?

Considering the numerous inflammatory and coagulation derangements associated with CPB, it was hoped that off-pump techniques would reduce the complications associated with heart surgery—especially those related to neurologic injury. There have been a number of studies that have suggested or failed to suggest that off-pump techniques offer some advantages. Bucerius et al. looking at a large database found a reduced incidence of postoperative stroke and delirium in patients who underwent beating heart surgery compared with those on CPB.[7] On the other hand, Nahoe et al. in a prospective trial of relatively healthy patients randomized to on- or off-pump surgery found no difference in cardiac surgery outcomes at 1 year including freedom from death, stroke, myocardial infarction, or additional coronary intervention.[8] Khan et al. randomized a small number of patients (roughly 50 in each group) to on- or off-pump surgery and assessed graft patency 3 months postoperatively.[9] The investigators noted that although there was a lower degree of myocardial damage as measured by troponin T levels following off-pump surgery, graft patency was lower in off-pump patients compared to those patients operated upon using on-pump techniques. Because off-pump surgery is performed on the beating heart with the use of myocardial stabilization devices, it is possible that grafts performed under these conditions may be technically inferior and, thus, have lower patency and longevity rates compared to those completed in the arrested heart following cardioplegia.

A study in 2203 randomly assigned patients to undergo off-pump or on-pump revascularization, found that the off-pump group had worse outcomes (death or complications like reoperation, new mechanical support, cardiac arrest, coma, stroke, or renal failure before discharge or within 30 days from surgery) and poorer graft patency than did patients in the on-pump group. There were no significant differences between the techniques in neuropsychological outcomes or use of major resources.[10] Recent studies have demonstrated improved long-term survival in coronary artery bypass patients managed with on-pump versus those managed with off-pump techniques.[11] However, a review of 65,097 patients who underwent isolated coronary artery bypass grafting in the Veterans Affairs Surgical Quality Improvement Program demonstrated that patients operated upon using on-pump techniques had higher perioperative morbidity compared with those patients operated upon using off-pump management.[12] Nevertheless, these authors reported no significant difference in operative deaths between the on-pump and off-pump patient cohorts. In a similar cohort, Bakaeen et al. also report that off-pump coronary artery bypass may be associated with reduced long term survival.[13] Diegeler et al. noted that in patients 75 and older there was no benefit of off-pump versus on-pump coronary artery bypass grafting at 30 days or one year.[14] Lamy et al. examined outcomes at 5 years in patients randomized to off-pump and on-pump coronary artery bypass.[15] These investigators did not note any difference in death, stroke, myocardial infarction, renal failure, or repeat revascularizations between the on-pump and off-pump groups. However, in a recent meta-analysis Smart et al. reported that on-pump coronary artery bypass grafting provided a statistically superior survival advantage compared with off-pump surgery.[16] Shaefi et al. in a 2018 review have summarized the major clinical trials of off-pump versus on-pump CABG (Tables 13–1 and 13–2).[17]

Puskas et al., in a meta-analysis of 102 clinical trials comparing on- and off-pump coronary artery bypass grafting, noted that off-pump coronary artery bypass grafting may improve short-term outcomes such as blood transfusion, renal dysfunction, stroke, atrial fibrillation, and length of stay.[18]

Table 13–1. Details and Methodology of Major Prospective Randomized Controlled Trials Examining Clinical Outcomes of Coronary Artery Bypass Grafting Versus Off-Pump Coronary Artery Bypass Grafting

Trial	Author, date, and journal	Title	Design	Primary outcome	Major findings	Commentary
BHACAS I and II	Angelini et al, 2002, Lancet	Early and midterm outcome after off-pump and on-pump surgery in Beating Heart Against Cardioplegic Arrest Studies (BHACAS 1 and 2): a pooled analysis of 2 randomized controlled trials	Single surgeon 401 randomized patients BHACAS I excluded patients with LVEF < 30% and/ or disease in circumflex branch, among other exclusions associated with high perioperative risk BHACAS II included patients with circumflex disease but still excluded low EF patients	Pooled analysis of BHACAS I and II; all-cause mortality or cardiac-related events 1-3 y after surgery	No significant difference in all-cause mortality at 24 mo between CABG and OPCAB groups (HR 0.57, 0.17-1.96) nor significant cardiac-related events	Pooled analysis showed reduced risk of transfusion, ICU stay > 1 d, and total hospital stay > 7 in OPCAB group compared with CABG group
SMART	Puskas et al, 2003, J Thorac Cardiovasc Surg	Off-pump coronary artery bypass grafting provides complete revascularization with reduced myocardial injury, transfusion requirements, and length of stay: a prospective randomized comparison of two hundred unselected patients undergoing off-pump versus conventional coronary artery bypass grafting	Single surgeon 197 randomized patients Excluded only patients in cardiogenic shock or those with intra-aortic balloon pumps	Index of completeness of revascularization (number of grafts performed/ number of grafts intended)	CABG and OPCAB groups had similar completeness of revascularization indices (1.01 ± 0.09 v 1.00 ± 0.18, respectively, p = 0.219)	Index of revascularization was similar between groups even with respect to circumflex territory. OPCAB groups required fewer transfusions and had shorter length of stay. No difference in stroke rate between groups.

(*Continued*)

327

Table 13–1. Details and Methodology of Major Prospective Randomized Controlled Trials Examining Clinical Outcomes of Coronary Artery Bypass Grafting Versus ABG Versus Off-Pump Coronary Artery Bypass Grafting (*Continued*)

Trial	Author, date, and journal	Title	Design	Primary outcome	Major findings	Commentary
Octopus	Nathoe et al, 2003, N Engl J Med	A comparison of on-pump and off-pump coronary bypass surgery in low-risk patients	Multileft, multiple surgeons 281 randomized patients, excluding patients with poor left ventricular function	Composite of death from any cause, stroke, myocardial infarction, or need for repeat revascularization	At 1 y, no significant difference between OPCAB and CABG groups (90.6% of CABG patients did not meet composite outcome v 88% of OPCAB patients, 95% CI −4.6 to 9.8)	No significant difference between groups in individual components of primary composite outcome. OPCAB group had lower total costs at 1-y follow-up.
Al-Ruzzeh trial	Al-Ruzzeh et al, 2006, BMJ	Effect of off-pump coronary artery bypass grafting on clinical, angiographic, neurocognitive, and quality of life outcomes: randomized controlled trial	Single surgeon 168 randomized patients Excluded patients with LVEF < 30% and those with only single-vessel CAD	Angiographic graft patency at 3 mo and neurocognitive function within 6 mo of surgery	No significant difference in graft patency rates (92.7% patency in CABG group v 92.1% in OPCAB, OR 1.08, 95% CI 0.54-2.15) OPCAB group performed significantly better in 3 memory subtests at 6 wk and in 2 memory subtests at 6 mo	OPCAB group had shorter length of stay, shorter duration of mechanical ventilation, and fewer transfusions than did the CABG group.

ROOBY	Shroyer et al, 2009, N Engl J Med	On-pump versus off-pump coronary artery bypass surgery	Multileft, multiple surgeons in which residents were primary operator in many instances 2,203 total patients randomized, excluding only those with anatomic limitations precluding an OPCAB approach	Primary short-term: composite of death or major complications (redo surgery, mechanical support, cardiac arrest, coma, stroke, or need for dialysis) within 30 d of surgery or before discharge, whichever was later Primary long-term: death from any cause, MI, or repeat revascularization within 1 y	No significant difference between CABG and OPCAB with composite short-term outcome (5.6% v 7.0% respectively, p = 0.19) Rate of the long-term composite outcome was higher in the OPCAB group than in the CABG group (9.9% v 7.4%, p = 0.04), with a trend toward more mortality from cardiac causes in the OPCAB group (2.7% v 1.3%, p = 0.03)	Graft patency rate lower in the OPCAB group. No difference in resource use or neuropsychological outcomes between groups. Nonsignificant trend toward reduced transfusion requirement in OPCAB group.
PROMISS	Sousa Uva et al, 2010, Eur Heart J	Early graft patency after off-pump and on-pump coronary bypass surgery: a prospective randomized study	Single surgeon 150 randomized patients, including those with poor ventricular function	Graft patency rates at 5 wk, analyzed using multidetector CT scan	OPCAB group had significantly lower graft patency rate than did the CABG group (89.9% v 95.0%, OR 2.2, 95% CI 1.07-4.44; p = 0.03) After adjusting by dose of heparin, graft patency was not statistically different between groups (OR 0.87, 95% CI 0.25-2.98, p = 0.83)	At 1 y, no difference in neurocognitive function between groups, even though neurocognitive function in the CABG group tended to be higher at baseline preoperatively, thus actually may have had a more precipitous decline.

(Continued)

Table 13–1. Details and Methodology of Major Prospective Randomized Controlled Trials Examining Clinical Outcomes of Coronary Artery Bypass Grafting Versus Off-Pump Coronary Artery Bypass Grafting (*Continued*)

Trial	Author, date, and journal	Title	Design	Primary outcome	Major findings	Commentary
Best Bypass Surgery	Moller et al, 2010, Circulation	No major differences in 30-d outcomes in high-risk patients random-ized to off-pump versus on-pump coronary bypass surgery	Multiple surgeons, single left 341 randomized patients Included only patients with a preoperative EuroSCORE > 4 who had three-vessel CAD, excluding patients with LVEF < 30%	Composite of adverse cardiac and cerebrovas-cular events (all-cause mortality, acute MI, cardiac arrest with suc-cessful resuscita-tion, cardiogenic shock, stroke, coronary reinter-vention) at 30 d	There were no sig-nificant differences in the composite primary outcome between OPCAB and CABG groups (15% v 17%; p = 0.48) or the individual components	Comparable num-ber of grafts per patient between groups, although the OPCAB group had significantly fewer grafts to the lateral wall.
MASS III	Hueb et al, 2010, Circulation	5-year follow-up of a ran-domized comparison between off-pump and on-pump stable multi-vessel coronary artery bypass grafting. The MASS III trial	Multiple surgeons, single left 308 randomized patients, excluding those with LVEF < 40%	Composite of mortality, stroke, MI, or need for additional revas-cularization at 5-y follow-up	No significant dif-ference between CABG and OPCAB groups with respect to composite out-come (HR 0.71, 95% CI 0.41-1.22, p = 0.21) or its individual components	No significant difference between groups with regard to in-hospital complications. OPCAB group had fewer anastomoses/ patient com-pared with CABG group.

DOORS	Houlind et al, 2012, Circulation	On-pump versus off-pump coronary artery bypass surgery in elderly patients: results from the Danish on-pump versus off-pump randomization study	Multiple surgeons, multileft 900 randomized patients, including those with poor ventricular function All patients were > 70 y old	Composite of mortality, MI, or stroke within 30 d postoperatively	No significant difference between CABG and OPCAB groups (10.2% v 10.7%, respectively, 95% CI −3.6 to 4.4, p = 0.83 for equality, and for noninferiority p = 0.49)	No significant difference in mortality at 6 mo follow-up. CABG group had 3.1 grafts/patient, OPCAB 2.9 (p = 0.007). Blood loss greater in CABG group (p < 0.001), but transfusion rates comparable between groups.
CORONARY	Lamy et al, 2012, N Engl J Med	Off-pump or on-pump coronary-artery bypass grafting at 30 d	Multiple surgeons, multileft 4,752 total patients, including only those older than 70 y, with PAD, cerebrovascular disease, carotid stenosis, renal insufficiency, or age 60-69 with diabetes, LVEF < 35%, recent smoking history, or need for urgent procedure, or age 55-59 with at least 2 of those risk factors	First coprimary outcome: composite of death, stroke, MI, or new dialysis within 30 d Second co-primary outcome: composite of first co-primary outcome or repeat coronary vascularization within 5 y of follow-up	No significant difference in rate of first co-primary outcome between OPCAB and CABG (9.8% v 10.3%, HR 0.95, 95% CI 0.79-1.14, p = 0.59) or any of its components No significant difference in rate of second co-primary outcome between OPCAB and CABG (23.1% v 23.6%, HR 0.98, 95% CI 0.87-1.10, p = 0.72) or in the rate of revascularization between groups	OPCAB required significantly fewer transfusions, redo surgeries for significant bleeding, rates of new acute kidney injury, and respiratory complications.

(Continued)

Table 13–1. Details and Methodology of Major Prospective Randomized Controlled Trials Examining Clinical Outcomes of Coronary Artery Bypass Grafting Versus Off-Pump Coronary Artery Bypass Grafting *(Continued)*

Trial	Author, date, and journal	Title	Design	Primary outcome	Major findings	Commentary
GOPCABE	Diegeler al, 2013, N Engl J Med	Off-pump versus on-pump coronary-artery bypass grafting in elderly patients	Multiple surgeons, multileft 2,539 randomized patients, including those with poor ventricular function All patients were at least 75 y old	Composite of death or major adverse event (MI, stroke, new dialysis, or repeat revascular-ization) within 30 d and 12 mo	At 30 d, no significant difference between rates of primary outcome in OPCAB and CABG groups (7.8% v 8.2%, OR 0.95, 95% CI 0.71-1.28, p = 0.74) Of the individual components of the primary outcome, only repeat revascularization was significantly different between groups, occurring more frequently in the OPCAB	OPCAB group required fewer transfusions than did the CABG group.

Reproduced with permission from Shaefi S, Mittel A, Loberman D, et al: Off-Pump Versus On-Pump Coronary Artery Bypass Grafting-A Systematic Review and Analysis of Clinical Outcomes, *J Cardiothorac Vasc Anesth*. 2019 Jan;33(1):232-244.

Table 13–2. Summary of Short-Term and Long-Term Clinical Outcomes Affected by Off-Pump Coronary Artery Bypass Grafting Versus Coronary Artery Bypass Grafting Approach to Revascularization

Short-Term Outcomes	
Discussion	
Perioperative myo-cardial injury	Even though small studies have supported the notion that OPCAB is associated with less inflammation, there is no strong evidence suggesting that OPCAB reduces the rate of myocardial infarction or otherwise harms immediate postoperative cardiac function.
Stroke	No RCTs have identified a decreased rate of stroke in OPCAB compared with CABG. The influence of particular approaches to OPCAB anastomoses to the aorta for vein grafting is not well established.
Length of stay and in-hospital complications	Several RCTs have found reduced duration of mechanical ventilation, length of ICU and total hospital stays, and severity of acute kidney injury (although not rates of need for dialysis) after OPCAB.
Bleeding and transfusion requirements	Many high-quality RCTs, including CORONARY and GOPCABE (the largest and most recent trials), have found significantly reduced requirements for transfusion in OPCAB compared with CABG groups.
Perioperative costs	Decreased need for specialized personnel, equipment, transfusions, and postoperative complications tends to reduce immediate costs associated with OPCAB compared with CABG.
Neurocognitive function	Some studies, specifically the RCT by Al-Ruzzeh and the CORONARY trial, have identified less neurocognitive deterioration in OPCAB patients compared with CABG patients in the immediate postoperative period. The clinical significance of these findings is likely small.

Long-Term Outcomes	
Discussion	
Mortality	The ROOBY trial found that OPCAB was associated with a slightly increased risk of death at 1-5 y postoperatively compared with CABG. However, no other high-quality RCT has identified a mortality risk associated with OPCAB, with the exception of patients in the MASS III trial who required lateral wall revascularization.
Effective revascularization	Revascularization appears to be highly dependent on surgical expertise. Studies with experienced surgeons generally have had comparable need for repeat revascularization at 1 to 5 y of follow-up between OPCAB and CABG groups. The ROOBY trial, which included a large percentage of relatively inexperienced surgeons, required notably more repeat revascularization at long-term follow-up compared with the similarly designed CORONARY trial. However, some revascularization targets (e.g., small target vessels or circumflex-based disease) are challenging even for experienced personnel. The MASS III trial, in particular, found less effective revascularization in circumflex distributions (and an increase in mortality in these patients). Many other trials have found a decreased number of grafts performed per OPCAB patient compared with CABG patients, lending credence to the conclusion that OPCAB poses a risk of less effective revascularization.

(Continued)

Table 13–2. Summary of Short-Term and Long-Term Clinical Outcomes Affected by Off-Pump Coronary Artery Bypass Grafting Versus Coronary Artery Bypass Grafting Approach to Revascularization (*Continued*)

Neurocognitive function	At 1- to 5-y follow-up, a difference in neurocognitive function between OPCAB and CABG groups generally has failed to be identified. The SMART trial did find some subtle benefit of OPCAB over CABG in this respect, although not enough to be clinically meaningful.
Quality of life	Similar to neurocognitive outcomes, quality of life has not been definitively shown to be enhanced after OPCAB compared with CABG.
Healthcare costs	Even though short-term costs are reduced in OPCAB, the added risk of needing repeat revascularization in OPCAB patients mitigates this difference in long-term follow-up.

Abbreviations: CABG, coronary artery bypass grafting; ICU, intensive care unit; OPCAB, off-pump coronary artery bypass grafting; RCT, randomized controlled trial.
Reproduced with permission from Shaefi S, Mittel A, Loberman D, et al: Off-Pump Versus On-Pump Coronary Artery Bypass Grafting-A Systematic Review and Analysis of Clinical Outcomes, *J Cardiothorac Vasc Anesth*. 2019 Jan;33(1):232-244.

Cognitive dysfunction as measured using psychometric testing is present in up to 50% of patients following cardiac surgery. Interestingly, in the long term there appears to be little difference in the presence of cognitive dysfunction in on- versus off-pump cardiac patients.[19] Of course, unlike stroke or delirium, which are clinical diagnoses, cognitive dysfunction must be assessed before and after cardiac surgery by psychological testing. At times, these testing methods themselves have come into question, making assessments as to the benefit of off-pump surgery in this setting difficult.

Different surgeons have varying experiences with off-pump and minimally invasive procedures and that may determine the use of a particular approach in a given institution. Certainly, selective use of off-pump surgery using the internal mammary arteries without cross clamp of the aorta can be helpful when the aorta is highly calcified or the patient's condition is especially susceptible to the deleterious effects from CPB. On the other hand, the patient with severe heart failure, cardiomegaly, and low ejection fraction may become too hemodynamically unstable to tolerate surgery without institution of CPB.

Whenever minimally invasive techniques are to be employed, communication between surgeon and anesthesiologist should be close. Lifting the heart to gain surgical exposure and the application of stabilization devices may adversely affect hemodynamic performance. Snare ligature of coronary arteries can quickly result in the development of myocardial ischemia and hemodynamic collapse. Likewise, the anesthesiologist should inform the surgeon if they must use heroic efforts to support the circulation for the patient to tolerate coronary occlusion or heart manipulation. On-pump minimally invasive procedures require a closely coordinated perioperative team and skilled perioperative echocardiographers to ensure correct placement of required catheters and cannulas.

CASE SCENARIO

A 73-year-old man presents for coronary artery bypass grafting. He has a severely calcified aorta.

What are his options?

Assuming that catheter-mediated PCI therapies have been ruled out, this patient is a candidate for off-pump surgery if he has no coexisting valvular disease in need of repair and can tolerate manipulations of the heart to facilitate completion of the graft anastomoses.

The surgeon lifts the heart to position it prior to completion of the first bypass graft. The blood pressure falls to 60 mm Hg systolic. How should the anesthesia team respond?

The anesthesiologist notes no new ST-T wave abnormalities and administers vasopressors and intravenous fluids and places the patient in slight Trendelenburg position to ensure adequate preload to offset the decrease in venous return. Blood pressure improves to 90 mm Hg systolic. Following heparinization and graft harvest, the surgeon places snares across the left circumflex artery. The patient remains hemodynamically stable. The anastomosis is completed uneventfully.

While the surgeon is completing the final bypass graft to the right coronary, the patient becomes asystolic. What should be done now?

The surgeon places an epicardial pacemaker wire and temporary VVI pacing is begun. Should the patient become hemodynamically unstable, the off-pump approach can be abandoned and the patient placed on CPB.

REFERENCES

1. Wasnick J, Acuff T. Anesthesia and minimally invasive thoracoscopically assisted coronary artery bypass: a brief clinical report. *J Cardiothorac Vasc Anesth*. 1997;11(5):552-555.

2. Wasnick J, Hoffman W, Acuff T, et al. Anesthetic management of coronary artery bypass via minithoracotomy with video assistance. *J Cardiothorac Vasc Anesth*. 1995;9:731-733.

3. Rasoli S, Zeinah M, Athanasiou T, Kourliouros A. Optimal intraoperative anticoagulation strategy in patients undergoing off-pump coronary artery bypass. *Interact Cardiovasc Thorac Surg*. 2012;12: 629-633.

4. Giambruno V, Jones P, Khaliel F, et al. Hybrid coronary revascularization versus on-pump coronary artery bypass grafting. *Ann Thorac Surg*. 2018;105:1330-1335.

5. Leyvi G, Vivel K, Sehgal S, et al. A comparison of inflammatory response between robotically enhanced coronary artery bypass grafting: implications for hybrid revascularization. *J Cardiothorac Vasc Anesth*. 2018;32:251-258.

6. Wang G, Gao C. Robotic cardiac surgery: an anaesthetic challenge. *Postgrad Med J*. 2014;90:467-474.

7. Bucerius J, Gummert J, Borger M, et al. Stroke after cardiac surgery: a risk factor analysis of 16,184 consecutive adult patients. *Ann Thorac Surg*. 2003;75:472-478.

8. Nahoe H, van Dijk D, Jansen E, et al. A comparison of on-pump and off-pump coronary artery bypass surgery in low risk patients. *NEJM*. 2003;348(5):394-402.

9. Khan N, De Souza A, Mister R, et al. A randomized comparison of off-pump and on-pump multivessel coronary-artery bypass surgery. *NEJM*. 2004;350(1):21-28.

10. Shroyer AL, Grover FL, Hattler B, et al. On-pump versus off-pump coronary artery bypass surgery. *NEJM.* 2009;361(5):1827-1837.

11. Kim J, Yun S, Lim J, et al. Long term survival following coronary artery bypass grafting: off-pump versus on-pump strategies. *JACC.* 2014;63:2280-2288.

12. Bakaeen F, Chu D, Kelly R, et al. Perioperative outcomes after on and off-pump coronary artery bypass grafting. *Tex Heart Inst J.* 2014;41(2):144-151.

13. Bakaeen F, Chu D, Kelly R, et al. Performing coronary artery bypass grafting off-pump may compromise long term survival in a veteran population. *Ann Thorac Surg.* 2013;95(6):1952-1958.

14. Diegeler A, Borgermann J, Kappert U, et al. Off pump versus on-pump coronary artery bypass grafting in elderly patients. *NEJM.* 2013;368:1189-1198.

15. Lamy A, Devereaux P, Prabhakaran D, et al. Five year outcomes after off-pump or on-pump coronary artery bypass grafting. *NEJM.* 2016;375:2359-2368.

16. Smart N, Dieberg G, King N. Long term outcomes of on versus off-pump coronary artery bypass grafting. *JACC.* 2018;71(9):983-991.

17. Shaefi S, Mittel A, Loberman D, Ramakrishna H. Off pump versus on-pump coronary artery bypass grafting—a systemic review and analysis of clinical outcomes. *J Cardiothorac Vasc Anesth.* 2018; epub ahead of print.

18. Puskas J, Martin J, Cheng D, et al. ISMICS consensus conference and statement of randomized controlled trials of off-pump versus conventional coronary artery bypass surgery. *Innovations (Phila).* 2015;10(4):219-229.

19. van Dijk D, Jansen E, Hijman R, et al. Cognitive outcome after off-pump and on-pump coronary artery bypass graft surgery. *JAMA.* 2002;287(11):1405-1412.

REVIEWS

Kuo C, Chang H, Hsing H, et al. Robotic mitral valve replacement with bioprosthetic valves in 52 patients: experience from a tertiary referral hospital. *Eur J Cardiothoracic Surg.* 2018; doi: 10.1083/ejctz/ezy134.

Adams D, Chickwe J. On pump CABG in 2018: still the gold standard. *JACC.* 2018;71(8):992-993.

Bernstein W, Walker A. Anesthetic issues for robotic cardiac surgery. *Ann Card Anaesth.* 2015;18(1):58-68.

Rehfeldt K, Andre J, Ritter M. Anesthetic considerations in robotic mitral valve surgery. *Ann Cardiothorac Surg.* 2017;6(1):47-53.

Leyvi G, Forest S, Srinivas S, et al. Robotic CABG decrease 30-day complication rate, length of stay and acute care facility discharge rate compared to conventional surgery. *Innovations (Phila).* 2014;9(5):361-367.

The Postoperative Care of the Cardiac Surgery Patient

14

Upon completion of surgery, the cardiac patient is transported to the intensive care unit (ICU) for postoperative management. The role of the anesthesiologist or the anesthesiology department in postoperative care depends on institutional policies and procedures. Anesthesiologists trained in intensive care, non-anesthesiologist intensivists, and nurse practitioners in consultation with the patient's attending cardiac surgeon might manage the ICU care. In other settings, the patient's anesthesiologist will manage some elements of postoperative care (e.g., ventilation) while the surgeon attends to others (e.g., chest tube management). What must be emphasized for the practitioner new to cardiac anesthesiology is the need to be aware of the operating paradigm used in one's individual institution. Moreover, it is critically important that anesthesiologists carefully document their report and the time of transfer of care to the ICU team. Unfortunately, some patients survive the intraoperative period only to succumb minutes, hours, or days following arrival in the ICU.

This chapter reviews common problems encountered in the postoperative care of the cardiac surgery patient. It is by no means a comprehensive text on critical care but rather highlights some of the particular problems that appear in routine postoperative cardiac surgery recovery and ICU.

ROUTINE TRANSPORT AND REPORT

Following cardiac surgery, patients are transported fully monitored (ECG, arterial pressure, oxygen saturation) from the operating room to the ICU. As the transport of an unstable patient to the ICU can be challenging, every effort to improve hemodynamic stability should be undertaken in the operating room prior to moving the patient. Anesthesiologists must be prepared for the inadvertent extubation of the patient or the accidental disconnection of a central venous line during transport. Consequently, airway management equipment and redundant intravenous access should be readily available. Similarly, anesthesia providers must be prepared to treat hemodynamic instability. Blood pressure variations are common as patients begin to regain sympathetic tone once anesthetics are withdrawn. Propofol and/or dexmedetomidine infusions, when hemodynamically tolerated, can be used to mitigate the increases in blood pressure often seen in postoperative patients during patient transport. Additionally, dexmedetomidine may reduce the incidence of delirium in ICU patients. Intravenous infusion of nicardipine or other anti-hypertensive agents can also be employed to blunt emergence hypertension. In particular, patients with noncompliant vasculature (common among cardiac surgery patients) will frequently develop severe hypertension during emergence requiring the administration of propofol, narcotics, and vasodilators postoperatively. At the same time, because these patients may be hypovolemic, when hypertension is treated there is often a tendency to overshoot transforming hypertension into severe hypotension.

Patients are routinely transported from the operating room to the ICU with any one of many vasoactive infusions running. Care must be taken to be sure that during transport all expected infusions are flowing at the desired rate and are correctly labeled. As patients awaken, the need for vasoconstrictors such as vasopressin and norepinephrine decreases as vascular tone is restored. Using hemodynamic and echocardiographic guidance, vasoconstrictors, inotropes, and volume loading are adjusted to ensure ideal right and left heart performance.

Patients following transport to the ICU may continue to require pacing initially necessary to separate from CPB. Should the patient arrive in the ICU in normal sinus rhythm, the DDD pacemaker can be set for a slow backup rate (e.g., 55-60 bpm). Many patients develop varying degrees of heart block following cardiac surgery, and some will require permanent pacemaker placement postoperatively. Should patients have complete heart block and be totally pacemaker dependent, the ICU team must be specifically informed to be sure that a secondary temporary pulse generator is available and that pacemaker battery reserves are sufficient.

Upon arrival in the ICU, the majority of patients are placed on a mechanical ventilator. Ventilator settings are dependent upon local policies regarding "preferred" modes of postoperative ventilation. Usually a volume-controlled mode is employed in adult patients with a tidal volume from 400 to 600 mL (6 mL/kg) delivered at a rate of 8 to 12 breaths per minute depending upon patient size. Positive end-expiratory pressure (PEEP) is also used as indicated (customary PEEP is 5-8 mm Hg). The anesthesiologist confirms that the ventilator is actually delivering oxygen through observation of the rise and fall of the chest, auscultation, oxygen saturation, and/or respiratory gas analysis before leaving the patient's bedside.

Assuming the patient is hemodynamically stable and ventilation acceptable, the anesthesiologist provides report to the ICU team. Report includes a brief summary of the patient's preexistent medical conditions, intraoperative course, the surgery completed, the results of the last intraoperative laboratory values, and any special concerns that the anesthesiologist might have (e.g., difficult airway). Efforts to control postoperative bleeding are reviewed including a summary of any and all blood products administered in the operating room.

Once report is completed, the anesthesiologist's duties are predicated upon the operative policy of the ICU.

Many patients following routine cardiac surgery will simply awaken from anesthesia and can be rapidly weaned from ventilatory support. So-called fast track approaches to ICU ventilator management permit ventilatory weaning within 2 to 4 hours of ICU arrival. Selected cardiac surgery patients can be extubated in the operating room. Appropriate consideration should be given to the potential for hemodynamic instability and airway compromise during patient transport when performing "in the OR" extubations of heart surgery patients. Enhanced recovery for cardiac surgery care bundles are increasingly being implemented as an extension of fast track programs. In addition to facilitating early extubation, such programs employ multimodal analgesia (see Chapter 18), goal-directed fluid therapy, early mobilization, and avoidance of delirium.

Ventilatory weaning of the "routine" cardiac surgery patient in the ICU can be advanced when the patient is awake and responsive and maintains adequate respiratory parameters [tidal volume 300-500 mL, acceptable oxygen saturation, and arterial blood gas on 0.4 fraction of inspired oxygen (FiO_2), with a respiratory rate < 30 breaths per minute]. The patient should have a normal breathing pattern, and the postoperative chest radiograph (CXR) should be acceptable.

Following extubation, the patient is ambulated as soon as possible, invasive monitors are discontinued, and the patient is expeditiously discharged from the ICU. Simply put, the patient with an uneventful operation, an uneventful anesthetic, and an uneventful medical history can have an uneventful ICU experience. Unfortunately, nowadays cardiac surgery patients have complicated medical histories and their surgical procedures are more often than not complicated. Consequently, many patients do not experience the uneventful recovery described above. Rather, they are at risk for lengthy ICU stays with single or multiorgan system failure.

INFLAMMATION AND THE CARDIAC SURGERY PATIENT

Much of the morbidity and mortality associated with prolonged ICU stays following cardiac surgery has been associated with the inflammatory process.[1] Inflammatory markers (e.g., C-reactive protein, IL-6, IL-8) increase during and after cardiac surgery. Proposed mechanisms for the inflammatory state associated with cardiac surgery include: contact activation of the inflammatory system through interaction of blood with the cardiopulmonary bypass machine, ischemia-reperfusion injury secondary to aortic cross clamping, and endotoxemia.[2] Endotoxin is considered a major initiator of the inflammatory response associated with cardiac surgery.

During cardiac surgery it is possible that intestinal ischemia reperfusion leads to endotoxin release. Once present, endotoxin can activate the complement cascade and neutrophils leading to a systemic inflammatory response including coagulopathy and microvascular thrombosis producing organ dysfunction. Moretti et al. have demonstrated an association between low preoperative endotoxin antibody levels and patient mortality.[2] Consequently, those patients with a reduced baseline immunity to endotoxin may be at increased risk for morbidity secondary to endotoxin release during cardiac surgery. Efforts are ongoing to identify therapies that would antagonize the contribution of endotoxin to systemic inflammation in the cardiac surgery patient.[1]

Similarly, efforts have been undertaken to mitigate the inflammatory response to CPB (Chapter 17). Complement activation is associated with CPB and with multiorgan injury. The inhibition of complement component 5 (C5) during CPB has been studied and shown to decrease the production of terminal complement cascade components and reduce inflammation tissue injury.[3] Complement-mediated activation of leukocytes results in tissue injury. Complement activation also promotes neutrophil accumulation in the lungs resulting in perioperative respiratory failure.[4] Activated neutrophils generate oxygen-free radicals and proteases producing inflammation-mediated tissue injury in many organ systems.

The inflammatory response has also been shown to be modulated by the use of perioperative statin therapy.[5,6] Statins were initially employed to lower serum cholesterol concentrations through 3-hydroxy-3-methyl-glutaryl-CoA (HMG-CoA) reductase inhibition. The overwhelming majority of patients presenting for cardiac anesthesia and surgery are on preoperative statin therapy. Although effective in lowering cholesterol, statins have also been shown to decrease inflammation, reduce thrombosis, and minimize ischemia-reperfusion injury. Patients on statins are at risk of increased morbidity if the statins are discontinued perioperatively. Statins inhibit generation of isoprenoids, which bind to Rho and Ras guanosine triphosphatases. Therefore, through the inhibition of Rho, statins have direct anti-inflammatory effects and lead to a reduction in inflammatory cytokines, an increase in anti-inflammatory cytokines, and an up-regulation of endothelial nitric oxide (NO) synthetase.[5] Consequently, statins result in less inflammation but increased NO production. Moreover, statins increase thrombomodulin expression and reduce tissue factor expression on endothelial cells resulting in an antithrombotic effect. Because inflammatory and thrombotic effects can contribute to neurologic, cardiac, and renal injury perioperatively, preoperative statin therapy may reduce all these. Discontinuation of statin therapy results in down-regulation of endothelial nitric oxide synthetase reducing production of vasodilating nitric oxide.

Investigations of various agents to modulate the inflammatory response to cardiac surgery are ongoing and likely to become increasingly important in the management of the cardiac surgery patient.[7] However, prophylactic methylprednisolone has not been shown to have beneficial outcome effects when given for prophylaxis of inflammation in patients requiring CPB according to the Steroids in caRdiac Surgery trial.[8] A trial using intraoperative dexamethasone similarly did not demonstrate any reduction in 30-day adverse events in adults undergoing cardiac surgery.[9] However, the Dexamethasone for Cardiac Surgery trial did demonstrate fewer respiratory complications and a reduced length of stay.

GENETIC ASSOCIATIONS AND CARDIAC SURGERY OUTCOMES

Whereas inflammation and thrombosis may contribute to adverse outcomes secondary to organ failure following cardiac surgery, ultimately the degree of the inflammatory response and the propensity toward a thrombotic state are determined by the patient's genotype. Gene association studies performed on cardiac surgery patients have attempted to identify the risk factors associated with perioperative organ injury.[10-13]

These studies attempt to identify genotypes associated with adverse cardiac, renal, and neurological events perioperatively. Even though these studies may illustrate why and how certain patient populations respond to cardiac surgery, individualized anesthetic management based upon genotype may never become manifest. However, knowledge of the genotypes associated with adverse outcomes provides insight as to the disease mechanisms at work leading to poor outcomes. So far, genetic influences have been demonstrated to impact inflammation, response to endotoxin, perioperative dysrhythmias, neurocognitive dysfunction, kidney failure, and thrombosis.[11,12]

Although it is currently not possible to identify the propensity for an adverse outcome in routine patient management, it is increasingly likely that common allelic variations associated with poor outcomes will become at some point part of preoperative screening and may ultimately be factored into clinical decision making and risk/benefit discussions prior to undertaking surgery. At the same time, the fact that such analyses could be used to deny patients therapy based upon genotype certainly raises ethical questions well beyond the scope of this text.

PERIOPERATIVE NEUROLOGICAL INJURY

There is little as discouraging to cardiac anesthesiologists and surgeons as to conduct what is thought to be an "uneventful" case only to find that the patient emerges from anesthesia with a postoperative neurological deficit. The landmark study of Roach et al. identified the problem of adverse cerebral outcomes following coronary bypass surgery.[14] They noted that 6.1% of patients experienced an adverse neurological outcome. These outcomes were identified as being either type I or type II injuries. Type I injuries (3.1% of the study population) were comprised of focal injuries, stupor, or coma at the time of hospital discharge. An additional 3% had a type II injury defined as deterioration in intellectual function, memory deficit, or seizures. Since 1996, numerous studies have been undertaken to better identify and reduce the incidence of type I and type II injury.

Moderate-to-severe proximal aortic atherosclerosis is associated with an incidence of type I adverse cerebral outcomes at least four times of that among patients without the condition.[15] Manipulation of the atheromatous aorta during cardiac surgery can produce multiple emboli leading to neurological injury. Consequently, many efforts to reduce neurological injury perioperatively are directed at minimizing embolic load during aortic manipulation. TEE and epiaortic ultrasound (EUA) as well as direct palpation have been employed to avoid manipulation of areas of the aorta with significant atheromatous disease. Manipulation of the atherosclerotic aorta can be avoided through so-called no-touch approaches.[16] Also, selective aortic cannulation is used to avoid a "sandblast" effect of the aortic perfusion cannula. Other risk factors associated with type I neurological injury include prior neurological abnormality (stroke or transient ischemic abnormality), diabetes mellitus, and the use of a left ventricular vent or an intra-aortic balloon pump. Patients undergoing "open chamber" cardiac procedures such as valve replacement are also at higher risk for type I neurologic injuries.[17] Maintenance of a perfusion pressure of more than 70 mm Hg and avoidance of hypoperfusion during CPB may minimize areas of potential cerebral underperfusion and promote washout of microemboli from the cerebral vasculature. Off-pump techniques may reduce but do not eliminate the risk of perioperative focal neurological injury.[18] Although reduction in the incidence of stroke with off-pump techniques has been suggested, studies remain inconclusive. Recent studies have failed to show a reduction in adverse neurologic outcomes with off-pump compared to on-pump coronary surgery.[19]

Type II injury is more difficult to identify and often requires psychometric testing to detect.[20,21] Cognitive function is assessed through tests of verbal memory and language comprehension, abstraction, attention, concentration, and visual memory.[18] At hospital discharge following cardiac surgery nearly 50% of patients show a decline from baseline in at least one of the domains of cognitive function.[20] Risk factors associated with the development of type II neurologic injuries are a history of alcohol abuse, peripheral vascular disease, cerebral hypoperfusion during CPB and hyperthermia during rewarming from CPB.

Allelic variation has also been associated with an increased incidence of cognitive dysfunction.[21,22] Mathew et al. examined gene candidates associated with inflammation, cell adhesion, thrombosis, lipid metabolism, and vascular reactivity and looked for associations with cognitive dysfunction at 6 weeks postoperatively.[12] They identified allelic variations in the genes coding for P-selectin and C-reactive protein (CRP), which were associated with a reduced incidence of postoperative cognitive dysfunction. Similarly, Grocott et al.[21] showed that genetic variants coding for CRP and interleukin-6 (IL-6) may be associated with an increased incidence of type I injury through their effects on the inflammatory response.

Many patients present to surgery with preoperative cognitive impairment,[23] and cognitive impairment detected on postoperative analysis may merely reflect a preoperative condition.

Nonetheless, irrespective of a patient's genetic predisposition toward an exaggerated inflammatory response or whatever their unknown preoperative condition, adverse neurological results have deleterious health, economic, and legal ramifications. Patients with focal neurological signs are generally evaluated by neurologists and receive supportive and rehabilitative care.

Type II injuries are often more subtle to detect, and frequently it is a patient's family and friends who detect that their loved one is not as "sharp" as they were prior to surgery. Unfortunately, cognitive deficit present at hospital discharge represents a predictor of cognitive dysfunction 5 years later.[20] Selnes et al. conclude that the pathogenesis of any adverse neurological outcome during coronary surgery is likely of a multifactorial nature and that patient-related risk factors such as cerebrovascular disease have a greater effect on neurological outcome than variables related to the procedure.[19]

RESPIRATORY FAILURE

Most patients following cardiac anesthesia and surgery can be readily separated from ventilatory support either in the operating room or within a few hours postoperatively.[24] Although intraoperative extubation at the end of surgery can be performed in patients with relatively well preserved ventricular function and limited pulmonary disease, such individuals are increasingly rare in cardiac anesthesia practice.

Nonetheless, many patients can be awakened fairly quickly following surgery and weaned from ventilatory support. Prior to weaning the patient from the ventilator, the ICU team confirms that the CXR is free of any overt pathology (e.g., a collapsed lobe, pneumothorax, hemothorax) and any lung-related problem is corrected (bronchoscopy, chest tube, etc.). The arterial blood gas should be adequate for extubation. Additionally, the patient should require a FiO_2 < 50% with minimal positive end-expiratory pressure (PEEP ≤ 5 cm H_2O), adequate tidal volume (approximately 4-5 mL/kg), and respiratory rate less than 30 breaths per minute. The chest is auscultated to rule out the presence of bronchospasm. The patient's neurological examination should be intact with the patient capable of airway protection at the time of extubation. Lastly, the patient should be hemodynamically stable such that the probability for return to the operating room and hemodynamic collapse is considered low.

Failure to wean from the ventilator following cardiac surgery has many etiologies including:

- Impaired pulmonary compliance secondary to fluid overload or inflammatory lung disease
- Bronchospasm, airway compromise
- Ventricular failure
- Neuromuscular blockade, anesthetic effects
- Delirium, stroke
- Metabolic acidosis
- Pain

Each of these etiologies must be considered and corrected before weaning can be successful. Failure to wean is often heralded by tachypnea, desaturation, hypertension, and tachycardia.

Many patients who present for cardiac surgery have associated pulmonary disease following many years of smoking. Other patients have no pulmonary history but nonetheless can develop respiratory failure following heart surgery.[4] Inflammation following heart surgery with CPB is secondary to activation of the complement cascade, ischemia-reperfusion injury, and endotoxemia from the potentially hypo-perfused gut. The inflammatory response to CPB can lead to acute lung injury. Neutrophils accumulate in the lung and contribute to lung tissue injury producing an increasing alveolar-arterial oxygen gradient, lung edema, reduced pulmonary compliance, increased pulmonary vascular resistance, and right heart dysfunction. Although most patients tolerate CPB-induced inflammatory lung injury, up to 1% of cardiac surgery patients[4] develop life-threatening acute respiratory distress syndrome. It has been suggested that the practice of discontinuing lung ventila-tion during CPB could contribute to the development of lung injury secondary to atelectasis, and inadequate bronchial arterial blood flow leading to pulmonary ischemic injury.[25]

Noninvasive ventilation is increasingly employed postoperatively following car-diac surgery.[26] Whereas noninvasive positive pressure ventilation enables ventila-tion without endotracheal tube placement in patients with acute respiratory failure, it has a failure rate greater than 30% to 50%.

ACUTE KIDNEY INJURY

Patients with impaired preoperative kidney function are at increased risk for worsened postoperative kidney dysfunction.[27,28] More than 8% of the patients undergoing cardiac surgery experience kidney injury, and up to 1% develop kidney failure requiring dialysis.[29-31] Using Acute Kidney Injury Network definitions, the incidence of kidney injury after heart surgery may exceed 30% of patients.[32,33] Glomerular filtration rate (GFR) can decrease from greater than 100 mL/min to less than 20 mL/min secondary to ischemic or nephrotoxic kidney injury. Emboli and hypoperfusion can injure the kidney during cardiac surgery. Indeed, patients with postoperative stroke have an increased peak of creatinine levels postopera-tively compared to patients with uneventful surgery.[29] Contrast dyes, antibiotics, angiotensin-converting enzyme (ACE) inhibitors, and nonsteroidal anti-inflammatory agents can all contribute to the development of kidney injury (see Figure 14–1).

Genome-wide association studies continue to identify genetic risk factors that possibly contribute to the development of perioperative kidney injury.[34,35]

Acute kidney injury is defined as an increase in serum creatinine concentration of 0.3 mg/dL, an increase in serum creatinine more than 50% of baseline, and a reduction in urine output to less than 0.5 mL/kg/h developing over the course of 48 hours. Biomarkers such as neutrophil gelatinase-associated lipocalin (NGAL) and others can provide earlier postoperative diagnosis of kidney injury. Reduced postoperative platelet count has also been associated with increased risk of acute kidney injury.[36] Platelet activation during cardiac surgery may lead to microag-gregates that may affect kidney vasculature leading to injury.

Low urine output should be addressed by correcting any pre- or post-renal causes. Hypovolemia, ventricular failure, and hypotension should be corrected. Kinked or occluded bladder catheters need to be managed accordingly. Patients manifesting a small increase in serum creatinine perioperatively may in reality have significant decreases in GFR. Consequently, kidney dysfunction should be suspected in the postcardiac surgery patient with a rising creatinine and a nephrology consultation

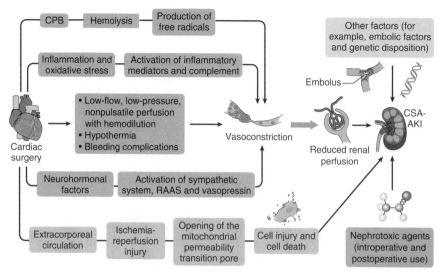

Figure 14–1. Cardiac surgery–associated acute kidney injury (CSA-AKI) can be caused by reduced renal perfusion that results from vasoconstriction after cardiac surgery. A number of pathophysiological pathways can lead to vasoconstriction. CSA-AKI can also be caused by ischemia–reperfusion injury that occurs in the extracorporeal circulation, leading to the opening of mitochondrial permeability transition pores in the kidneys and to cell injury or cell death. In addition, nephrotoxic agents and other factors can contribute to CSA-AKI. CPB, cardiopulmonary bypass; RAAS, renin-angiotensin-aldosterone system. [Reproduced with permission from Wang Y, Bellomo R: Cardiac surgery-associated acute kidney injury: risk factors, pathophysiology and treatment, *Nat Rev Nephrol.* 2017 Nov;13(11):697-711.]

obtained. Of course, many cardiac surgery patients demonstrate a mild creatinine increase on the second postoperative day. Consequently, biomarkers are useful to stratify kidney injury.

Operative patients with preoperative serum creatinines greater than 2.5 mg/dL have a 30% chance of developing acute renal failure.[33] Additional factors that contribute to the development of perioperative acute kidney injury include: duration of CPB, presence of diabetes mellitus, presence of a carotid bruit as an indicator of atherosclerosis and peripheral vascular disease, reduced ejection fraction, and increased body weight. These factors as well as genetic associations may permit anesthesiologists to better identify those patients at risk for perioperative kidney dysfunction.

When AKI occurs, management is supportive in consultation with a nephrologist. Renal replacement therapy may be required to correct acid/base and electrolyte concentrations in addition to removing excess fluid accumulated during cardiac surgery. Patients on dialysis taken to surgery often require immediate postoperative dialysis to remove excessive potassium following repeated administrations of potassium-rich cardioplegia solution during the bypass run. Unfortunately, hemodialysis can lead to hemodynamic instability perioperatively necessitating close attention by the ICU team. Continuous renal replacement therapy (CRRT) may avoid the hemodynamic instability associated with intermittent dialysis, and its early use in critically ill patients with severe AKI is suggested.[37]

Postoperative kidney injury contributes to perioperative mortality especially when combined with other organ system failures.[38] The search for "renoprotective" medications during cardiac surgery remains ongoing (e.g., erythropoietin). One certain strategy is to first prevent kidney injury. Thiele et al. suggest the following recommendations to mitigate perioperative acute kidney injury[39]:

- Delay surgery 24 to 48 hours after contrast administration.
- Hold angiotensin converting enzyme inhibitors.
- Optimize glucose control in patients with diabetes.
- Minimize cardiopulmonary bypass and cross clamp times.
- Base red blood cell transfusions on physiological data.
- Favor vasopressin over alpha agonists to combat vasodilation.
- Target moderate glucose control.
- Hemodynamic management guided by goal-directed therapy.

ICU HEMODYNAMICS

Postoperative hypertension can be particularly problematic following cardiac surgery. More than 50% of cardiac surgery patients require intravenous antihypertensive medications.[40] Uncontrolled postoperative hypertension can lead to cerebral edema, stroke, bleeding at aortic suture lines, and aortic dissections. However, when treating hypertensive episodes, consideration should be given to the autoregulation of organ blood flow in patients with chronic hypertension. Ideally, mean arterial pressure should be maintained within 20% of the patient's baseline to prevent decreases in organ blood flow associated with shifted autoregulatory thresholds. However, in the postoperative cardiac surgery patient mean arterial pressure may need to be reduced by greater than 20% of the patient's baseline should postoperative conditions (e.g., aortic dissection, anastomotic bleeding at surgical suture lines) be of concern.

There are many agents available for blood pressure control postoperatively. Propofol can be administered along with narcotics when indicated in patients requiring ongoing ventilatory support.

Intravenous antihypertensive agents employed include the following:

1. Sodium nitroprusside (SNP) is well associated with the release of cyanide and cyanide toxicity. SNP produces both arterial and venous dilation and can lead to dramatic swings in blood pressure leading to potentially reduced organ perfusion.

2. Nicardipine is a calcium antagonist that provides more selective arterial vasodilation. Clevidipine,[41,42] a rapid-acting calcium antagonist, has been shown to be an effective, direct acting, arterial vasodilator. Unlike nicardipine, clevidipine has a very short half-life (1 min), which makes it useful for rapid titration to effect.

3. Fenoldopam is a vasodilatory dopamine agonist useful for blood pressure control.
4. Beta-blockers are generally administered to patients following cardiac surgery if tolerated to avoid dysrhythmias. However, in the immediate postoperative period, there may be reluctance to administer intravenous beta-blockers in patients with limited ventricular function.

The management of heart failure and hypotension in the immediate postoperative period continues from the operating room. Inotropes, vasoconstrictors, and fluids are administered in response to the interpretation of hemodynamic monitors and perioperative echocardiography (see Chapter 5).

Atrial fibrillation (AF) complicates the postoperative course in 10% to 65% of the patients.[43,44] Risk factors associated with postoperative AF include advanced age, previous history of AF, male gender, decreased left-ventricular ejection fraction, left atrial enlargement, valvular heart surgery, chronic obstructive pulmonary disease, chronic kidney failure, diabetes mellitus, and rheumatic heart disease. Atrial fibrillation occurs most frequently within 2 to 4 days postoperatively. Re-entrant atrial mechanisms are thought primarily responsible for the development of AF and may be associated with inflammation, ischemia, increased sympathetic tone, and atrial suture lines. Postoperative hypomagnesemia may also contribute to the development of AF supporting routine intravenous magnesium replacement. Numerous drugs have been studied regarding prophylaxis of AF. The present data suggest that beta-blockers are effective and safe and should not be discontinued before cardiac surgery. Intravenous amiodarone also reduces the incidence of postoperative AF and may be used in high-risk patients.

Patients who develop postoperative AF are generally treated with beta-blockers and often convert to sinus rhythm. Patients who are hemodynamically unstable require synchronized cardioversion. Intravenous amiodarone can be administered to convert atrial fibrillation to sinus rhythm and can be continued orally in patients who require antiarrhythmic prophylaxis following hospital discharge. Patients with persistent AF should be started on anticoagulant therapy after 48 hours of AF and should have a TEE examination to rule out the presence of an atrial clot prior to attempts at cardioversion.

Ventricular tachyarrhythmias also frequently complicate the immediate postoperative period. Ventricular fibrillation (VF) requires immediate defibrillation. Altered sympathetic tone, inflammation, embolic phenomena, electrolyte abnormalities, mechanical effects, pacemaker dysfunction, myocardial ischemia, ventricular scarring, and a legion of other possible etiologies can contribute to the development of postoperative VF. Usually, it is impossible to identify the cause of VF in a particular patient when it occurs. Ventricular tachycardia occurs most frequently postoperatively in patients having both coronary bypass and concurrent valve surgery.[45] Low ventricular ejection fraction is considered the strongest risk factor for the development of sustained ventricular tachycardia and VF. Nonetheless, ventricular tachycardia and ventricular fibrillation can occur in any cardiac surgery patient. Amiodarone also is useful in suppressing ventricular arrhythmias postoperatively.

Patients may also experience varying degrees of heart block perioperatively. Placement of epicardial pacemaker leads is routine in cardiac surgery, and patients often require atrial or atrial-ventricular pacing depending upon the degree of heart block present. Temporary pacing as established in the operating room (Chapter 4) is continued to the ICU. Usually, a DDD mode (dual-chamber pacing, dual-chamber sensing, dual-chamber inhibition) is selected. If the patient has an appropriate intrinsic rhythm and rate, the pacemaker is set as a backup at a low heart rate (usually 60 bpm).

ANALGESIA, ELECTROLYTES, GLUCOSE

Postoperative pain is usually controlled with multimodal methods including parenteral opioids. There are potential complications from the use of NSAIDs related to gastrointestinal bleeding, platelet function, and renal function. Intrathecal morphine has been advocated to improve postoperative analgesia.[46,47] However, intrathecal morphine in combination with large doses of systemic narcotics may increase requirements for postoperative ventilatory support. Thoracic epidural analgesia has also been employed; however, the risk of epidural hematoma formation following catheter placement in patients who are to be administered large doses of heparin has retarded the use of neuraxial techniques in cardiac surgery patients. Enhanced recovery care bundles also include ketamine, gabapentin/pregabalin, lidocaine infusions, and nerve blocks. Postoperative analgesia is discussed in greater detail in Chapter 18.

Electrolyte disturbances are very common following cardiac surgery, and arterial blood gas, serum electrolytes, and blood glucose should be closely monitored during the immediate postoperative period.

Hypokalemia is often secondary to diuresis and requires potassium replacement. Hyperkalemia also occurs perioperatively, particularly, in patients with kidney dysfunction. Regular insulin and glucose can be given to shift potassium intracellularly. Increasing ventilation and/or administering sodium bicarbonate can correct acidosis. However, hemodialysis should be strongly considered in patients with significant kidney dysfunction as potassium shifts can occur as the patient is weaned off mechanical ventilation or inotropic support. Hypocalcemia is usually self-correcting following cardiac surgery and is often associated with a decreased serum albumin concentration (if total calcium is measured) or blood product transfusions. Reduced ionized calcium if symptomatic is treated with calcium chloride administration. Likewise, hypomagnesemia is corrected by the administration of parenteral magnesium sulphate.

Perioperative glucose control with insulin is often required. Regular insulin infusions are continued perioperatively. Most institutions have an established protocol for perioperative management of blood glucose with the goal of avoiding both deleterious hypoglycemia (from overly tight control) and hyperglycemia.

Postoperative bleeding and coagulopathy are discussed in detail in Chapter 16. Chest tube drainage of greater than 300 mL/h must be closely watched and may require surgical reexploration. Supplemental protamine can be given in the ICU to treat so-called residual heparin or heparin rebound, and blood products are administered as clinically indicated. Deep venous thrombosis prophylaxis should be initiated in the perioperative period.

ECHOCARDIOGRAPHY IN THE ICU

The role of transthoracic echocardiography (TTE) and TEE in the ICU is primarily evaluation of hemodynamic instability. Causes of hemodynamic instability in the immediate postoperative period are numerous including graft thrombosis with resultant ischemia, right or left heart dysfunction, pericardial tamponade, valvular dehiscence, and hypovolemia. In all these instances, TEE/TTE can potentially identify the cause of instability in a matter of minutes.

Pericardial tamponade[48] often presents with nonspecific signs and symptoms. Tachycardia, increased pressor requirements, hypotension, rising central venous pressures, and pulsus paradoxus can all herald its presence. Patients with chronic pericardial fluid accumulations often tolerate large amounts of fluid before clinical tamponade is overt. In the immediate postoperative period, localized collections of clot compressing cardiac chambers can impair cardiac function (**Videos 14–1 and 14–2**). Reopening of the sternum and removal of clot restores the normal chamber geometry and hemodynamic stability.

Anesthetic management of the patient with postoperative pericardial tamponade depends on the time course of its development and the degree of hemodynamic compromise. Intubated patients with acute pericardial tamponade are brought emergently to the operating room. In this scenario the patient needs to be transported to the operating room for reexploration, removal of any compressing clots, and correction of any source of surgical bleeding. Transport to the operating room can be problematic as these patients often have increasing pressor requirements and are unstable. At times, the sternum must be opened in the ICU if transport is not deemed feasible due to patient instability. Full monitoring, airway equipment, and resuscitative drugs must accompany the patient from the ICU to the operating room in the presence of the anesthesiology and surgery staff.

Patients with chronic effusions from either pericardial disease processes (malignancy, infection, uremia) may require creation of a pericardial window. Some of these patients might have had a pericardiocentesis prior to the presentation for the creation of pericardial window with subsequent amelioration in their symptoms. These patients usually tolerate general anesthesia induction uneventfully. Other patients will present with unrelieved, symptomatic tamponade and may become hemodynamically unstable following the induction of anesthesia and institution of positive pressure ventilation. Invasive arterial pressure monitoring and reliable venous access should be secured prior to induction of anesthesia. The surgical staff should be present and ready to emergently open the chest and relieve the tamponade immediately following induction should severe, irreversible hemodynamic instability ensue. TEE is useful to guide therapy and to ensure that all areas of localized cardiac compression are free of clot and fluid. TEE can also demonstrate the presence of left and right pleural effusions (**Video 14–3**). The presence of fluid in the chest following surgery can decrease pulmonary compliance. Prior to chest closure in the operating room the pleural spaces should be examined and thoroughly suctioned of any residual fluid. TEE is also employed in the ICU for the examination of the atria prior to attempts at elective cardioversion for AF. TTE can likewise be employed in the ICU management of the cardiac surgery patient. However, obtaining suitable echo windows via the thorax can be difficult secondary to the presence of chest tubes and pacemaker wires.

SUMMARY

This chapter provides an overview of many of the acute postoperative events, which can occur in the ICU following cardiac surgery. Patients with prolonged ICU stays may develop additional problems related to infections, skin breakdown, and nutritional concerns. Review of any ICU manual will touch on approaches to the management of ICU-acquired infections and nutritional support. Patients with sternal wound infection often require return to the operating room for debridement and stabilization, days to weeks postoperatively. General anesthesia is required and invasive arterial pressure monitoring advised particularly if the patient manifests signs of systemic sepsis.

The involvement of cardiac anesthesiologists in the postoperative care of the cardiac surgery patient varies between institutions. Irrespective of the local operating paradigm, the cardiac anesthesiologist will find much professional satisfaction in visiting all patients postoperatively.

REFERENCES

1. Bennett-Guerrero E, Grocott H, Levy J, et al. A phase II, double blind, placebo controlled, ascending dose study of eritoran (e5564), a lipid A antagonist, in patients undergoing cardiac surgery with cardiopulmonary bypass. *Anesth Analg.* 2007;104(2):378-383.
2. Moretti E, Newman M, Muhlbaier L, et al. Effects of decreased preoperative endotoxin core antibody levels on long term mortality after coronary artery bypass graft surgery. *Arch Surg.* 2006;141:637-641.
3. Shernan S, Fitch J, Nussmeier N, et al. Impact of pexelizumab, an anti-C5 complement antibody, on total mortality and adverse cardiovascular outcomes in cardiac surgical patients undergoing cardiopulmonary bypass. *Ann Thorac Surg.* 2004;77:942-950.
4. Asimakopoulos G, Smith P, Ratnatunga C, et al. Lung injury and acute respiratory distress syndrome after cardiopulmonary bypass. *Ann Thorac Surg.* 1999;68:1107-1115.
5. Le Manach Y, Coriat P, Collard C, Riedel B. Statin therapy within the perioperative period. *Anesthesiology.* 2008;108(6):1141-1146.
6. Katznelson R, Djaiani G, Borger M, et al. Preoperative use of statins is associated with reduced early delirium rates after cardiac surgery. *Anesthesiology.* 2009;110:67-73.
7. Hall R. Identification of inflammatory mediators and their modulation by strategies for the management of the systemic inflammatory response during cardiac surgery. *J Cardiothorac Vasc Anesth.* 2013;27(5):983-1033.
8. Whitlock R, Devereaux P, Teoh K, Lamy A, et al. Methylprednisolone in patients undergoing cardiopulmonary bypass (SIRS): a randomized, double blind placebo controlled trial. *Lancet.* 2015;386:1243-1253.
9. Dieleman J, de Wit G, Nierich A, et al. Long term outcomes and cost effectiveness of high dose dexamethasone for cardiac surgery: a randomized trial. *Anaesthesia.* 2017;72:704-713.
10. Ziegeler S, Tsusaki B, Collard C. Influence of genotype on perioperative risk and outcome. *Anesthesiology.* 2003;99:212-219.
11. Fox A, Shernan S, Body S, Collard C. Genetic influences on cardiac surgical outcomes. *J Cardiothorac Vasc Anesth.* 2005;19(3):379-391.
12. Mathew J, Podgoreanu M, Grocott H, et al. Genetic variants in P-selectin and C-reactive protein influence susceptibility to cognitive decline after cardiac surgery. *JACC.* 2007;49(19):1934-1942.

13. Hirschhorn J. Genomewide association studies—illuminating biological pathways. *NEJM.* 2009;360(17): 1699-1701.

14. Roach G, Kanchuger M, Mora Mangano C, et al. Adverse cerebral outcomes after coronary bypass surgery. *NEJM.* 1996;335(25):1857-1863.

15. Gold J, Torres K, Maldarelli W, et al. Improving outcomes in coronary surgery: the impact of echo-directed aortic cannulation and perioperative hemodynamic management in 500 patients. *Ann Thorac Surg.* 2004;78:1579-1585.

16. Newman M, Mathew J, Grocott H. Central nervous system injury associated with cardiac surgery. *Lancet.* 2006;368:694-703.

17. Bucerius J, Gummert J, Borger M, et al. Stroke after cardiac surgery: a risk factor analysis of 16,184 consecutive adult patients. *Ann Thorac Surg.* 2003;75:472-478.

18. Newman M. Open heart surgery and cognitive decline. *Cleve Clin J Med.* 2007;74(S1):s52-s55.

19. Selnes O, Gottesman R, Grega M, et al. Cognitive and neurologic outcomes after coronary artery bypass surgery. *NEJM.* 2012:366(3):250-257.

20. Hogue C, Selnes O, McKhann G. Should all patients undergoing cardiac surgery have preoperative psychometric testing: a brain stress test? *Anesth Analg.* 2007;104(5):1012-1014.

21. Grocott H, White W, Morris R, et al. Genetic polymorphisms and the risk of stroke after cardiac surgery. *Stroke.* 2005;36:1854-1858.

22. Ti L, Mathew J, Mackensen G, et al. Effect of apolipoprotein E genotype on cerebral autoregulation during cardiopulmonary bypass. *Stroke.* 2001;32:1514-1519.

23. Silbert B, Scott D, Evered L, et al. Preexisting cognitive impairment in patients scheduled for elective coronary artery bypass graft surgery. *Anesth Analg.* 2007;104(5):1023-1028.

24. Boles J, Bion J, Connors A, et al. Weaning from mechanical ventilation. *Eur Respir J.* 2007;29:1033-1056.

25. John L, Ervine I. A study assessing the potential benefit of continued ventilation during cardiopulmonary bypass. *Interact Cardiovasc Thorac Surg.* 2008;7:14-17.

26. Landoni G, Sangrillo A, Cabrini L. Noninvasive ventilation after cardiac and thoracic surgery in adult patients: a review. *J Cardiothorac Vasc Anesth.* 2012;26(5):917-922.

27. Byers J, Sladen R. Renal function and dysfunction. *Curr Opin Anaesth.* 2001;13(6):699-706.

28. Star R. Treatment of acute renal failure. *Kidney Int.* 1998;54:1817-1831.

29. Swaminathan M, McCreath B, Phillips-Bute B, et al. Serum creatinine patterns in coronary bypass surgery patients with and without post operative cognitive dysfunction. *Anesth Analg.* 2002;95:1-8.

30. Mackensen G, Swaminathan M, Ti L, et al. Preliminary report on the interaction of apolipoprotein E polymorphisms with aortic atherosclerosis and acute nephropathy after CABG. *Ann Thorac Surg.* 2004;78:520-526.

31. Chew S, Newman M, White W, et al. Preliminary report on the association of apolipoprotein E polymorphisms with postoperative peak serum creatinine concentrations in cardiac surgical patients. *Anesthesiology.* 2000;93:325-331.

32. Alsabbagh M, Asmar A, Ejaz N, et al. Update on clinical trials for the prevention of acute kidney injury in patients undergoing cardiac surgery. *Am J Surg.* 2013;206:86-95.

33. Conlon P, Stafford-Smith M, White W, et al. Acute renal failure following cardiac surgery. *Nephrol Dial Transplant.* 1999;14:1158-1162.

34. Stafford-Smith M, Yi-Ju L, Mathew J, et al. Genome wide association study of acute kidney injury after coronary bypass graft surgery identifies susceptibility loci. *Kidney Int.* 2015;88(4):823-832.

35. Zhao B, Lu Q, Cheng Y, et al. A genome wide association study to identify single nucleotide polymorphisms for acute kidney injury. *Am J Respir Crit Care Med.* 2017;195(4):482-490.

36. Kertai M, Zhou S, Karhausen J. et al. Platelet counts, acute kidney injury and mortality after coronary artery bypass grafting surgery. *Anesthesiology.* 2016;124(2):339-352.

37. Karvellas C, Farhat M, Sajjad I, et al. A comparison of early versus late initiation of renal replacement therapy in critically ill patients with acute kidney injury: a systematic review and meta-analysis. *Crit Care.* 2011;15(1):R72.

38. Mentzer R, Oz M, Sladen R, et al. Effects of perioperative nesiritide in patients with left ventricular dysfunction undergoing cardiac surgery. *JACC.* 2007;49:716-726.

39. Thiele R, Isbell J, Rosner M. AKI associated with cardiac surgery. *Clin J Am Soc Nephrol.* 2015;10(3):500-514.

40. Cheung A. Exploring an optimum intra/postoperative management strategy for acute hypertension in the cardiac surgery patient. *J Card Surg*. 2006;21:s8-s14.

41. Singla N, Warltier D, Gandhi S, et al. Treatment of acute postoperative hypertension in cardiac surgery patients: an efficacy study of clevidipine assessing its postoperative antihypertensive effect in cardiac surgery-2 (escape-2), a randomized, double blind, placebo controlled trial. *Anesth Analg*. 2008;107(1):59-67.

42. Aronson S, Dyke C, Stierer K, et al. The eclipse trials: comparative studies of clevidipine to nitroglycerin, sodium nitroprusside and nicardipine for acute hypertension treatment in cardiac surgery patients. *Anesth Analg*. 2008;107(4):1110-1121.

43. Maisel W, Rawn J, Stevenson W. Atrial fibrillation after cardiac surgery. *Ann Internal Med*. 2001;135:1061-1073.

44. Echahidi N, Pibarot P, O'Hara G, et al. Mechansims, prevention, and treatment of atrial fibrillation after cardiac surgery. *JACC*. 2008;51:793-801.

45. Yeung-Lai-Wah J, Qi A, Mcneill E, et al. New-onset sustained ventricular tachycardia and fibrillation early after cardiac operations. *Ann Thorac Surg*. 2004;77:2083-2088.

46. Zarate E, Latham P, White P, et al. Fast track cardiac anesthesia use of remifentanil combined with intrathecal morphine as an alternative to sufentanil during desflurane anesthesia. *Anesth Analg*. 2000;91:283-287.

47. Lena P, Balarac J, Arnuf J, et al. Intrathecal morphine and clonidine for coronary artery bypass grafting. *Br J Anesth*. 2003;90(3):300-303.

48. Tsang T, Barnes M, Hayes S, et al. Clinical and echocardiographic characteristics of significant pericardial effusions following cardiothoracic surgery and outcomes of echo-guided pericardiocentesis for management. *Chest*. 1999;116(2):322-331.

REVIEW

Wang Y, Bellomo R. Cardiac surgery associated acute kidney injury: risk factors, pathophysiology and treatment. *Nat Rev Nephrol*. 2017;13:697-711.

Anesthesia for Electrophysiology, Hybrid, and Catheterization Procedures

TOPICS

The number of diagnostic and therapeutic interventions performed outside of the operating room requiring anesthesia services has increased exponentially over the past 10 years. Anesthesiologists are engaged in doctor's offices, ambulatory surgery centers, and endoscopy suites. Although cardiac anesthesiologists are most often involved with highly invasive heart surgery procedures, they too find an increasing part of their practice spent outside of the traditional heart surgery operating theater. Evermore complicated catheter-mediated procedures are completed in ever-sicker patients in the cardiac catheterization and electrophysiological laboratories. Increasingly, hybrid suites have been constructed to facilitate combined open and catheter-based surgeries. Common procedures include: diagnostic coronary angiography, coronary stenting, percutaneous closure of septal defects, electrophysiology studies, arrhythmia ablations, and implantations of pacemakers and cardioverter defibrillators. Also, as was previously discussed, catheter-based valve replacements and aortic aneurysm repairs are performed in hybrid procedural suites (see Chapters 6 and 9).

ELECTROPHYSIOLOGY AND OTHER CATHETER-BASED PROCEDURES OVERVIEW

Cardiac electrophysiology (EP) is the medical specialty devoted to the diagnosis and treatment of abnormal heart rhythms. It involves diagnostic EP testing, radiofrequency catheter ablation, and implantation of antiarrhythmic devices such as pacemakers and cardio-defibrillators.

Advanced medical research, new technology, an aging population, and the prolonged survival of very ill patients have added to the complexity of procedures performed and management of patients requiring EP therapies.[1-5] The anesthesiologist is frequently consulted in both the cardiac catheterization and EP laboratories to help manage patients with severe coronary, valvular, and vascular diseases. Patients can experience hemodynamic perturbations secondary to arrhythmias, poor baseline ventricular function, or procedurally related iatrogenic myocardial perforation and tamponade. Anesthesiologists are called upon not only to maintain patient comfort during these procedures but also to be available to resuscitate the patient should hemodynamic or airway complications present.[1] Procedures that might involve the anesthesia team include:

1. Coronary artery stenting: Coronary artery stents are used in the treatment of ST-elevation myocardial infarction, in-stent restenosis, stenting of saphenous vein grafts, and treatment of chronic coronary artery occlusions. Most of these procedures are performed under moderate sedation given by the nursing staff of the catheterization laboratory. Involvement of the anesthesia team typically is requested when the patient is hemodynamically unstable or there is a need for emergent airway management.

2. Percutaneous ventricular assist devices (VADs): Until recently, intra-aortic balloon counterpulsation with inotropic support was the main therapeutic option for supporting the failing ventricle. During the past few years, a number of percutaneous VAD designs have appeared that can be employed in the catheterization laboratory to provide emergent support for the failing heart (see Chapter 11).

   Examples of percutaneous ventricular assist devices (PVADs) that can be placed in the cardiac catheterization laboratory include the TandemHeart (Cardiac Assist, Inc., Pittsburg, PA) and the Impella devices (Abiomed Inc., Danvers, MA). Anesthesia staff are often called upon to provide hemodynamic management when percutaneous VADs are employed. High-risk percutaneous coronary interventions are at times undertaken with the patient's ventricular function "protected" by a PVAD during the procedure.

3. Percutaneous closure of septal defects: Increasingly closure of atrial septal defects is accomplished through the placement of a variety of catheter-delivered occluding devices. Left atrial appendage (LAA) occlusion devices are also increasingly placed to prevent clot formation in patients with atrial fibrillation (AF).

4. Percutaneous valve repair and replacement: Percutaneous valvuloplasty or valvotomy has been performed for decades, but current interventions permit percutaneous valve repair and replacement.

   The introduction of nonsurgical catheter-based approaches to the management of valvular disease is in a phase of rapid development. Initially, the patient population considered suitable for percutaneous aortic valve replacement was thought limited to those believed to be at high risk for surgery or nonsurgical candidates with significant comorbidities. Although early mortality with this approach was high, rapid improvements continue to better patient outcomes. A 2013 review of

7710 transcatheter aortic valve replacement (TAVR) patients enrolled in the Society of Thoracic Surgeons/American College of Cardiology Transcatheter Valve Therapy Registry demonstrated that the device was successfully placed in 92% of cases. Overall, in-hospital mortality was 5% with a 2% stroke rate.[6] Usually the transcatheter valve is placed into the aortic position via arterial femoral, subclavian, transaortic, or even carotid approach.[7] Stroke and paravalvular leaks are complications of TAVR, but the technique offers benefits to patients who are not considered candidates for surgical valvular repair (Figure 15–1, **Video 15–1**).[8]

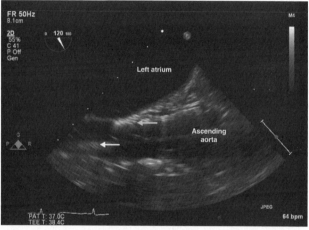

A.

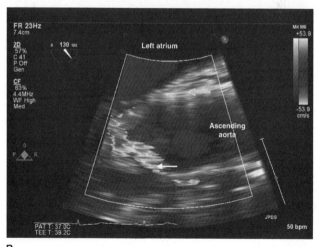

B.

Figure 15–1. (A) Mid-esophageal aortic valve long-axis view showing the transcatheter aortic valve (gray arrows point toward the valve cage). A guide wire (white arrow) is seen crossing the valve. (B) Mid-esophageal aortic valve long axis with color flow Doppler shows an anterior moderate paravalvular leak (white arrow) with turbulent flow. The gray arrows point toward the valve cage.

Indications for TAVR as an alternative to open aortic valve replacement are likely to continue to expand.

Catheter-based approaches to the mitral valve are quite complex as there is no single therapeutic approach for repair for every etiology of mitral regurgitation.[9] Catheter-based treatments for mitral regurgitation include clipping together the anterior and posterior leaflets of the mitral valve at the midpoint yielding a double-barrel mitral orifice for both patients with degenerative disease as well as chronic secondary mitral regurgitation. In high-risk surgical patients with mitral regurgitation due to degenerative disease, the Endovascular Valve Edge to Edge Repair Study (EVERST) demonstrated that percutaneous mitral valve repair resulted in reduced mitral regurgitation and symptoms in patients not thought likely to be offered surgical repair.[10] A recent trial by Stone et al. in patients with moderate to severe mitral regurgitation due to left ventricle dysfunction who failed medical therapy showed encouraging results with trans- catheter mitral valve repair resulting in a lower rate of hospitalization for heart failure and lower all-cause mortality with 24 months of follow-up.[11]

EP PROCEDURES

Indications for EP studies include:

1. Determine the precise mechanism of tachyarrhythmia.
2. Perform catheter ablation for treatment of a medically refractory arrhythmia.
3. Evaluate the need for placement of implantable defibrillators in patients with or at risk of life-threatening ventricular arrhythmias.
4. Risk stratification for sudden cardiac death (SCD) syndrome.

EP procedures include percutaneous catheter-based therapy/ablation for atrial and ventricular arrhythmias, pacemaker, and/or defibrillator implantation.

Electrophysiology studies are performed in specialized EP laboratories, equipped with a fluoroscopy (x-ray) machine. During an EP study, peripherally inserted catheters are advanced into the heart to identify areas of altered cardiac electrical conduction.

Intracardiac measurements of electrical activity are recorded at different parts of the heart at baseline or following electrical stimulation or administration of chronotropic agents.

During an EP procedure, two to four temporary electrode catheters are inserted and positioned into the heart chambers (with the x-ray guidance) via a large vein either in the groin or in the neck.

These wires permit electrical stimulation and recording of electrical responses. An important part of the EP study is to induce the arrhythmia to locate the abnormal circuit.

Treatment options for cardiac arrhythmias include the following[2,3]:

1. Antiarrhythmic drug therapy
2. Catheter ablation therapy
3. Implantable device therapy (pacemakers, defibrillators)

The decision of choosing one option over another depends on the severity of cardiac arrhythmia and the impact of therapy options upon the patient's quality of life.

Catheter-Based Ablation

Until 20 to 35 years ago, the only viable treatment for most arrhythmias was medication. On rare occasions open-heart surgeries with mapping and ablation or high-energy direct current internal ablation were performed.

In the 1990s, radiofrequency (RF) catheter ablation was developed. Catheter ablation has evolved over the past decades to become first-line therapy for many cardiac arrhythmias. Catheter ablation often eliminates the need for chronic drug therapy and can result in significant long-term cost savings.[12,13]

Tachyarrhythmias amenable to RF catheter ablation include:

AV nodal reentrant tachycardia

AV reciprocating tachycardia (WPW syndrome)

Some forms of atrial tachycardia and flutter

Selected patients with paroxysmal AF

Some forms of ventricular tachycardias

Catheter ablation in the setting of reentrant supraventricular tachycardia (SVT) and atrial flutter is associated with both low complication and high success rates. It can be safer, more effective, and less expensive than chronic medical therapy for all age groups. Catheter ablation has expanded to include the treatment of more complex arrhythmias such as AF, unstable ventricular tachycardia (VT), and epicardial VT.

Catheter-based EP studies first identify the area responsible for arrhythmia generation. Using radio frequency (RF) energy, the small focus of heart tissue responsible for initiating the arrhythmia is ablated. Catheter-based ablation is limited by: inability to precisely localize (map) the area responsible, difficulty in positioning the catheter tip at the critical site, or inability to deliver adequate energy to the target.

Catheter ablation procedures are tripartite by nature involving:

1. Placement of electrode catheters inside the heart through veins and arteries
2. Performance of an EP study to detect the mechanism of arrhythmia and localize the responsible area
3. Performance of the actual RF ablation to destroy the target tissue

Atrial fibrillation is one of the more common arrhythmias successfully treated by RF catheter ablation and is the most common sustained cardiac rhythm disturbance associated with an increased risk of stoke, heart failure, and death.

The pulmonary veins (PV) have been demonstrated to play an important and mischievous role in generating AF. Because of their critical role in AF, a variety of surgical and catheter ablation techniques are used to isolate the PV within the left atrium (Figure 15–2).[14]

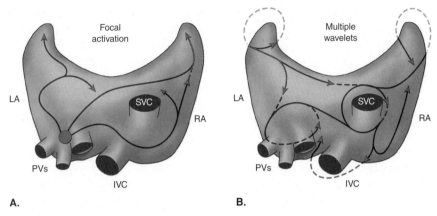

Focal activation

Multiple wavelets

LA

SVC

RA

PVs

IVC

A.

LA

SVC

RA

PVs

IVC

B.

Figure 15–2. Posterior view of principal electrophysiological mechanisms of atrial fibrillation. (A) Focal activation. The initiating focus (indicated by the dot) often lies within the region of the pulmonary veins. The resulting wavelets represent fibrillatory conduction, as in multiple-wavelet reentry. (B) Multiple-wavelet reentry. Wavelets (indicated by arrows) randomly reenter tissue previously activated by the same or another wavelet. The routes the wavelets travel vary. ICV, inferior vena cava; LA, left atrium; PV, pulmonary vein; RA, right atrium; SCV, superior vena cava. [Adapted with permission from Fuster V, Rydén LE, Cannom DS, et al: ACC/AHA/ESC 2006 Guidelines for the Management of Patients with Atrial Fibrillation: a report of the American College of Cardiology/American Heart Association Task Force on Practice Guidelines and the European Society of Cardiology Committee for Practice Guidelines (Writing Committee to Revise the 2001 Guidelines for the Management of Patients With Atrial Fibrillation): developed in collaboration with the European Heart Rhythm Association and the Heart Rhythm Society, *Circulation*. 2006 Aug 15; 114(7):e257-e354.]

Before the procedure, computerized tomography (CT) scan of the heart with three-dimensional reconstruction is performed to define the anatomy of the (PV).

The procedure involves positioning a catheter in the right atrium via the femoral vein. The patient is anticoagulated with heparin, and transeptal catheterization of the left atrium is achieved after systemic anticoagulation to a target activated clotting time (ACT) of 250 to 350 seconds. Angiograms of the four pulmonary veins are performed. Once identified, PV isolation is performed by the delivery of RF energy at the pulmonary vein's ostium for a target temperature of 52°C and a maximum power of 30 to 35 watts (W) for 30 to 45 seconds. Elimination of all ostial PV potentials and complete entrance block into the pulmonary veins are considered indicative of complete PV electrical isolation. Cryoballoon ablation is alternatively used for PV isolation.

Potential limitations of PV ablation include technical failure due to variations in anatomy and difficulty in mapping the focus. The procedure may result in complications, including PV stenosis (up to 45%), hemopericardium (1%), and chronic thromboembolic events (1%).

Most ablative procedures can be performed with moderate sedation and standard monitoring. However, some of the percutaneous ablation procedures can be very lengthy (6-8 h). Also, coughing or partial airway obstruction with abdominal paradoxical motion can interfere with the procedure, so moderate to deep sedation or even general anesthesia with controlled respiration might be required. In patients with compromised ventricular function, inotropic/pressor support with invasive monitoring may be necessary.

Implantation of Cardioverter Defibrillators (ICD/Biventricular Pacemakers)

The placement and testing of ICDs has increased exponentially in recent years, mostly secondary to an expanded list of indications. Biventricular pacing and cardiac resynchronization therapy (CRT) permit better timing of global left ventricular depolarization and improve mechanical contractility and mitral regurgitation in selected patients with heart failure. Many clinical trials have shown that CRT results in improved quality of life,[15] lower mortality rate, and improved functional class in heart failure patients.[16] Moreover, biventricular pacing has been shown to be superior to right ventricular pacing in patients with left ventricular failure and atrioventricular heat block.[17]

Standard indications for ICD therapy include[4,16,18]:

1. Primary prevention of SCD for patients who have not yet sustained a clinical event, but who are at risk for SCD:
   a. Prior myocardial infarction with left ventricular ejection fraction (LVEF) of less than 35% (by cardiac imaging, echocardiography, nuclear study, or cardiac catheterization)
   b. Nonischemic cardiomyopathy (CMP) with LVEF less than 35%
   c. Hypertrophic cardiomyopathy and risk for SCD
   d. Primary electrical disorders (long QT, Brugada syndrome)

2. Secondary prevention of SCD for patients who have already had a clinical event:
   a. Survived cardiac arrest due to ventricular tachycardia (VT) or ventricular fibrillation (VF)
   b. Sustained VT
   c. Syncope in the setting of high-risk disorders

3. Cardiac resynchronization therapy through biventricular pacing in selected patients[5,15,19]:
   a. CHF class III-IV
   b. LVEF less than 35%
   c. QRS duration more than 120 milliseconds

The majority of these devices are placed percutaneously with mild to moderate sedation; however, the placement of a biventricular pacemaker can be a lengthy procedure. Testing of the device [defibrillating threshold (DFT) testing] requires deep sedation or general anesthesia to keep the patient comfortable. Particular attention should be paid to patients undergoing biventricular lead placement for CRT. They typically have very poor cardiac function, so sedation must be titrated carefully, since these patients may poorly tolerate deep sedation or general anesthesia.

Lead Extraction

As evermore patients are having pacemakers and ICDs implanted, the need for explantation of these devices is likewise increasing. Pacemaker leads can fracture, insulations can become worn, and leads can dislodge or become infected. All of these complications require lead extraction. Over time, pacemaker leads become attached to the heart and tissue grows around them. Consequently, they simply cannot just be pulled out easily and their removal has the potential for morbidity and mortality. Powered sheaths have been introduced to facilitate the removal of leads that are adherent to the superior vena cava, tricuspid valve, or right ventricle. These powered sheaths burn through scar tissue with either *laser* or electrocautery. Many patients requiring lead extraction have low ejection fractions, coronary artery disease, and rhythm disturbances. Extracting the lead can be very difficult even with laser or electrocautery and can cause severe hypotension, blood loss, tamponade, and arrhythmias.[1,20]

Short Procedures

Elective cardioversion is a short procedure performed under brief general anesthesia for the treatment of cardiac arrhythmias. It is frequently performed in areas outside the operating room often at the patient's bedside in the ICU or postanesthesia care unit. Before administering general anesthesia for elective cardioversion, it is paramount to ensure the ability of providing full resuscitation and airway management. In patients who are not anticoagulated and are considered at risk of embolism following cardioversion, a TEE examination is performed prior to cardioversion to examine the LAA for the presence of clot.

ANESTHETIC MANAGEMENT OF EP PROCEDURES

With the expansion of the number and complexity of procedures in the cardiac catheterization and EP laboratories, the once occasional involvement of the anesthesiologist (mostly for monitoring and managing of patients with difficult airway or morbid obesity) has become quite frequent.[1,5,21] Out-of-the-OR demand for cardiac anesthesiologists is ever increasing to provide assistance for increasingly sicker patients who are treated by percutaneous modalities. Anesthesia personnel working in these locations often find themselves in corners of dark rooms, which have not been designed to accommodate the presence of anesthesia equipment and personnel. Consequently, there is often too little space for the anesthesia machine and supply cart. Anesthesia staff should make sure that they have adequate access to the airway during all phases of the procedure as well as adequate oxygen and suction before they agree to provide sedation or general anesthesia in any out-of-the-OR location.

1. Preoperative assessment: In addition to the routine anesthetic assessment, a targeted cardiovascular review is required, with particular attention to history of dyspnea, orthopnea, or any signs or symptoms of ventricular failure.

The ability of the patient to breathe comfortably while lying flat should be assessed, although sedation often facilitates recumbent breathing.

2. Preoperative medication: Mild sedation of the patient before induction may be performed with the use of benzodiazepines, but close monitoring of the patient is warranted. The cardiology team may discontinue antiarrhythmic medications before electrophysiological studies as they may prevent detection of accessory conducting pathways and arrhythmogenic foci. Consequently, it is advised that should the anesthesia team administer any medication in the pre-procedure holding area, they constantly monitor the patient since the discontinuation of routine medications may make the patient at increased risk for arrhythmia in the holding area.

3. Monitoring: Standard monitors recommended by the American Society of Anesthesiologists (ASA) should be used for all procedures.

   Additional monitors should be tailored to the specific procedure, patient status, and possible complications associated with either the procedure itself or the anesthesia technique.

   Arterial lines are occasionally placed in patients with compromised ventricular function who undergo lengthy procedures (where there may be a need for blood gases monitoring) or for procedures with the potential for blood loss or hemodynamic compromise.

   External defibrillation pads are placed on the patient, as a "backup" in case the internal catheters or ICD fail to terminate the induced arrhythmia during the device testing or catheter manipulation.

   Temperature monitoring is important since hypothermia can be a problem. Esophageal temperature monitoring specific for PV ablation of AF is desirable to alert physicians to the possibility of thermal injury to the esophagus and danger of creation of an atrio-esophageal fistula.

4. Anesthesia techniques: These range from local anesthesia alone[22] to sedation (mild to deep) or general anesthesia, depending on the procedure and patient characteristics.

   1. Sedation

      Most cases can be performed under monitored anesthesia care and/or deep sedation with supplemental oxygen.

      A variety of agents, including benzodiazepines, propofol, etomidate, ketamine, dexmedetomidine, and opioids have been used to sedate patients during cardiac catheterization and EP laboratory procedures. Dexmedetomidine may make the induction of arrhythmias more difficult secondary to its sympatholytic effects as an alpha 2 agonist.

      Propofol is associated with a high incidence of hypotension[23]; however, it is an effective sedative. A prolonged procedure time requires a higher dose of sedative agents, which may over time lead to more pronounced hemodynamic consequences. Propofol should be used with caution in patients with the combined risk factors of advanced heart failure, poor ejection fraction, and severe renal dysfunction.[24] Although the incidence of propofol infusion syndrome is not known in the context of sedation during lengthy EP procedures, the high incidence of metabolic acidosis detected by arterial blood gases during these procedures suggests that it is not rare.[24-26]

During ICD placement, there is a need for deepening the sedation during device testing. A variety of intravenous anesthetics can be used to produce a deeper level of sedation when necessary. There are advantages and disadvantages associated with each agent, such as delay in recovery of arterial pressure after device testing with propofol.[27,28]

Radiofrequency treatment during ablation therapy generates short, acute pain during the heating process, and it is very important that adequate sedation and patient immobility be ensured during such periods. No single anesthetic drug or sedation regimen has been demonstrated to be superior to any other. Patients sedated primarily with propofol have been shown to have higher sedation scores; however, some require supplementation with opioids and airway control. Other patients managed primarily with a remifentanil infusion can experience apneic episodes.[29]

2. General anesthesia

General anesthesia is at times preferred for management of the EP or out-of-the-OR patient when the procedure is lengthy or painful and performed on very young patients or on patients at risk for airway collapse under sedation. The choice of induction technique is dictated by cardiac function, expected procedure duration, and the usual anesthesia concerns. A variety of anesthesia induction and maintenance agents can be employed. Both laryngeal mask airway (LMA) and/or general endotracheal anesthesia with muscle relaxation can be used. In patients with poor ventricular function, hemodynamic instability can occur secondary to anesthesia induction and maintenance. Sudden, sustained loss of blood pressure during performance of a catheter-based procedure should raise the immediate specter of cardiac perforation and tamponade in addition to the usual hemodynamic variations associated with general anesthesia in a patient with poor ventricular function.

3. Postoperative care

The patient should be monitored and observed after all sedation and general anesthesia procedures in a postoperative care unit or ICU if indicated, and the puncture or procedure site should be observed for signs of bleeding. A chest x-ray may be required to confirm correct placement of devices and exclude possible complications such as pneumothorax or CHF exacerbation.

RISKS AND COMPLICATIONS OF OUT-OF-THE-OR CARDIAC PROCEDURES

The risks and complications of out-of-the-OR cardiac procedures are related to the procedure itself, the patient's characteristics, and the usual anesthesia problems associated with care of the patient with poor cardiac function. Additionally, there are risks associated with exposure to radiation secondary to the fluoroscopy used in these procedures.

Complications Related to the Anesthetic Management

Patients treated in the cardiology suite frequently have multiple and significant comorbidities such as coronary artery disease, valvular disease, heart failure, diabetes, renal insufficiency, obstructive lung disease, and morbid obesity. Consequently, anesthetic management is challenging, as almost all patients are ASA class III or higher. Many of the procedures can be performed under minimal or moderate sedation, but many others require deep sedation or even general anesthesia, often of prolonged duration.

Possible complications associated with anesthetic management include airway obstruction, hypoxemia, hypercarbia, aspiration, and hypotension. Studies suggest[30] that a large percentage of patients undergoing electrophysiologic procedures (40%) require some type of airway intervention, from nasal/oral airway insertion to LMA or endotracheal tube placement.

Also, of note are the effects of anesthetic agents on cardiac conduction. Volatile agents can affect the sinoatrial node automaticity, shorten cardiac potential, and prolong atrioventricular conduction time.

Factors such as increased patient weight and prolonged anesthesia time increase the chance of conversion from sedation to general anesthesia.

Complications Related to the Procedure

Nearly all procedures in the EP laboratory require percutaneous intravenous access with sizable catheters.

Potential complications related to the percutaneous access (common to most procedures) include bleeding, hematoma, pneumothorax, and occasional arrhythmias.

Some risks and complications are procedure specific:

1. Cardioverter defibrillator placement and testing requires the induction of ventricular arrhythmias that are recognized and converted by the device. The effect of multiple trials of VF with electrical conversion can produce hypotension during or immediately after testing.[31]
2. Intraoperative complications related to catheter-based RF ablation are relatively uncommon. They include esophageal rupture, atrial-esophageal fistula, PV stenosis, thromboembolism, left atrial flutter, and atrial perforation.[32,33]

When using RF ablation for AF, the goal is to create a series of lesions in the atrium. The probe is set to deliver energy to a preset temperature and time, but the depth of the lesion is not easily controlled, hence the possibility of through the atrial wall injuries to adjacent structures. The esophagus sits behind the atria and as such can be injured leading to life-threatening mediastinitis.[34]

In this era of increased interventional cardiology, acute tamponade from cardiac perforation is encountered more frequently. Perforation of either the atrium or the ventricle is potentially fatal. The incidence of perforation is about 1% during PV isolation.[35,36]

Cardiac tamponade is life threatening. The rapid accumulation of blood in the pericardial sac leads to compression of all chambers as a result of increased intra-pericardial pressure, which ultimately leads to a severely diminished filling of the heart. The clinical picture depends on the rate of fluid accumulation and the effectiveness of compensatory mechanisms. Therefore, the intrapericardial hemorrhage from cardiac perforation can become very dangerous, very fast.

Clinical findings include tachypnea and dyspnea, which are difficult to evaluate in the anesthetized or sedated patient. Physical findings are nonspecific. Tachycardia, hypotension, and diminished heart sounds may be suggestive. Hypotension is almost always present, and any change in blood pressure downward should raise the alert of the possibility of tamponade and myocardial perforation. A key finding is pulsus paradoxus, defined as an inspiratory systolic fall in arterial pressure of 10 mm Hg or more during normal breathing. This may be difficult to assess in the EP laboratory.

Echocardiography is of great importance in the diagnosis of pericardial tamponade. Among some of the echocardiographic signs, characteristic, although not very specific, are right atrial collapse during late diastole and right ventricle collapse during early diastole.[37,38] Intracardiac echocardiography has been advocated as a method to prevent serious or fatal complications.

The treatment of cardiac tamponade involves drainage of the pericardial contents, preferably by needle pericardiocentesis, with the use of echocardiographic guidance.

Surgical exploration or intervention is indicated when complete control of the bleeding is in question or hemodynamic stability is not rapidly restored with pericardiocentesis alone.

The use of laser-assisted lead extractions techniques for chronically implanted pacemaker and ICDs leads are associated with potentially fatal complications from cardiac perforation, as well, and in addition to superior vena cava disruption and subclavian vein injury. The literature cites mortality from laser-lead extraction ranging from 1.9% to 3.4%.[20]

Given the severity and acuteness of the pericardial tamponade secondary to perforation of the above-mentioned chamber/structures, it is not always possible to perform needle pericardiocentesis in a timely manner, and emergent surgical intervention may be required.

The ASA has published guidelines regarding the management of implantable cardiac rhythm devices.[39]

The management of patients with implanted devices is a three-step process:

1. Preoperative management centers upon:
   - Establishing whether or not a patient has a cardiac rhythm management device (CRMD), by focused history, review of chest radiography (CXR), electrocardiogram (ECG), and physical examination
   - Defining the type of device by reviewing the manufacturer's card, interrogating it with a CRMD programming device, CXR, or querying the manufacturer's databases

- Determining whether a patient is device dependent for antibradycardia pacing by patient history and device interrogation
- Determining the device's function through consultation with a cardiologist or CRMD service

Next the preoperative preparation should include the following steps:

- Determine whether electromagnetic interference will be present during the planned procedure.
- Determine whether reprogramming the device to asynchronous pacing mode or disabling the rate responsiveness function is needed.
- Suspend the device's anti-tachyarrhythmia functions, if present.
- Advise the use of bipolar electrocautery system if the patient is pacemaker dependent. If monopolar electrocautery must be used, recommend the use of short, irregular bursts.
- Ensure the availability of temporary pacing and external defibrillation equipment.

The task force recommends changing to an asynchronous pacing mode for all patients who are pacer dependent. This can be accomplished either by programming or magnet application.

CAUTION: There is no reliable way to assess proper magnet placement.

- Magnet application to a combined ICD/pacemaker may disable the tachyarrhythmia therapy function depending on the manufacturer of the device but not alter the pacing mode to an asynchronous mode. Therefore, in these devices only a consultant can change the pacing mode by using a device programmer.

2. Intraoperative management includes managing potential sources of electromagnetic interference:

- Electrocautery: Position the return pad in such a way that the current pathway does not pass through or in the vicinity of the device; suggest the use of short, intermittent bursts of cautery; suggest the use a bipolar cautery that reduces the current flow through the body.
- RF ablation: Keep the RF current path as far away from the device as possible.
- Lithotripsy: Avoid focusing of the lithotripsy beam near the generator; disable atrial pacing if the lithotripsy triggers on the R wave.
- Magnetic resonance imaging: Various protocols in different institutions have been established to allow MRI in some circumstances in patients with implanted cardiac devices. Additionally, newer devices are designated "MRI conditional" increasing the possibility of MR imaging in device patients

The external defibrillation pads should be placed as far away from the generator as possible to minimize damaging the device in case of emergency defibrillation. Before attempting emergency defibrillation or cardioversion in patients with disabled ICDs, the magnet should be removed to re-enable the tachyarrhythmia therapy function of the device. If the device does not deliver the appropriate shock, then external defibrillation or cardioversion should be immediately performed.

3. Postoperative management

The postoperative management should include interrogation of the device and restoration of the tachyarrhythmia therapy function of the device in the post-anesthesia care unit or intensive care unit. Until the defibrillating function of the device is restored, the function should be monitored with continuous ECG. *No patient should be discharged from a monitored area until the device has been interrogated postoperatively.* However, some consider this warning too restrictive especially if bipolar cautery has been used and the device is more than 15 cm from the surgical site.

REFERENCES

1. Shook DC, Gross W. Offsite anesthesiology in the cardiac catheterization lab. *Curr Opin Anesthesiol.* 2007;20(4):352-358.

2. Blomstrom-Lundqvist C, Scheinman MM, Aliot E (committee members). ACC/AHA/ESC guidelines for management of patients with supraventricular arrhythmias: a report of the American College of Cardiology/American Heart Association Task Force and the European Society of Cardiology Committee for Practice Guidelines. *Circulation.* 2003;108(15):1871-909.

3. Zipes D, Camm A, Borggrefe M, et al. ACC/AHA/ESC Guidelines for management of patients with ventricular arrhythmias and the prevention of sudden cardiac death: a Report of the American College of Cardiology/American Heart Association Task Force and the European Society of Cardiology Committee for Practice Guidelines. *J Am Coll Cardiol.* 2006;48(5):e247-346.

4. Gregoratos G, Abrams J, Epstein AE, et al. ACC/AHA/NASPE 2002 guideline update for implantation of cardiac pacemakers and antiarrhythmia devices: summary article: a report of the Cardiac College of Cardiology/American Heart Association Task Force on Practice Guidelines (ACC/AHA/NASPE Committee to Update the 1998 Pacemeker Guidelines). *Circulation.* 2002;106:2145-2161.

5. Reddy K, Jaggar S, Gillbe C. The anesthetist and the cardiac catheterization laboratory. *Anesthesia.* 2006;61:1175-1186.

6. Mack M, Brennan J, Brindis R, et al. Outcomes following transcatheter aortic valve replacement in the United States. *JAMA.* 2013;310(19):2069-2077.

7. Webb JG, Chandavimol M, Thompson CR, et al. Percutaneous aortic valve implantation retrograde from the femoral artery. *Circulation.* 2006;113:842-850.

8. Tang G, Lansman S, Cohen M, et al. Transcatheter aortic valve replacement: current developments, ongoing issues, future outlook. *Cardiology in Review.* 2013;21(2):55-76.

9. Webb JG, Harneck J, Munt BI, et al. Percutaneous transvenous mitral annuloplasty: initial human experience with device implantation in the coronary sinus. *Circulation.* 2006;113:851-855.

10. Glower D, Kar S, Trento A, et al. Percutaneous mitral valve repair for mitral regurgitation in high risk patients: results of the EVERST II study. *JACC.* 2014;64(2):172-181.

11. Stone GW, Lindenfeld J, Abraham W, Kar S, et al. Transcatheter mitral valve repair in patients with heart failure. *NEJM.* 2018;379:2307-2318.

12. Lin D, Marchlinski FE. Advances in ablation therapy for complex arrhythmias; atrial fibrillation and ventricular tachycardia. *Curr Cardiol Rep.* 2003;5:407-414.

13. Natale A, Newby K, Pissano E, et al. Prospective randomized comparison of antiarrhythmic therapy versus first-line radiofrequency ablation in patients with atrial flutter. *J Am Coll Cardiol.* 200;35:1898-1904.

14. Oral H, Pappone C, Chugh A, Good E, et al. Circumferential pulmonary-vein ablation for chronic atrial fibrillation. *N Engl J Med.* 2006;354(9):934-941.

15. Abraham WT, Fisher WG, Smith AL, et al. Cardiac resynchronization in chronic heart failure. MIRACLE Study group. Multicenter Insync Randomized Clinical Evaluation. *NEJM.* 2002;46:1845-1853.

16. Kadish A, Dyer A, Daubert JP, et al. Prophylactic defibrillator implantation in patients with nonischemic dilated cardiomyopathy. *N Engl J Med.* 2004;350:2151-2158.

17. Curtis A, Worley S, Adamson P, et al. Biventricular pacing for atrioventricular block and systolic dysfunction. *NEJM.* 2013;368(17):1585-1593.

18. Moss AJ, Hall WJ, Cannon DS, et al. Improved survival with an implanted defibrillator in patients with coronary disease at high risk for ventricular arrhythmia. Multicenter automatic defibrillator implantation trial investigation. *N Engl J Med.* 1996;335:1933-1940.

19. Leon AR, Abraham WT, Curtis AB, et al. Safety of transvenous cardiac resynchronization system implantation in patients with chronic heart failure. *J Am Coll Cardiol.* 2005;46:2348-2356.

20. Gaca JG, Lima B, Milano CA, et al. Laser-assisted extraction of pacemaker and defibrillator leads: The role of cardiac surgeon. *Ann Thorac Surg.* 2009;87(5):1446-1450.

21. Conlay L. Special concerns in the cardiac catheterization lab. *Int Anesthesiol Clin.* 2003;41(2):63-67.

22. Tung RT, Bajaj AK. Safety of implantation of a cardioverter-defibrillator without general anesthesia in an electrophysiology laboratory. *Am J Cardiol.* 1995;75:908-912.

23. Canessa R, Lema G, Urzua J, et al. Anesthesia for elective cardioversion: a comparison of four anesthetics. *J Cardiothoracic Vasc Anesth.* 1991;5(6):566-568.

24. Pandya K, Patel B, Natla J, et al. Predictors of hemodynamic compromise with propofol during defibrillator implantation; a single center experience. *J Interv Card Electrophysiol.* 2009;25(2):141-151.

25. Cravens GT, Packer DL, Johnson ME. Incidence of propofol infusion syndrome during noninvasive radiofrequency ablation for atrial flutter or fibrillation. *Anesthesiology.* 2007;106(6):1134-1138.

26. Lippmann M, Kakazu C. Hemodynamics with propofol: is propofol dangerous in classes III-IV patients? *Anesth Analg.* 2006;103(1):260.

27. Camci E, Kolta K, Sungur Z, et al. Implantable cardioverter-defibrillator placement in patients with mild-to-moderate left ventricular dysfunction: hemodynamics and recovery profile with two different anesthetics used during deep sedation. *J Cardiothorac Vasc Anesth.* 2003;17(5):613-616.

28. Keyl C, Tassani P, Kemkes B, et al. Hemodynamic changes due to intraoperative testing of the automatic implantable cardioverter-defibrillator: implications for anesthesia management. *J Cardiothoracic Vasc Anesth.* 1993;7:442-447.

29. Lena P, Mariottini CJ, Balarac N, et al. Remifentanil versus propofol for radiofrequency treatment of atrial flutter. *Can J Anesth.* 2006;53(4):357-362.

30. Trentman TL, Fasset SL, Mueller JT, Altemose GT. Airway interventions in the cardiac electrophysiology laboratory: a retrospective review. *J Cardiothoracic Vasc Anesth.* 2009;23(6):841-845.

31. Gilbert TB, Gold MR, Shorofsky SR, et al. Cardiovascular responses to repetitive defibrillation during implantable cardioverter-defibrillator testing. *J Cardiothoracic Vasc Anesth.* 2002;16(2):180-185.

32. Tsai MT, Fisher JM, Norotsky M, et al. Perforation of the right atrium during radiofrequency ablation. *J Cardiothoracic Vasc Anesth.* 2008;22(3):426-427.

33. Oral H, Chugh A, Ozaydin M, et al. Risk of thromboembolic events after percutaneous left atrial radiofrequency ablation of atrial fibrillation. *Circulation.* 2006;114:759-765.

34. Gillinov AM, Petterson G, Rice TW. Esophageal injury during radiofrequency ablation for atrial fibrillation. *J Thorac Cardiovasc Surg.* 2001;122:1239-1240.

35. Hindricks G. The Multicenter European Radiofrequency Survey (MERFS): complications of radiofrequency catheter ablation of arrhythmia. *Eur Heart J.* 1993;14(120):1644-1653.

36. Hsu LF, Jais P, Hocini M, et al. Incidence of cardiac tamponade complicating ablation for atrial fibrillation. *Pacing Clin Electrophysiol.* 2005;28(s1):S106-S109.

37. Spodick DH. Acute cardiac tamponade. *N Engl J Med.* 2003;349(70):684-690.

38. Tsang TSM, Freeman WK, Barnes ME, et al. Rescue echocardiographically guided pericardiocentesis for cardiac perforation complicating catheter-based procedures. The Mayo clinic experience. *J Am Coll Cardiol.* 1998;32(5):1345-1350.

39. American Society of Anesthesiologists Task Force on Perioperative Management of Patients with Cardiac Rhythm Management Devices. Practice advisory for the perioperative management of patients with cardiac rhythm management devices: pacemakers and implantable cardioverter-defibrillators. *Anesthesiology.* 2005;103:186-198.

REVIEWS

The American College of Cardiology and the American Heart Association provide extensive guidelines for the management of arrhythmias. See Chapter 3.

Calkins H, Hindricks G, Cappato R, et al. 2017 HRS/EHRA/ECAS/APHRS/SOLAECE expert consensus statement on catheter and surgical ablation of atrial fibrillation. *Heart Rhythm.* 2017;14(10):e275-e444.

Bleeding frequently complicates both elective and emergency cardiac surgery. Innumerable surgical database analyses undertaken in recent years have demonstrated the deleterious effects of blood and blood component transfusion in cardiac surgery patients. Conversely, there are other studies that highlight the negative effects of failing to transfuse. This chapter will examine the causes, prevention, and management of perioperative bleeding in cardiac surgery. Additionally, since many cardiac surgical emergencies are associated with increased bleeding these too will be reviewed.

HEMOSTASIS AND CARDIAC SURGERY

Hemostasis during and after cardiac surgery begins with surgical control of active bleeding sites. Unfortunately, control of bleeding in cardiac surgery is far more complicated than the mere application of suture to a bleeding vessel. Rather, the effects of hypothermia and hemodilution perturb the entire coagulation system, which balances clot formation and clot degradation. Anticoagulation required for cardiopulmonary bypass (CPB) coupled with the activation of the coagulation, fibrinolytic, and inflammatory systems further disrupts hemostatic mechanisms.[1,2]

Primary hemostasis occurs when the subendothelial layer of a bleeding vessel is exposed to injury. The endothelial cell of the normal vessel wall is antithrombogenic. However, the subendothelial layer is replete with thrombogenic tissue factor (TF) to

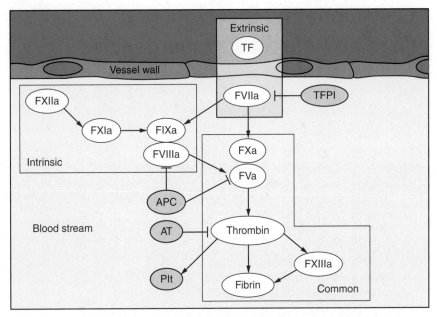

Figure 16–1. The coagulation pathway. The extrinsic pathway consists of tissue factor (TF) and FVIIa. The intrinsic pathway develops from factors FXIIa, FXIa, FIXa, and FVIIIa. The common pathway to fibrin involves FXa, FVa, and thrombin. Factor FXIIIa links fibrin. Thrombin activates platelets (PLT). Regulation of the clotting cascade is provided by tissue factor pathway inhibitor (TFPI), which inhibits the tissue factor VIIa complex. Activated protein C (APC) inactivates factors FVa and FVIIIa. Lastly antithrombin (AT) inhibits thrombin. [Adapted with permission from Mackman N: The role of tissue factor and factor VIIa in hemostasis, *Anesth Analg.* 2009 May;108(5):1447-1452.]

initiate coagulation (Figure 16–1). Platelets adhere to subendothelial collagen–von Willebrand factor (vWF) via their glycoprotein (GP) Ib receptors to begin local clot formation. Fibrinogen links adjacent platelets through their GP IIb/IIIa receptors and a clot is born.

Coagulation follows through activation of the well-known coagulation cascades and is limited and regulated by various proteins and mechanisms (Figure 16–2). Tissue factor and factor VIIa through the extrinsic pathway activate factor X leading to the generation of thrombin and then the conversion of fibrinogen to fibrin via the common pathway. The intrinsic pathway follows from the activation of factors XII, IX, and XI and results in activation of factor X and finally generation of thrombin through the common pathway. Various inhibitory proteins moderate the clotting cascade. Tissue factor pathway inhibitor (TFPI) inhibits the initiation of the extrinsic pathway, and protein C and protein S inactivate factor VIIIa and factor Va. Antithrombin III (AT III) inhibits thrombin as well as factors IX, XI, XII, and X.

The final phase of normal hemostasis is fibrinolysis. Fibrinolysis involves the production of plasmin through the conversion of plasminogen to plasmin by plasminogen activators. Fibrinolysis remodels the fibrin clot and ultimately leads to the dissolution of the clots.

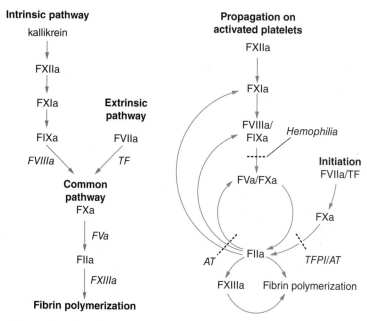

Figure 16–2. (A) A simplified, classical approach to the coagulation cascade. (B) Propagation of thrombin generation. Initiation of coagulation by the FVIIa/TF complex. Antithrombin (AT) and tissue factor pathway inhibitor (TFPI) regulate thrombin production. Thrombin itself activates factors FXIa, FVIIIa/FIXa, and FVa to further increase thrombin production. [Modified with permission from Tanaka KA, Key NS, Levy JH: Blood coagulation: hemostasis and thrombin regulation, *Anesth Analg.* 2009 May;108(5):1433-1446.]

Manipulation of the normal coagulation system is a critical part of the perioperative management of the heart surgery patient. Complete anticoagulation is required while the patient is on CPB. Likewise, cardiologists frequently employ various degrees of anticoagulation. Patients following percutaneous coronary interventions (PCIs) are often treated with abciximab or eptifibatide. These agents antagonize platelet GP IIb/IIIa-mediated binding and prevent platelet aggregation. Often patients presenting for emergency heart surgery in the setting of a failed stent will be treated with these agents and are likely to need platelet transfusion perioperatively. An ever-increasing number of patients are treated with the oral agent clopidogrel, which blocks the platelet's ADP receptor and likewise inhibits platelet aggregation. Clopidogrel use is ever more increasing as it is taken not only to prevent thrombosis of cardiac stents but for a variety of vascular conditions where antiplatelet activity is desired. Discontinuation of clopidogrel perioperatively carries risk of stent thrombosis, and as such perioperative discontinuation of this agent should be preceded by a conversation between the cardiologist, the surgeon, and the anesthesiologist. However, patients treated with antiplatelet agents are at risk for increased bleeding when taken to heart surgery. Conversely, aspirin has not been shown to increase perioperative bleeding in cardiac surgical patients[3] in spite of its antiplatelet effects. Nonetheless, many surgeons will discontinue aspirin use 7 days before surgery. Patients presenting emergently for surgery may have been treated with factor X_a inhibitors (e.g., apixaban) or the direct thrombin inhibitor dabigatran. Idarucizumab can reverse the effects of dabigatran. A factor X_a specific reversal agent (e.g., andexanet alfa) is also becoming available. Andexanet binds factor X_a inhibitors. Idarucizumab inhibits the ability of dabigatran to bind to thrombin.

Heparin is frequently administered to preoperative cardiac surgical patients at risk for coronary thrombosis. As was discussed in Chapter 4, heparin resistance can occur in patients previously heparinized who are brought to surgery and are required to have an activated clotting time (ACT) of 480 seconds or higher for the initiation of CPB. Reduced concentrations of AT III are associated with prolonged heparin use. Recombinant AT III concentrates and fresh frozen plasma (FFP) can be used to treat heparin resistance secondary to AT III deficiency.

Other patients may come for surgery with various coagulation disorders, platelet deficiencies, or cold agglutinin disease. Consultation with a hematologist is recommended to aid in management of those patients with established clotting disorders or hematological diseases (e.g., sickle cell disease). Patients with uremia or hepatic failure are at increased risk for bleeding perioperatively.

However, many patients bleed without any history of anti-hemostatic agent drug use or other contributing medical conditions. Cardiac surgery with CPB is associated with a major inflammatory reaction secondary to the contact of blood with the surface of the bypass circuit. Inflammation impairs protein C and protein S regulation of clot formation and increases expression of TF, which can lead to coagulation activation.[4] Microvascular thrombosis may occur as a consequence of this inflammatory pathway. Consumption of clotting factors and fibrinolysis can lead to impaired clotting, perioperative bleeding, blood product delivery, and potential morbidity and mortality.

There are many methods employed to monitor the patient's hemostatic system perioperatively.[5] The combination of hemodilution of platelets and clotting factors, factor and platelet activation, and fibrinolysis makes close monitoring of the patient's coagulation status essential to avoid unnecessary transfusion of allogenic blood products. Traditional laboratory monitors of the coagulation system (e.g., prothrombin time, partial thromboplastin time, platelet count, hematocrit, and fibrinogen concentration) are usually provided preoperatively and can be ordered intra-operatively as well. However, there is frequently a time delay making such laboratory tests too slow to aid in immediate clinical decision making. Point-of-care (POC) measures of coagulation are employed in certain institutions to varying degrees. Rotational thromboelastometry has been shown to be able to predict thrombocytopenia and hypofibriginonemia in patients after 5 minutes.[6] Thromboelastography is also routinely employed as a POC test to assess the coagulation system (Figures 16–3 and 16–4).

When blood contacts the surfaces of the bypass circuit, the coagulation, inflammatory, and fibrinolytic pathways are activated. As discussed in Chapter 4, activated clotting time (ACT) and heparin concentration assays are routinely employed to determine a safe degree of anticoagulation status during CPB. Thromboelastography

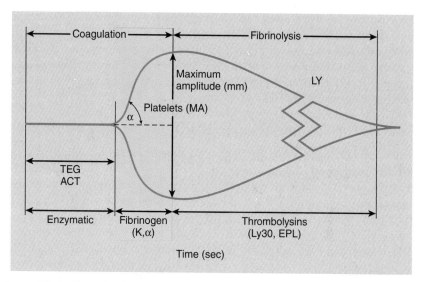

Figure 16–3. Thromboelastograph (TEG). The graph begins as a straight line until clot formation begins (the enzymatic stage of clotting). As a clot forms, increasing resistance develops on the strain gauge, creating a splaying of the graph. The pattern of the graph suggests the status of fibrinogen stores (α angle) and platelet function (maximum amplitude, MA). Eventually, fibrinolysis will occur as demonstrated by decreasing MA. Deficiencies of various clotting components will affect each phase of the TEG, whereas increased fibrinolysis will be demonstrated by an earlier decline in the maximum amplitude. ACT, activated clotting time; EPL, Ly30, K, R, values related to rate of clot breakdown. [Reproduced with permission from Kashuk JL, Moore EE, Sawyer M, et al: Postinjury coagulopathy management: goal directed resuscitation via POC thrombelastography, *Ann Surg.* 2010 Apr;251(4):604-614.]

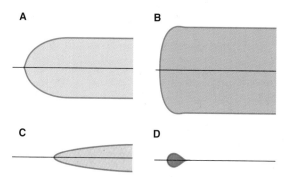

Figure 16–4. Examples of typical thromboelastograph tracings. (A) Normal. (B) Hypercoagulation. (C) Hypocoagulation (e.g., thrombocytopenia). (D) Fibrinolysis. (Adapted with permission from Johansson PI, Stissing T, Bochsen L, et al: Thrombelastography and tromboelastometry in assessing coagulopathy in trauma, *Scand J Trauma Resusc Emerg Med.* 2009 Sep 23;17:45.)

(TEG) permits the diagnosis of various coagulopathic states including factor deficiency, platelet dysfunction, and fibrinolysis. TEG is employed in some institutions to aid in the postoperative management of bleeding through identification of the source of the coagulation deficit.[7] Efforts to provide for bedside determination of platelet function and not just platelet count are ongoing through the use of whole blood aggregometry.[8]

PREVENTION OF BLOOD LOSS DURING CARDIAC SURGERY

Because so many patients present with or develop impaired hemostatic function during cardiac surgery, all efforts are undertaken to minimize blood loss. The Society of Thoracic Surgeons has prepared extensive guidelines to promote blood conservation and minimize blood transfusion in the cardiac surgery patient.[9] In 2017 the European Association for Cardio-Thoracic Surgery and the European Association of Cardiothoracic Anaesthesiology reported guidelines on patient blood management for adult cardiothoracic surgery. Their recommendations with the associated class and level of evidence are summarized in Tables 16–1 to 16–8.

The authors of the Joint Effort Patient Blood Management Guidelines for Adult Cardiac Surgery have summarized their key messages (see Figure 16–5).

The use of antifibrinolytic agents has been at the center of efforts to reduce perioperative blood loss in the cardiac surgery patient. Aminocaproic acid and tranexamic acid are so-called lysine analogues.[10] These drugs attach to the lysine-binding site of

Table 16–1. Classes of Recommendations

Classes of recommendations	Definition	Suggested wording to use
Class I	Evidence and/or general agreement that a given treatment or procedure is beneficial, useful and effective	Is recommended/is indicated
Class II	Conflicting evidence and/or a divergence of opinion about the usefulness/efficacy of the given treatment or procedure	
Class IIa	Weight of evidence/opinion is in favor of usefulness/efficacy.	Should be considered
Class IIb	Usefulness/efficacy is less well established by evidence/opinion.	May be considered
Class III	Evidence/general agreement that the given treatment/procedure is not useful/effective and may sometimes be harmful.	Is not recommended

Classes of recommendations based on the Methodology Manual for European Association for Cardio-Thoracic Surgery clinical guidelines.
Reproduced with permission from Task Force on Patient Blood Management for Adult Cardiac Surgery of the European Association for Cardio-Thoracic Surgery (EACTS) and the European Association of Cardiothoracic Anaesthesiology (EACTA), et al: 2017 EACTS/EACTA Guidelines on patient blood management for adult cardiac surgery, *J Cardiothorac Vasc Anesth.* 2018 Feb;32(1):88-120.

Table 16–2. Laboratory and Point-of-Care Tests to Predict Perioperative Bleeding

Recommendations	Class[a]	Level[b]
Preoperative fibrinogen levels may be considered to identify patients at high risk of bleeding.	IIb	C
Routine use of viscoelastic and platelet function testing is not recommended to predict bleeding in patients without antithrombotic treatment.	III	C
Platelet function testing may be considered to guide the decision on the timing of cardiac surgery in patients who have recently received P2Y12 inhibitors or who have ongoing DAPT.	IIb	B

[a]Class of recommendation.
[b]Level of evidence
DAPT: dual antiplatelet therapy.
Reproduced with permission from Task Force on Patient Blood Management for Adult Cardiac Surgery of the European Association for Cardio-Thoracic Surgery (EACTS) and the European Association of Cardiothoracic Anaesthesiology (EACTA), et al: 2017 EACTS/EACTA Guidelines on patient blood management for adult cardiac surgery, *J Cardiothorac Vasc Anesth.* 2018 Feb;32(1):88-120.

plasminogen and plasmin, displacing it from fibrin. Thus, they impair fibrinolysis. Aprotinin is a serine protease inhibitor, which prevents plasmin-mediated fibrinolysis and many of the enzymatic intermediaries that contribute to the systemic inflammatory response associated with CPB.[11-14]

Some studies have demonstrated that patients treated with aprotinin have an increased incidence of mortality, stroke, and/or renal dysfunction. However, the lysine analogues were not associated with such outcomes.[15] Tranexamic acid (TXA) is associated with increased risk of perioperative seizures, and both aminocaproic acid and TXA should be used only after careful consideration in patients with history of thrombosis. Antifibrinolytic agents are summarized in Table 16–9.

WHEN TO TRANSFUSE

There is much variability in cardiac surgery and cardiac anesthesia practice as to when transfusion of blood products is indicated. There is no support for a specific "transfusion trigger"[9]; however, transfusion for a hemoglobin less than 6 g/dL is considered "reasonable since this can be life-saving" by the Society of Thoracic Surgeons/Society of Cardiovascular Anesthesiologists guidelines. In determining when to transfuse, the risks of anemia must be balanced against the risks associated with blood product administration. Karkouti et al. have found that severe anemia during CPB presents an increased risk of renal failure, stroke, and death.[17-19] Preoperative anemia has likewise been found to be associated with adverse outcomes in cardiac surgery patients. Moreover, the degree of acute anemia that cardiac surgery patients can tolerate is inversely related to their baseline hemoglobin concentration.[20] Indeed, a decrease in baseline hemoglobin concentration greater than 50% was associated with a 50% increase in the composite risk of death, stroke, or renal failure.[19] Consequently, the suggested transfusion threshold of hemoglobin 6.0 g/dL may be too low for a person with a baseline Hb concentration of 18 g/dL.

Table 16–3. Management of Preoperative Anticoagulant and Antiplatelet Drugs

Recommendations	Class[a]	Level[b]
In patients undergoing CABG, ASA should be continued throughout the preoperative period.	IIa	C
In patients at high risk of bleeding[c] or refusing blood transfusions and undergoing noncoronary cardiac surgery, stopping ASA should be considered at least 5 days preoperatively.	IIa	C
It is recommended that ASA be re(started) as soon as there is no concern over bleeding (within 24 h) after isolated CABG.	I	B
In patients taking DAPT who need to have non-emergent cardiac surgery, postponing surgery for at least 3 days after discontinuation of ticagrelor, 5 days after clopidogrel and 7 days after prasugrel should be considered.	IIa	B
It is recommended that GPIIb/IIIa inhibitors be discontinued at least 4 h before surgery.	I	C
To reduce the risk of bleeding, preoperative bridging of oral anticoagulation with UFH/LMWH is only indicated in patients at high risk of thrombotic events.[d]	I	B
It is recommended that prophylactic LMWH be discontinued 12 h before surgery and fondaparinux 24 h before surgery. A longer interval may be necessary for patients with impaired renal function and/or therapeutic doses.	I	B
It is recommended that OACs be bridged with UFH.	I	B
Bridging OACs with subcutaneous LMWH should be considered an alternative to bridging with UFH.	IIa	B
Elective cardiac surgery should be performed if the INR is < 1.5 in patients taking VKAs. When surgery cannot be postponed, coagulation factors should be used to reverse the effect.	IIa	C
In patients having elective cardiac surgery, DOACs should be stopped at least 48 h before surgery. A longer interval may be necessary for patients with impaired renal function.	IIa	C

[a]Class of recommendation.
[b]Level of evidence.
[c]Complex and redo operation, severe renal insufficiency, hematological diseases and hereditary deficiencies in platelet function.
[d]Mechanical prosthetic heart valve, atrial fibrillation with rheumatic valvular disease, an acute thrombotic event within the previous 4 weeks and atrial fibrillation with a CHA_2DS_2-VASc score > 4.
ASA, acetylsalicylic acid; CABG, coronary artery bypass grafting; CHA_2DS_2-VASc, congestive heart failure, hypertension, age ≥ 75 (2 points), diabetes, prior stroke (2 points)–vascular disease, age 65–74, sex category (female); DAPT, dual antiplatelet therapy; DOAC, direct oral anticoagulant; GP, glycoprotein; INR, international normalized ratio; LMWH, low-molecular-weight heparin; OAC, oral anticoagulants; UFH, unfractionated heparin; VKA, vitamin K antagonist.
Reproduced with permission from Task Force on Patient Blood Management for Adult Cardiac Surgery of the European Association for Cardio-Thoracic Surgery (EACTS) and the European Association of Cardiothoracic Anaesthesiology (EACTA), et al: 2017 EACTS/EACTA Guidelines on patient blood management for adult cardiac surgery, *J Cardiothorac Vasc Anesth.* 2018 Feb;32(1):88-120.

Efforts to establish a physiologic guide to transfusion have also been suggested.[21] The oxygen extraction ratio is a measure of global oxygenation. It is a ratio between tissue oxygen delivery and uptake. Transfusion based upon low Hb concentration in patients with a normal oxygen extraction ratio (< 30%) may not be warranted. Additionally, the so-called storage lesion of packed cells due to decreased

Table 16–4. Cardiopulmonary Bypass

Recommendations	Class[a]	Level[b]
Implementation of institutional measures to reduce hemodilution by fluid infusion and CPB during cardiac surgery to reduce the risk of bleeding and the need for transfusions is recommended.	I	C
The use of a closed extracorporeal circuit may be considered to reduce bleeding and transfusions.	IIb	B
The use of a biocompatible coating to reduce perioperative bleeding and transfusions may be considered.	IIb	B
The routine use of cell salvage should be considered to prevent transfusions.	IIa	B
(Modified) ultrafiltration may be considered as part of a blood conservation strategy to minimize hemodilution.	IIb	B
Retrograde and antegrade autologous priming should be considered as part of a blood conservation strategy to reduce transfusions.	IIa	A
Normothermia during CPB (temperature > 36°C) and maintenance of a normal pH (7.35–7.45) may contribute to a reduced risk of postoperative bleeding.	IIb	B

[a]Class of recommendation.
[b]Level of evidence.
CPB, cardiopulmonary bypass.
Reproduced with permission from Task Force on Patient Blood Management for Adult Cardiac Surgery of the European Association for Cardio-Thoracic Surgery (EACTS) and the European Association of Cardiothoracic Anaesthesiology (EACTA), et al: 2017 EACTS/EACTA Guidelines on patient blood management for adult cardiac surgery, *J Cardiothorac Vasc Anesth.* 2018 Feb;32(1):88-120.

Table 16–5. Intraoperative Anticoagulation

Recommendations	Class[a]	Level[b]
Heparin level-guided heparin management should be considered over ACT-guided heparin management to reduce bleeding.	IIa	B
Heparin level-guided protamine dosing may be considered to reduce bleeding and transfusions.	IIb	B
Protamine should be administered in a protamine-to-heparin dosing ratio[c] < 1:1 to reduce bleeding.	IIa	B
AT supplementation is indicated in patients with AT deficiency to improve heparin sensitivity.	I	B
AT supplementation is not recommended to reduce bleeding following CPB.	III	C
In patients with HIT antibodies for whom surgery cannot be postponed, anticoagulation with bivalirudin should be considered when the bleeding risk is acceptable. The use of heparin in the pre- and postoperative periods should be avoided.	IIa	C

[a]Class of recommendation.
[b]Level of evidence.
[c]Protamine-to-heparin dosing ratio based on the initial heparin dose.
ACT, activated clotting time; AT, antithrombin; CPB, cardiopulmonary bypass; HIT, heparin-induced thrombocytopenia.
Reproduced with permission from Task Force on Patient Blood Management for Adult Cardiac Surgery of the European Association for Cardio-Thoracic Surgery (EACTS) and the European Association of Cardiothoracic Anaesthesiology (EACTA), et al: 2017 EACTS/EACTA Guidelines on patient blood management for adult cardiac surgery, *J Cardiothorac Vasc Anesth.* 2018 Feb;32(1):88-120.

Table 16–6. Intravascular Volume

Recommendations	Class[a]	Level[b]
The use of goal-directed hemodynamic therapy to reduce transfusions is not recommended.	III	C
The use of modern low-molecular weight starches in priming and nonpriming solutions to reduce bleeding and transfusions are not recommended.	III	C
Limitation of hemodilution is recommended as part of a blood conservation strategy to reduce bleeding and transfusions.	I	B
Preoperative autologous blood donation in patients with high hemoglobin levels (> 110 g/L) may be considered to reduce postoperative transfusions.	IIb	B
Acute normovolemic hemodilution may be considered to reduce postoperative transfusions.	IIb	B

[a]Class of recommendation.
[b]Level of evidence.
Reproduced with permission from Task Force on Patient Blood Management for Adult Cardiac Surgery of the European Association for Cardio-Thoracic Surgery (EACTS) and the European Association of Cardiothoracic Anaesthesiology (EACTA), et al: 2017 EACTS/EACTA Guidelines on patient blood management for adult cardiac surgery, *J Cardiothorac Vasc Anesth.* 2018 Feb;32(1):88-120.

Table 16–7. Procoagulant Interventions

Recommendations	Class[a]	Level[b]
Antifibrinolytic therapy (TXA, aprotinin and EACA) is recommended to reduce bleeding and transfusions of blood products and reoperations for bleeding (TXA and aprotinin).	I	A
The prophylactic use of FFP to reduce bleeding is not recommended.	III	B
The use of PCC or FFP may be considered to reverse the action of VKAs.	IIb	B
In patients with factor XIII activity < 70% after CPB, the administration of factor XIII may be considered to reduce bleeding.	IIb	B
Prophylactic fibrinogen administration is not recommended.	III	B
In the bleeding patient with a low fibrinogen level (< 1.5 g/L), fibrinogen substitution may be considered to reduce postoperative bleeding and transfusions.	IIb	B
In patients where bleeding is related to coagulation factor deficiency, PCC or FFP administration should be considered to reduce bleeding and transfusions.	IIa	B
The prophylactic use of DDAVP to reduce bleeding is not recommended.	III	B
In bleeding patients with platelet dysfunction on the basis of an inherited or acquired bleeding disorder, the use of DDAVP should be considered to reduce bleeding and the requirement for transfusions.	IIa	C
The prophylactic use of rFVIIa to prevent bleeding is not recommended.	III	B
In patients with refractory, non-surgical bleeding, off-label use of rFVIIa may be considered to reduce bleeding.	IIb	B

Bleeding is defined as persistent, non-surgical microvascular blood loss.
[a]Class of recommendation.
[b]Level of evidence.
CPB, cardiopulmonary bypass; DDAVP, desmopressin; EACA, ε-aminocaproic acid; FFP, fresh-frozen plasma; PCC, prothrombin complex concentrate; rFVIIa, recombinant activated factor VII; TXA, tranexamic acid; VKAs, vitamin K antagonists.
Reproduced with permission from Task Force on Patient Blood Management for Adult Cardiac Surgery of the European Association for Cardio-Thoracic Surgery (EACTS) and the European Association of Cardiothoracic Anaesthesiology (EACTA), et al: 2017 EACTS/EACTA Guidelines on patient blood management for adult cardiac surgery, *J Cardiothorac Vasc Anesth.* 2018 Feb;32(1):88-120.

Table 16–8. Transfusion Strategies

Recommendations	Class[a]	Level[b]
Implementation of a PBM protocol for the bleeding patient is recommended.	I	C
The use of PRBCs of all ages is recommended, because the storage time of the PRBCs does not affect the outcomes.	I	A
The use of leucocyte-depleted PRBCs is recommended to reduce infectious complications.	I	B
Pooled solvent detergent FFP may be preferred to standard FFP to reduce the risk of TRALI.	IIb	B
Perioperative treatment algorithms for the bleeding patient based on visco-elastic POC tests should be considered to reduce the number of transfusions.	IIa	B
It is recommended that one transfuse PRBCs on the basis of the clinical condition of the patient rather than on a fixed haemoglobin threshold.	I	B
A hematocrit of 21%–24% may be considered during CPB when an adequate DO_2 (> 273 ml O_2/min/m^2) level is maintained.	IIb	B
Platelet concentrate should be transfused in bleeding patients with a platelet count below 50 (10^9/L) or patients on antiplatelet therapy with bleeding complications.	IIa	C

[a]Class of recommendation.
[b]Level of evidence.
CPB, cardiopulmonary bypass; FFP, fresh-frozen plasma; PBM, patient blood management; POC, point of care; PRBCs, packed red blood cells; TRALI, transfusion-related acute lung injury.
Reproduced with permission from Task Force on Patient Blood Management for Adult Cardiac Surgery of the European Association for Cardio-Thoracic Surgery (EACTS) and the European Association of Cardiothoracic Anaesthesiology (EACTA), et al: 2017 EACTS/EACTA Guidelines on patient blood management for adult cardiac surgery, *J Cardiothorac Vasc Anesth*. 2018 Feb;32(1):88-120.

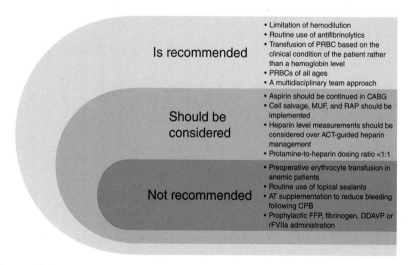

Figure 16–5. Key messages of the Joint Effort Patient Blood Management Guidelines for Adult Cardiac Surgery. ACT, activated clotting time; AT, antithrombin; CABG, coronary artery bypass grafting; CPB, cardiopulmonary bypass; DDAVP, desmopressin; FFP, fresh-frozen plasma; MUF, modified ultrafiltration; PRBC, packed red blood cells; RAP, retrograde autologous priming; rFVIIa, recombinant factor VIIa. [Reproduced with permission from Task Force on Patient Blood Management for Adult Cardiac Surgery of the European Association for Cardio-Thoracic Surgery (EACTS) and the European Association of Cardiothoracic Anaesthesiology (EACTA), et al: 2017 EACTS/EACTA Guidelines on patient blood management for adult cardiac surgery, *J Cardiothorac Vasc Anesth*. 2018 Feb;32(1):88-120.]

Table 16-9. Antifibrinolytic Agents: Drugs Description, Doses, and Mechanisms of Action

Drugs	Composition	Mechanism of action	Elimination	Pharmacodynamics	Suggested dosing in adults	Approval
Aprotinin	Protein, isolated from bovine lung tissue	Protease inhibitor; reversibly complexes with the active sites of plasmin, kallikrein, and trypsin; inhibition of fibrinolysis, activated factor XIIa, thrombin-induced platelet activation, and inflammatory response	Predominantly proteolysis, < 10% renal	Initial plasma half-life 150 min and terminal half-life 10 h	1. "Full dose": 2×10^6 KIU bolus patient, 2×10^6 KIU bolus CPB, continuous infusion of 5×10^5 KIU. 2. Half dose: 1×10^6 KIU bolus patient, 1×10^6 KIU bolus CPB, continuous infusion of 2.5×10^5 KIU	Suspended since 2008; suspension lifted in Canada in 2011 and Europe in 2012; In the United States still suspended
Tranexamic acid	Synthetic lysine analog	Antifibrinolytic; competitive inhibition of the activation of plasminogen to plasmin	Renal	Plasma half-life 3 h	1. "High dose": 30 mg/kg bolus patient, 2 mg/kg CPB, and continuous infusion of 16 mg/kg; 2. "Low dose": 10 mg/kg bolus patient, 1-2 mg CPB, and continuous infusion of 1 mg/kg	United States, Canada, Europe
ε-Aminocaproic acid	Synthetic lysine analog	Antifibrinolytic: competitive inhibition of the activation of plasminogen to plasmin	Renal	Plasma half-life 2 h	100 mg/kg bolus patient, 5 mg/kg CPB, and continuous infusion of 30 mg/kg	United States, Canada

CPB = cardiopulmonary bypass; KIU = Kallikrein International Unit.
Reproduced with permission from Koster A, Faraoni D, Levy JH: Antifibrinolytic Therapy for Cardiac Surgery: An Update, *Anesthesiology.* 2015 Jul;123(1):214-221.

concentrations of 2,3-diphosphoglycerate (DPG) may render transfused cells less useful in delivery of oxygen to the tissues than might otherwise be expected.

Irrespective of what methods are used to determine when to transfuse the cardiac surgical patient, there is no doubt that wide variations in practice patterns exist.[22] More than 20% of all blood products given nationally find their way to cardiac surgery patients. However, it is possible to predict which patients will likely require greater than 5 units of RBCs on the day of surgery.[23,24] Ultimately, efforts should be undertaken to employ multiple modalities of perioperative blood conservation to reduce the need for allogenic transfusion.[25] These modalities include: preoperative autologous blood donation, use of erythropoiesis stimulating agents, antifibrinolytic use intraoperatively, and perhaps intraoperative acute normovolemic hemodilution. Routine use of desmopressin acetate (DDAVP) to promote the release of endogenous factor VIII precursors is not recommended.[9]

The risk of blood conservation techniques in cardiac surgery must be balanced against the risk of transfusion. The Society of Thoracic Surgeons (STS) and the Society of Cardiovascular Anesthesiologists guidelines are intermittently updated as new evidence develops as to best transfusion practices in the heart surgery patient.[26]

OUTCOMES FOLLOWING TRANSFUSION

Should red cell transfusion be considered necessary, it is important to note that an increasing number of studies have demonstrated that exposure to even one to two units of red blood cells is associated with decreased survival following cardiac surgery.[27] Suggested mechanisms by which red cell transfusion decreases survival include transfusion-related immunosuppression and congestion or damage of the microvascular circulation secondary to the altered morphology of the transfused red blood cells. Blood transfusion has similarly been associated with a reduced quality of life following cardiac surgery.[28] Other analyses of large surgical populations associate red blood cell transfusion with increased risk for postoperative atrial fibrillation[29] and heart failure.[30] Because development of postoperative atrial fibrillation is believed related to an inflammatory mechanism, it is suggested that the modulation of inflammation due to the blood transfusion may contribute to post-cardiac surgery atrial fibrillation. Use of statin drugs which have anti-inflammatory effects may decrease the incidence of atrial fibrillation in transfused patients.[29] Surgenor et al.[30] suggest that the increased risk of postoperative low-output heart failure following transfusion occurs secondary to a number of possibilities including:

- Increased systemic inflammatory response leading to hypotension requiring various mechanical or inotropic supports
- Packed cell storage lesion whereby decreased 2,3-DPG hinders the unloading of oxygen to the tissue from the red cells
- Pulmonary capillary sludging secondary to the deformed morphology of stored red blood cells leading to impaired capillary transit

The suppression of the immune system associated with blood transfusion was thought by Surgenor et al. to more likely manifest in an increased infection risk in transfused patients rather than impact their immediate separation from CPB.

Transfusion of packed cells stored for more than 2 weeks has also been shown to worsen outcomes[31] following cardiac surgery. Because the storage lesion of banked blood becomes manifest after 2 weeks, Koch et al. suggest that decreased cell deformability can impede microvascular flow.[31] Karkouti suggests that each unit of perioperative blood transfusion is associated with a 10% to 20% increase in risk of acute kidney injury following cardiac surgery utilizing CPB.[32] Additionally, the biochemical changes associated with blood stored greater than 2 weeks may likewise contribute to the increased morbidity and mortality associated with transfusion. Transfusion of platelets has not been shown to contribute to postoperative mortality.[33]

However, Murphy et al. demonstrated that a restrictive (hemoglobin < 7.5 g/dL) or a liberal (hemoglobin < 9 g/dL) transfusion did not impact morbidity or healthcare costs postoperatively[34] Likewise a Cochrane review concluded that restrictive or liberal transfusion strategies did not impact 30-day morbidity or mortality[35] Nakamura et al. suggest that a restrictive transfusion strategy may contribute to a greater incidence of cardiogenic shock in patients aged 60 years or greater.[36] More recently, the Transfusion Requirements in Cardiac Surgery (TRICS III) trial found that in patients undergoing cardiac surgery who were at moderate to high risk for death, a restrictive strategy (<7.5 g/dL) regarding red cell transfusion was noninferior to a liberal strategy (< 9.5 g/dL in the operating room or intensive care unit, or < 8.5 g/dL in a non–intensive care unit ward) with respect to the composite outcome of death from any cause, myocardial infarction, stroke, or new-onset renal failure with dialysis, with less blood transfused.[37]

So what to do? Permitting too low a hemoglobin concentration will lead to potential patient risks. Administering even one unit of transfused blood likewise carries risk. Certainly, transfusion of red cells should not be automatic or primed to a set transfusion trigger. Each patient should be considered individually and an appropriate plan for blood cell conservation employed. Hemodilution from excessive crystalloid fluid administration should be avoided. When to begin transfusion for a particular patient remains problematic; however, measures such as the oxygen extraction ratio may provide some additional insights along with clinical signs of inadequate oxygen tissue delivery. What is becoming clear is that red cell transfusion has significant risks well beyond classical transfusion reactions and infection. Thus, both surgeon and anesthesiologist should discuss the risks and benefits of red cell transfusion when considered in each patient perioperatively. Identification of patients at high risk according to the STS guidelines (advanced age, preoperative anemia, small body size, non coronary artery or urgent surgery, patients on preoperative antithrombotic drugs, patients with acquired or congenital clotting abnormalities, and patients with multiple comorbidities) should be identified and all possible perioperative efforts taken to promote blood conservation.

MASSIVE TRANSFUSION AND CARDIAC TRAUMA

Patients with cardiac trauma present emergently following penetrating or blunt chest wounds. Often these patients arrive with little additional workup, and many may have multiple other undetected injuries. Patients generally are brought to the

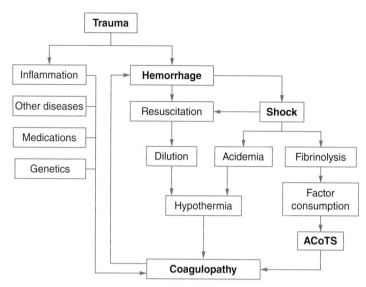

Figure 16–6. Traumatic injury results in coagulopathy through myriad mechanisms. Some patients are predisposed to coagulation problems secondary to other diseases, medications, and genetic influences. The shock state itself can produce an acute coagulopathy of trauma shock (ACoTS). Resuscitation efforts as well can lead to dilution and hypothermia which similarly potentiate coagulopathy. [Modified with permission from Hess JR, Brohi K, Dutton RP, et al: The coagulopathy of trauma: a review of mechanisms, *J Trauma*. 2008 Oct;65(4):748-754.]

operating room intubated, receiving fluids and blood through multiple venous lines. Patients frequently are exsanguinated, hypovolemic, hypotensive, and acidotic (Figure 16–6). The surgical team should be assembled to open the sternum immediately upon the induction of anesthesia as these patients generally do not tolerate loss of sympathetic tone associated with anesthesia induction. If the airway has not already been secured, in-line neck stabilization is generally necessary as there may be concomitant neck injury. A video-assisted laryngoscope can be useful in this emergency setting. Arterial pressure monitoring should be established as quickly as possible. Ketamine and muscle relaxants can be employed for rapid sequence induction and endotracheal tube placement. Often these patients will tolerate only very limited amounts of anesthetic agents due to severe hemodynamic instability, and as such there is a high risk of awareness in this patient population.

Massive hemorrhage can occur, and most institutions now have a massive transfusion protocol.[38] Coagulopathy is of concern in any patient with traumatic injury. Hemorrhage accounts for up to 40% of trauma-related deaths. Traumatized patients develop a systemic inflammatory response and develop an "acute coagulopathy of trauma shock."[39] The combination of tissue trauma, shock, hemodilution, hypothermia, acidemia, and inflammation contribute to an ongoing coagulopathic state. Shock also activates fibrinolytic pathways.[40] Thrombomodulin expression on endothelial cells is increased during periods of hypoperfusion. Thrombomodulin activates protein C, retarding clot development in the traumatized patient.

Consequently, shock in itself aggravates coagulopathy separate from fibrinolysis or hemodilution.

Massive transfusion protocols (MTPs) are designed to address the acute coagulopathy of trauma shock. MTPs approximate fluid resuscitation with whole blood by using a 1:1:1 ratio of red cells, fresh frozen plasma, and platelets. Whole blood is increasingly available outside of military settings.

Recombinant activated factor VII (rFVIIa)[41-43] can be used in massive hemorrhage following both trauma and uncontrollable postcardiac surgery bleeding. Recombinant activated factor VII is a thrombogenic agent, which enhances thrombin generation at the injury site. The dose of rFVIIa has not been clearly established, but ranges from 20 to 90 µg/kg have been suggested. Prothrombin complex concentrates (PCCs) are concentrates of vitamin K–dependent coagulation factors II, VII, IX, X and are also being used in the treatment of refractory coagulopathy following cardiac surgery.[44] Point-of-care coagulation testing can be incorporated in MTPs and can guide hemostatic therapy using a combination of plasma (or PCCs), platelets, cryoprecipitate (or fibrinogen concentrate), and antifibrinolytic agents (TXA or aminocaproic acid).

The right heart is located anteriorly in the chest and is a frequent site of knife injuries. Often such injuries can be controlled without the need for institution of CPB.

Penetrating wounds of the heart can also occur iatrogenically following electrophysiological and cardiac catheterization laboratory procedures. These patients often are brought with cardiac tamponade directly to the OR accompanied by the cardiologist. Management is centered upon immediate release of tamponade physiology and control of the site of perforation. Many times such patients will be in cardiac arrest with cardiopulmonary resuscitation (CPR) in progress. Unfortunately, CPR in a heart with tamponade is probably ineffective. Prompt release of tamponade and defibrillation are essential. The availability of various percutaneous ventricular assist devices (VADs) makes possible the placement of patients in cardiac arrest on circulatory support while they are transported to the operating room. Such patients will be anticoagulated and may or may not have received antiplatelet agents. These patients are likely to require multiple blood products to control hemorrhage should they survive resuscitation and emergency surgery.

OPTIONS FOR PATIENTS WHO REFUSE BLOOD PRODUCT ADMINISTRATION

Many patients have successfully undergone cardiac surgery without the need for blood product administration.[45] Patients may refuse blood components such as red blood cells, platelets, and plasma. Cell salvage techniques should be discussed and may be acceptable to individual patients if blood is kept in continuity with their own circulation. Minimizing crystalloid administration and the use of antifibrinolytics may be helpful. Most hospitals have established forms that delineate which techniques and products will and will not be accepted by an individual patient. Discussion of risk and benefits as well as appropriate documentation is mandatory.

THE EMERGENCY PATIENT FROM THE CARDIAC CATHETERIZATION LABORATORY

There are several reasons why patients from the cardiac catheterization laboratory present emergently to the cardiac surgery operating room. Many patients will simply have been diagnosed with critical coronary artery pathology not amenable to percutaneous coronary interventions (PCI). These patients may be hemodynamically stable yet have such tenuous coronary lesions that it is imprudent to delay surgical intervention. Other patients may have varying degrees of ongoing myocardial ischemia. Such patients may have had an intra-aortic balloon pump (IABP) placed for hemodynamic support. Patients from the catheterization laboratory will likely have been given heparin and as such are prone to bleeding during attempts at vascular access. Additionally, patients may have received antiplatelet agents potentially leading to bleeding following separation from CPB requiring multiple platelet transfusions.

Still other patients are likely to present in full cardiac arrest following a failed PCI. Dissection of a coronary vessel can lead to ventricular ischemia and dysfunction. Perforation of the heart can occur, which leads to tamponade and hemodynamic collapse. Management is directed at resuscitative efforts and expeditious surgical management.

As with any emergency anesthetic, efforts are initially directed at the ABCs of airway, breathing, and circulation. The awake patient with active ischemia and tight left main disease can be quite challenging. Should myocardial oxygen consumption outpace supply, this patient population can develop profound ventricular dysfunction. ECG signs of ischemia develop and PA pressures rise. Systemic and pulmonary artery pressures equilibrate. TEE can demonstrate striking dysfunction and acute mitral insufficiency. Restoration of the balance between supply and demand will improve systemic pressures, lower PA pressures, and improve LV contractility. By using the ECG, PA catheter, and TEE in combination, the anesthesiologist can detect and restore, if possible, hemodynamic stability. Some patients will present in cardiogenic shock on IABP or percutaneous VAD support. In these instances, the anesthesiologist attempts to maintain viability until the initiation of CPB. Complete hemodynamic collapse secondary to ventricular dysfunction and or fibrillatory cardiac arrest can occur at any moment and as such the surgeon and anesthesiologist should be prepared for the immediate institution of CPB.

PERIOPERATIVE TAMPONADE

Pericardial tamponade (see Chapter 14) develops secondary to postoperative bleeding and clot compression of the heart. Tamponade decreases venous return to the heart leading to a reduced stroke volume. Tamponade patients are progressively tachycardic, hypotensive, with decreased mixed venous oxygen saturation and a reduced cardiac output. Postoperative tamponade requires prompt return to the operating room for removal of the compressing clot and control of any bleeding sites. Patients are usually supported with vasoconstrictors to maintain blood pressure during transport to the operating room. TEE is very useful to identify clot amount and location and to confirm its removal. Upon opening of the sternum and release of tamponade the heart's chambers expand and ventricular filling is restored. Blood pressure usually rises rapidly with release of tamponade necessitating the rapid discontinuation of any vasoconstrictors previously required to support the patient.

If the patient returning to the operating room for postoperative tamponade has an endotracheal tube already in place, the anesthetic management can be done with muscle relaxants and anesthetic agents as tolerated. Hemodynamic compromise may prevent sufficient delivery of anesthetic agents to prevent perioperative awareness. Bispectral index monitoring to assess depth of anesthesia and minimize the risk of awareness may be particularly useful in this setting. Patients with tamponade tolerate positive pressure ventilation very poorly as venous return is further compromised. The surgical team should be ready and the patient prepared and draped to permit immediate surgical release of the tamponade should the patient develop hemodynamic collapse upon anesthetic induction.

Invasive arterial pressure monitoring and good venous access are essential in this instance.

Patients can also present for drainage of pericardial fluid with or without pericardial tamponade. Such patients can often be treated with a subxyphoid pericardial window. Uremia, malignancy, and infectious processes can all lead to the development of pericardial effusions.

REFERENCES

1. Levy J. Pharmacologic preservation of the hemostatic system during cardiac surgery. *Ann Thorac Surg.* 2001;72:S1814-S1820.
2. Lasne D, Jude B, Susen S. From normal to pathological hemostasis. *Can J Anesth.* 2006;53(6):S2-S11.
3. Tuman K, McCarthy R, O'Connor C, et al. Aspirin does not increase allogeneic blood transfusion in reoperative coronary artery surgery. *Anesth Analg.* 1996;83:1178-1184.
4. Dixon B, Santamaria J, Campbell D. Coagulation activation and organ dysfunction following cardiac surgery. *Chest.* 2005;128(1):229-236.
5. Shore-Lesserson L. Point of care coagulation monitoring for cardiovascular patients: past and present. *J Cardiothorac Vasc Anesth.* 2002;16(1):99-106.
6. Olde Engberinck R, Kuiper G, Wetzels R, et al. Rapid and correct prediction of thrombocytopenia and hypofibrinogenemia with rotational thromboelastometry in cardiac surgery. *J Cardiothorac Vasc Anesth.* 2014;28(2):210-216.
7. Tuman K, McCarthy R, Djuric M, et al. Evaluation of coagulation during cardiopulmonary bypass with a heparinase modified thromboelastographic assay. *J Cardiothorac Vasc Anesth.* 1994;8:144-149.
8. Velik-Salchner C, Maier S, Innerhofer P, et al. An assessment of cardiopulmonary bypass induced changes in platelet function using whole blood and classical light transmission aggregometry: the results of a pilot study. *Anesth Analg.* 2009;108(6):1747-1754.
9. The Society of Thoracic Surgeons Blood Conservation Guideline Task Force. Perioperative blood transfusion and blood conservation in cardiac surgery: the Society of Thoracic Surgeons and the Society of Cardiovascular Anesthesiologists clinical practice guideline. *Ann Thor Surg.* 2007;83:S27-S86.
10. Mannucci P, Levi M. Prevention and treatment of major blood loss. *NEJM.* 2007;356(22):2301-2311.
11. Mangano D, Miao Y, Vuylsteke A, et al. Mortality associated with aprotinin during 5 years following coronary artery bypass graft surgery. *JAMA.* 2007;297(5):471-479.
12. Mangano D, Tudor I, Dietzel C, et al. The risk associated with aprotinin in cardiac surgery. *NEJM.* 2006;354:353-365.

13. Greilich P, Okada K, Latham P, Kumar R, and Jessen M. Aprotinin but not epsilon-aminocaproic acid decreases interleukin-10 after cardiac surgery with extracorporeal circulation. *Circulation.* 2001; (12 Suppl 1):1265-1269.

14. Brown J, Birkmeyer N, O'Connor G. Meta-analysis comparing the effectiveness and adverse outcomes of antifibrinolytic agents in cardiac surgery. *Circulation.* 2007;115:2801-2813.

15. Schneeweiss S, Seeger J, Landon J, Walker A. Aprotinin during coronary artery bypass grafting and risk of death. *NEJM.* 2008;358(8):771-783.

16. Fergusson D, Hebert P, Mazer C, et al. Comparison of aprotinin and lysine analogues in high risk cardiac surgery. *NEJM.* 2008;358(22):2319-2331.

17. Karkouti K, Beattie WS, Wijeysundera D, et al. Hemodilution during cardiopulmonary bypass is an independent risk factor for acute renal failure in adult cardiac surgery. *J Thorac Cardiovasc Surg.* 2005;129:391-400.

18. Karkouti K, Djaini G, Borger M, et al. Low hematocrit during cardiopulmonary bypass is associated with increased risk of perioperative stroke in cardiac surgery. *Ann Thorac Surg.* 2005;80:1381-1387.

19. Karkouti K, Wijeysundera D, Beattie WS, et al. Risk associated with preoperative anemia in cardiac surgery: a multicenter cohort study. *Circulation.* 2007;117(4): 478-484.

20. Karkouti K, Wijeysundera D, Yau T, et al. The influence of baseline hemoglobin concentration on tolerance of anemia in cardiac surgery. *Transfusion.* 2008;48:666-672.

21. Orlov D, O'Farrell R, McCluskey S, et al. The clinical utility of an index of global oxygenation for guiding red blood cell transfusion in cardiac surgery. *Transfusion.* 2009;49:682-688.

22. Snyder-Ramos S, Mohnle P, Yi-Shin W, et al. The ongoing variability in blood transfusion practices in cardiac surgery. *Transfusion.* 2008;48:1284-1299.

23. Karkouti K, O'Farrell R, Yau T, et al. Prediction of massive blood transfusion in cardiac surgery. *Can J Anesth.* 2006;53(8):781-794.

24. Karkouti K, Wijeysundera D, Beattie WS, et al. Variability and predictability of large volume red blood cell transfusion in cardiac surgery; a multicenter study. *Transfusion.* 2007;47:2081-2088.

25. Karkouti K, McCluskey S. Perioperative blood conservation—the experts, the elephants, the clinicians, and the gauntlet. *Can J Anesth.* 2007;54(11):861-867.

26. Ferraris V, Brown J, Despotis G, et al. 2011 update to the Society of Thoracic Surgeons and the Society of Cardiovascular Anesthesiologists blood conservation clinical practice guidelines. *Ann Thorac Surge.* 2011;91:944-982.

27. Surgenor S, Kramer R, Olmstead E, et al. The association of perioperative red blood cell transfusions and decreased long term survival after cardiac surgery. *Anesth Analg.* 2009;108(6):1741-1747.

28. Koch CG, Khandwala F, Li L, et al. Persistent effect of red cell transfusion on health related quality of life after cardiac surgery. *Ann Thorac Surg.* 2006;82:13-20.

29. Koch CG, Li L, Van Wagoner D. Red cell transfusion is associated with an increased risk for postoperative atrial fibrillation. *Ann Thorac Surg.* 2006;82:1747-1757.

30. Surgenor S, DeFoe G, Fillinger M. Intraoperative red blood cell transfusion during coronary artery bypass graft surgery increases the risk of postoperative low output heart failure. *Circulation.* 2006; (1 Suppl):I43-I48.

31. Koch CG, Li L, Sessler D, et al. Duration of red cell storage and complications after cardiac surgery. *NEJM.* 2008;352(12):1229-1239.

32. Karkouti K. Transfusion and risk of acute kidney injury in cardiac surgery. *BJA.* 2012;109(suppl 1):i29-i38.

33. McGrath T, Koch CG, Xu M, et al. Platelet transfusion in cardiac surgery does not confer increased risk for adverse morbid outcomes. *Ann Thorac Surg.* 2008;86:543-553.

34. Murphy G, Pike K, Rogers C, et al. Liberal or restrictive transfusion after cardiac surgery. *NEJM.* 2015;372(11):997-1008.

35. Carson J, Stanworth S, Roubinian N, et al. Transfusion thresholds and other strategies for guiding allogeneic red blood cell transfusion. *Cochrane Database Syst Rev.* 2016;10:1-14.

36. Nakamura R, Vincent J-L, Fukushima J, et al. A liberal strategy of red blood cell transfusion reduces cardiogenic shock in elderly patients undergoing cardiac surgery. *J Thorac Cardiovasc Surg.* 2015;150:1314-1320.

37. Mazer C, Whitlock R, Fergusson D, et al. Restrictive or liberal red-cell transfusion for cardiac surgery. *NEJM.* 2017;377(22):2133-2144.

38. Shaz B, Dente C, Harris R, et al. Transfusion management of trauma patients. *Anesth Analg.* 2009;108(6):1760-1768.

39. Hess J, Brohi K, Dutton R, et al. The coagulopathy of trauma. *J Trauma.* 2008;65(4):748-754.

40. Brohi K, Cohen M, Ganter M, et al. Acute coagulopathy of trauma: hypoperfusion induces systemic anticoagulation and hyperfibrinolysis. *J Trauma.* 2008;64(5):1211-1217.

41. Karkouti K, Beattie WS, Ramiro A, et al. Comprehensive Canadian review of the off label use of recombinant activated factor VII in cardiac surgery. *Circulation.* 2008;118(4):331-338.

42. Al-Ruzzeh S, Ibrahim K, Navia J. The role of recombinant factor VIIa in the control of bleeding after cardiac surgery. *J Cardiothorac Vasc Anesth.* 2008;22(5):783-785.

43. Karkouti K, Beattie WS. The role of recombinant factor VIIa in cardiac surgery. *J Cardiothorac Vasc Anesth.* 2008;22(5):779-782.

44. Song H, Tibayan F, Kahl E, et al. Safety and efficacy of prothrombin complex concentrates for the treatment of coagulopathy after cardiac surgery. *J Thorac Cardiovasc Surg.* 2014;147:1036-1040.

45. Sniecinski R, Levy J. What is blood and what is not? Caring for the Jehovah's Witness patient undergoing cardiac surgery. *Anesth Analg.* 2007;104(4):753-754.

REVIEWS

Boer C, Meesters M, Milojevic M, et al. 2017 EACTS/EACTA guidelines on patient blood management for adult cardiac surgery. *J Cardiothorac Vasc Anesth.* 2018;12:88-120.

Ferraris V, Brown J, Despotis G, et al. 2011 Update to the Society of Thoracic Surgeons and the Society of Cardiovascular Anesthesiologists Blood Conservation Clinical Practice Guidelines. *Ann Thorac Surg.* 2011;91:944-982.

American Society of Anesthesiologists Task Force on Perioperative Blood Management. Practice guidelines for perioperative blood management. *Anesthesiology.* 2015;122(5):241-275.

Gerstein NS, Brierley J, Windsor J, et al. Antifibrinolytic agents in cardiac and noncardiac surgery: a comprehensive overview and update. *J Cardiothorac Vasc Anesth.* 2017;31(6):2183-2205.

Cardiopulmonary Bypass

17

TOPICS

Perfusion science is a unique discipline unto itself, and a full discussion of its many intricacies is far beyond the scope of this introduction to cardiac anesthesia and echocardiography. Still, much that is unique to cardiac anesthesia care can be in some degree related to the use of cardiopulmonary bypass (CPB). At the start it is important for practitioners new to cardiac anesthesia to establish a close working partnership with their perfusionist colleagues. Perfusionists are certified healthcare professionals who devote their careers to the management of circulatory support. In most institutions they work under the direct authority of the attending surgeon; however, from time to time they are under the medical direction of the anesthesiologist. At no times must they be considered a substitute for an appropriately qualified anesthesia practitioner in the operating room. Hence, during the "bypass run" a member of the patient's anesthesia team must be physically present in the operating room. During CPB, the anesthesiologist and the perfusionist work together to bypass the functions of the heart and the lungs so that cardiac surgery may proceed. The pump's flow becomes the patient's cardiac output (CO). The oxygenator of the CPB machine provides gas exchange. Simply put, the hemodynamic principles, which guide normal patient management, are operative when the bypass machine is in use. Blood pressure is still the product of CO and systemic vascular resistance (SVR)—except that the CPB machine now generates the CO in place of the heart's pumping function.

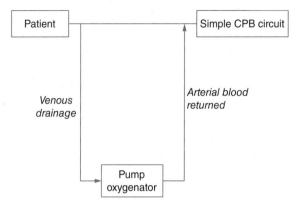

Figure 17–1. Venous blood is drained from the patient, flows through the pump oxygenator, and is returned oxygenated to the arterial system. Other functions of a simple CPB circuit are to deliver cardioplegia solution to the heart as well as suction blood from the surgical field to be oxygenated, filtered, and returned to the patient.

THE PLUMBING OF CPB

CPB has been in use in cardiac surgery for more than 50 years. It is likely that over that time successive generations of anesthesia trainees have been initially overwhelmed by the complexity of the bypass machine. Nonetheless, the basic circuit is straightforward enough (Figure 17–1). Anticoagulated venous blood is drained from the right atrium or directly from the superior and inferior venae cavae through the venous cannula and associated tubing to the pump reservoir. The deoxygenated venous blood is returned to the patient after passing through the oxygenator as well as a heat exchanger to deliver oxygenated blood at the desired temperature back to the patient. In the oxygenator, carbon dioxide is swept away by the oxygen gas flow across a gas permeable membrane. Oxygenated blood is then returned to the patient through a cannula most often placed in the ascending aorta or occasionally in a femoral artery. Along the oxygenated blood's course there are a number of filters and alarms to prevent the perfusionist from pumping air or clot into the aorta resulting in a perioperative embolic catastrophe.

Of course, the pump looks more formidable than the simple description just given and to be sure, it is. One very useful exercise is to visit with the perfusionist with whom one works and trace and examine the flow of blood to and from the patient with the particular equipment employed (Figure 17–2).

BYPASSING THE HEART

Before initiation of CPB, the CPB machine is "primed" with a volume of crystalloid, colloid, or blood. Following anticoagulation and cannula placement, release of clamps on the venous cannula commences CPB. Blood drains from the patient into the bypass machine, and the perfusionist starts the pump flow. Assuming the aortic valve is competent, following institution of CPB, the heart will be drained of blood by the venous cannula and emptied. At the same time, the normal arterial

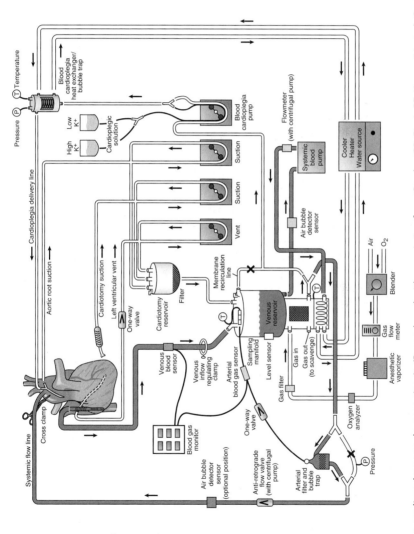

Figure 17–2. The **cardiopulmonary bypass circuit.** (Reproduced with permission from Gravlee GP, Davis RF, Kurusz M, et al: *Cardiopulmonary Bypass: Principles and Practice*, 2nd ed. Philadelphia, PA: Wolters Kluwer Health/Lippincott Williams & Wilkins; 2000.)

waveform loses pulsatility as the main driver of aortic blood flow becomes the non-pulsatile pump of the bypass machine. Consequently, full bypass flow is non-pulsatile. However, it is important to remember that the presence of a pulsatile aortic pressure wave does not preclude the patient's circulation being sustained by the CPB machine. As long as the heart has an electrical rhythm that can sustain a coordinated contraction, it will continue to beat and will eject any blood delivered to it. At times, the venous cannulae do not sufficiently drain venous blood into the bypass machine resulting in some venous return going to the heart—producing partial bypass. At other times, the surgeons will reduce venous return to the bypass machine intentionally leaving the patient on partial bypass. Patients with aortic insufficiency often fill their heart when on bypass and may develop distended hearts during CPB due to the incompetent aortic valve. Therefore, in these patients, until the aorta is cross-clamped, it is important to keep the heart ejecting to prevent the heart from overdistention and ischemic injury. If the heart is ejecting, the patient will have both a pulsatile waveform and be supported by partial bypass. Pulsatility on the arterial pressure trace during CPB can also be observed when an intra-aortic balloon pump is triggering. *When unsure whether the patient is or is not on full or partial bypass, ask the perfusionist and surgeon so as to avoid serious management errors.*

Hemodynamic basic principles apply equally to the patient on or off bypass support.

Recall,

$$BP = CO \times SVR$$

where,

$$CO = SV \times HR$$

When the patient is placed on CPB, CO is no longer provided by the patient's heart but by the bypass machine. If all the venous blood is delivered through the venous cannulae to the bypass machine, the patient is on total or "full flow" bypass. If on the other hand, some venous blood returns to the patient's heart, then the patient is on "partial" bypass. It is important to note that when the patient is on full flow the overwhelming majority of the blood flow will pass through the CPB machine's oxygenator and hence all the blood will be oxygenated. On the other hand, that part of the patient's blood flow that returns to the patient's heart will be oxygenated by the patient's own lungs. Because the lungs may be deflated during full bypass, it is important to remember to ventilate the lungs and oxygenate the patient if the patient is placed on partial bypass.

For example, if the patient's total bypass flow is 5 L/min, this would mean that the CPB machine is doing the work of a CO of 5 L/min. If, however, 2.5 L/min of venous blood flow returns to the patient's heart, then the machine only would pump 2.5 L/min of flow and the heart would provide the other 2.5 L of CO. Now if the 2.5 L/min of CO were to pass through lungs that were not ventilated, this would mean that the patient when on CPB would have a 50% pulmonary shunt—and a greatly reduced PaO_2. Therefore, it is always important to make sure that ventilation is ongoing when the patient is on partial bypass. Moreover, it has been suggested that maintenance of ventilation during CPB can reduce the incidence of postoperative pulmonary dysfunction.[1]

Blood pressure when on CPB is the product of CO and SVR just as in any patient. The CO when on total bypass or "full flow" is the pump flow—namely, how many liters per minute the bypass machine is delivering to the patient. As in any patient whether on or off CPB, SVR is determined by many factors including sympathetic tone, temperature, inflammatory mediators, and blood viscosity. SVR can be adjusted on CPB by the use of vasodilators and anesthetic agents to promote vasodilation or vasoconstrictors to increase vascular resistance.

The amount of flow that the perfusionist can deliver to the patient is dependent upon the venous return to the reservoir. If the patient is vasodilated, venous return may be reduced and the perfusionist will need to add volume to the reservoir to maintain flow. Restoring vascular resistance will increase venous return and increase blood pressure for the same pump flow.

Thus, when on CPB, the perfusionist can increase blood pressure by either increasing pump flow and/or SVR. Conversely, lowering pump flow or vasodilating the patient can reduce BP.

But what is the optimal blood pressure and flow when on CPB?

Murphy et al. provide some evidence-based guidance on best perfusion practices.[2] Some have advocated lower mean aortic pressure on CPB of 50 to 60 mm Hg. This has been suggested because a mean arterial pressure (MAP) of 50 mm Hg is thought to be the lower limit of cerebral autoregulation. Additionally, lower MAP is thought to reduce blood in the surgical field, improve myocardial protection by reducing collateral blood flow, and reducing emboli. Others have suggested that a MAP of 70 to 80 mm Hg should be employed.[3] In particular, the elderly patients now routinely being operated for cardiac disease often have hypertension and preexisting cerebral vascular disease. Such patients might do better with relatively higher MAPs during bypass. Sun et al. suggest in a retrospective cohort study that a sustained MAP less than 64 mm Hg during CPB was associated with postoperative ischemic stroke.[4] Conversely, Vedel et al. in a randomized trial found that targeting a higher (70-80 mm Hg) or lower (40-50 mm Hg) MAP during CPB did not affect the volume or number of new cerebral infarcts detected through diffusion weighted imaging.[5] Hori et al. note that MAP above the upper limit of cerebral autoregulation during CPB increased the incidence of postoperative delirium.[6] Consequently, MAP during CPB that is either too high or too low may have deleterious consequences. Similarly, there are differences as to what constitutes an "ideal" pump flow during CPB. Generally, flow is aimed at approximately 2.2 to 2.5 $L/min/m^2$ because this is similar to the normal cardiac index of a normal patient. Of course, oxygen delivery to the tissues is dependent on the pump flow and also on the blood oxygen-carrying capacity and tissue oxygen utilization. Reduced flows can be employed during hypothermic bypass. Moreover, deep hypothermic cardiac arrest permits periods of surgery with no pump flow at all (see Chapter 9). Anesthesiologists and perfusionists must work together to establish for each individual patient an appropriate blood pressure and pump flow during CPB.

Delivery of oxygenated blood to the tissues is the main function of the pump. Tissue oxygen delivery is dependent not only upon pump flow but also upon hematocrit. However, during CPB, hemodilution occurs due to the priming volume in the bypass reservoir. In patients who are profoundly anemic, the reservoir is primed with blood. Nonetheless, as was discussed in Chapter 16, even the use of one unit of homologous red cells can worsen perioperative outcomes. Of course, anemia during CPB and cardiac surgery can also lead to adverse outcomes as well. Hemodilution has benefits during CPB in that it can decrease blood viscosity and improve microcirculatory blood flow and oxygen delivery.[7] There are no clear guidelines as to what constitutes an appropriate hematocrit during CPB. Ideally, blood transfusion should be avoided if possible and all efforts undertaken to minimize red cell loss perioperatively. As with many decisions, the risks and benefits of transfusion during CPB must be determined on an individual basis. Generally, moderate anemia with a hematocrit of 21% to 25% is well tolerated in most cardiac surgery patients.[8]

Calculation of the systemic delivery of oxygen (DO_2) has also been suggested as a guide to determine the best combination of pump flow and blood's arterial oxygen content during CPB.[2]

$$DO_2 = \text{Pump flow} \times (\text{Hemoglobin concentration} \times \text{Hemoglobin saturation} \times 1.36) + (0.003 \times \text{Arterial saturation})^1$$

Normal DO_2 is 350 to 450 mL/min/m^2. A "critical" DO_2 of 330 mL/min/m^2 has been suggested in anesthetized patients as the point where maximal oxygen extraction occurs prior to the development of anaerobic metabolism.[2] If oxygen delivery does not meet oxygen consumption, patients develop tissue acidosis. Increased mean lactate concentration is a predictor of adverse outcome in patients undergoing coronary artery bypass grafting.[9]

Perfusionists also monitor venous oxygen saturation during CPB to determine if there is adequate delivery of oxygen globally to the tissues. A decrease in venous oxygen saturation is indicative of either a decrease in the oxygen-carrying capacity, an increase in oxygen utilization by the tissues, or inadequate tissue perfusion.

BYPASSING THE LUNGS

The pump oxygenator membrane provides the surface area over which gas exchange occurs during CPB. Much as hemodynamic principles are constant for the patient on or off bypass, so too the basics of oxygenation and ventilation hold true for the patient on CPB. As with any patient, an increased $PaCO_2$ can only occur because of either increased CO_2 production or decreased ventilation. A low PaO_2 only occurs secondary to absolute shunt or ventilation perfusion mismatch. During CPB all blood that passes through the gas exchanger is oxygenated. During partial bypass, some venous blood may pass by nonventilated alveoli resulting in a ventilation perfusion mismatch. The resulting mixture between 100% saturated blood from the oxygenator and poorly oxygenated blood returning from the heart could lead to a reduced arterial oxygen saturation. Recall, the p50 of normal hemoglobin occurs at a PaO_2 of 26 torr. Thus, hemoglobin A is saturated at 50% at a rather low arterial oxygen tension.

The membrane oxygenator employs a microporous membrane that separates the ventilating gas in the bypass machine from the venous blood. Gas exchange occurs by diffusion across the membrane. The ventilating gas mixture of oxygen, air, and inhalational anesthetics is delivered to the membrane. Increasing the gas mixture's FiO_2 will increase the PaO_2 of the blood following passage through the oxygenator. Thus, oxygenating blood on the pump is easy and blood returned to the patient should be well oxygenated. Ventilation (CO_2 removal) on the pump is dependent on the total gas flow in the oxygenator (the "sweep rate"). CO_2 is thus blown away from the oxygenator depending on the flow of gas. Increase the "sweep rate," and the $PaCO_2$ will decrease. This parallels the patient's lungs—increasing ventilation decreases $PaCO_2$.

Although oxygenating the blood is straightforward, the perfusionist's main challenge is to ensure adequate DO_2. Generally, perfusionists monitor the saturation of the venous return. They aim for a venous oxygen saturation SvO_2 of 65% to 80%. Anemia, reduced bypass flow, and increased oxygen consumption can all reduce SvO_2. Decreasing temperature and increasing bypass flow can improve SvO_2 by decreasing oxygen consumption and improving oxygen delivery. Increasing the patient's hemoglobin will improve hematocrit; however, the reduced 2,3-diphosphoglycerate found in stored blood may not readily lead to increased delivery of oxygen to the tissues due to reduced tissue release of O_2.

Hypothermia to 28°C is frequently employed in CPB to reduce tissue oxygen consumption. However, although hypothermia will decrease global oxygen consumption, the overall effect on tissue oxygen delivery can be clouded as hypothermia shifts the oxygen-hemoglobin dissociation curve leftward, meaning that the hemoglobin has a greater avidity for the oxygen it carries. Both normothermic bypass and hypothermic bypass are employed depending upon individual practice preferences. There is currently no established norm for the ideal temperature during bypass.[2] Should hypothermic bypass be used, the rate and degree of rewarming prior to separation from CPB has been associated with postoperative cognitive dysfunction.[10] Limiting the temperature of the arterial blood returned from the pump to 37°C may reduce the incidence of neurological injury. Often "mild" hypothermic bypass to 32°C is currently employed in many centers. Guidelines for temperature management during CPB have been established. In particular cerebral hyperthermia should be avoided by keeping arterial outlet blood temperature < 37°C.

Temperature during CPB also impacts the management of CO_2 during bypass. $PaCO_2$ during bypass is regulated in the same manner as CO_2 in the breathing patient. An increased $PaCO_2$ generally results from either the increased production or decreased ventilation of the gas. Causes of increased CO_2 production during CPB are the usual culprits: malignant hyperthermia, hyperalimentation, thyrotoxicosis, and any hypermetabolic state. Ventilation as previously mentioned is dependent on the rate of sweep gas over the oxygenator to carry away CO_2.

When hypothermia is used, however, $PaCO_2$ can be influenced by the temperature-dependent change in carbon dioxide solubility. During hypothermia, the solubility of oxygen and carbon dioxide in blood is increased reducing the partial pressure of the gas. The impact of temperature upon CO_2 solubility is at the center of the issue surrounding what is known as pH stat and alpha stat bypass management.

The increased solubility of CO_2 causes a reduction of $PaCO_2$ in the blood resulting in alkalosis. Because cerebral blood flow increases with increased $PaCO_2$ and decreases with decreased $PaCO_2$, many perfusionists have been concerned that the reduction in CO_2 gas tension can cause a deleterious decrease in cerebral blood flow during CPB. Consequently, when pH stat management is employed, the perfusionist cools the patient on CPB and determines what the pH and $PaCO_2$ are for the temperature measured. Because cooling causes the $PaCO_2$ to be reduced, the perfusionist adds CO_2 to the gas mixture to increase CO_2 to correct for the effect of temperature on carbon dioxide solubility.

During alpha stat management, the perfusionist similarly cools the patient as indicated but in this instance does not supplement the gas flow with additional carbon dioxide. Alpha stat management is based on the concept that the homeostatic mechanisms of the body adjust for changes associated with decreasing body temperature.[11]

Alpha stat management has been suggested to be beneficial because it preserves autoregulation of cerebral blood flow and prevents cerebral hyperfusion. pH stat management provides for more global cooling of the brain and for less desaturation of jugular venous blood during rewarming. However, since most neurologic injuries are of an embolic nature, it is possible that pH stat management by increasing cerebral blood flow merely increases the opportunity for emboli to be delivered to the brain. Aziz and Meduoye concluded in a review of patients undergoing deep hypothermic circulatory arrest that pH stat management improved results in the pediatric population and alpha stat management achieved better results in adults.[12] Jonas notes that alpha stat strategy is appropriate for normal flow bypass in adult patients because alpha stat management better matches cerebral blood flow with metabolic demand.[13] However, he reports that pH stat management better cools the brain and counteracts the leftward shift of the hemoglobin dissociation curve associated with hypothermia and may offer advantages in patients undergoing deep hypothermic circulatory arrest. Conversely, Broderick et al. suggest that alpha stat management avoids excessive brain edema from potential cerebral hyperperfusion.[14] Most routine adult cardiac surgeries are performed using alpha stat pH management.

PRESERVING THE HEART

Once the patient is placed on CPB, the heart is routinely isolated from the circulation by placement of the aortic cross clamp. The aortic cross clamp is placed below the aortic perfusion cannula. Once the cross clamp is positioned across the aorta, oxygenated blood no longer passes through the right and left coronary arteries. Without myocardial protection, the heart would become ischemic and die. However, myocardial preservation techniques permit the blood flow to the heart to be arrested and the myocardium to be protected, permitting cardiac surgery to proceed. Close coordination between the perfusionist and surgeon is necessary to successfully deliver myocardium protecting cardioplegia solution to the patient's heart. Failure to adequately protect the heart during the period of aortic cross clamp can produce ventricular dysfunction and extreme difficulty in separating the patient from CPB.

Cardioplegia solutions usually contain a relatively high potassium concentration to produce electrical silence of the heart and are administered to reduce myocardial metabolism. Various surgical teams incorporate other electrolytes and blood into the solution, which can be administered in an anterograde manner via the coronary arteries or retrograde via the coronary sinus. There is great variability in the composition of cardioplegia formulations.[15]

Anterograde cardioplegia is administered via a small cannula placed by the surgeon between the aortic cross clamp and the aortic valve. After application of the aortic cross clamp, anterograde cardioplegia is administered under considerable pressure using a separate pump on the CPB machine. Assuming the aortic valve is competent, pressure builds in the aortic root between the cross clamp and the aortic valve. Cardioplegia solution then flows through the left and right coronary arteries perfusing the myocardium in solution and arresting the heart. If the patient has significant aortic regurgitation, the heart will distend and the solution will not pass via the coronary arteries. Rather, it will leak into the left ventricle where a venting catheter under mild suction will eliminate it to prevent the heart from distending. In patients with severe coronary artery disease, blockages can impede delivery of cardioplegia solution and hinder myocardial protection during the aortic cross clamp. In procedures where the aorta is going to be opened, the surgeon can directly perfuse both the right and left coronary arteries with cardioplegia.

Retrograde cardioplegia is given via a cannula placed in the coronary sinus (Video 17–1). The coronary sinus drains venous blood from the heart. A balloon cuff at the distal end of the retrograde cardioplegia cannula seals the outflow from the coronary sinus. Cardioplegia solution is delivered, and a pressure builds in the sinus as cardioplegia flows back through the venous system of the heart to bathe the myocardium in cardioplegia solution. Pressure in the coronary sinus is measured so as not to exceed 45 mm Hg at the tip of the balloon catheter. Cold cardioplegia will produce myocardial cooling to 8°C to 10°C. Surgeons from time to time add cooled or frozen saline to the pericardium to further chill the heart externally.

Not all centers use cold cardioplegia and hypothermic bypass. Various combinations of temperature and solution mixtures are used. Clearly, one must learn the operating protocols of their institution. Additionally, not all cardiac procedures require the use of CPB and not all patients placed on CPB require cardioplegia. In patients having vein bypass grafts, additional cardioplegia can be delivered via these grafts once the distal anastomosis has been completed.

PROTECTING THE BRAIN

There are countless studies that examine neurologic injuries associated with heart surgery and CPB in general.[16-18] Roach et al. in 1996 identified the high incidence of neurological injury associated with cardiac surgery. Injuries range from cognitive dysfunction detected by sophisticated neuropsychological studies to frank stroke. Etiologies of neurological injury include: particulate embolism, air embolism, and inadequate perfusion. Genetic factors and their influence upon the inflammatory response may also play a role in the development of neurological injury secondary to CPB.

Genetic influences upon neurological outcomes are discussed in Chapter 14.

The grade of atherosclerotic plaque in the aorta has been associated with the development of stroke in patients requiring CPB. Patients with highly mobile plaque are at particular risk for the development of stroke in the CPB population.[19] Avoiding manipulation of the aorta in patients with aortic plaque can reduce the incidence of stroke. Additionally, higher MAP (> 70-80 mm Hg) during CPB has been suggested to reduce the incidence of overt postoperative stroke in CPB patients.

Transesophageal echocardiography (TEE) examination of the aorta and epiaortic ultrasound (EAU) can be employed to guide placement of aortic cannula and aortic cross clamp away from areas of potentially embolic plaque. Epiaortic ultrasound examination is particularly useful in patients because TEE often fails to visualize the ascending aorta in the area of cannula placement. TEE can also be used to diagnose aortic dissections that may occur as complications of aortic cannulation.

Blood glucose control during cardiac surgery has been previously discussed. During hypothermic CPB, blood glucose concentration often increases. Some cardioplegia solutions contain glucose making perioperative glucose management difficult. Maintenance of appropriate glucose control is the subject of ongoing debate. Both glucose control that is too tight or too loose has been associated with adverse outcomes in cardiac surgical patients.[20] Glucose control during CPB can be difficult; however, regular insulin should be infused to maintain glucose according to those protocols locally operative.

Rewarming temperature and rate of rewarming have similarly been associated with adverse neurological outcomes. Arterial temperatures not greater than 37°C have been suggested to avoid thermally mediated cerebral injury.

There are various methods suggested to monitor the brain during CPB. Cerebral saturation monitors provide a global measure of brain tissue saturation. Likewise, monitoring of jugular venous bulb saturation has been used as a measure of the adequacy of cerebral perfusion during CPB. Decreased cerebral or jugular saturations may be suggestive of higher oxygen extraction (e.g., hyperthermia) or be secondary to insufficient oxygen delivery to the brain (e.g., cerebral vasoconstriction, anemia, inadequate pump flow). However, since many neurological injuries are thought to be secondary to embolic processes rather than inadequate perfusion, the role of such monitors and how they should or should not be incorporated into routine patient management remains subject to debate and institutional preferences. Various neuroprotective schemes have appeared over the years to mitigate adverse neurological outcomes associated with CPB. Efforts have been directed to decrease cerebral oxygen consumption during CPB through pharmacologic means such as suppressing the electroencephalogram (EEG) with propofol or treatment with barbiturates. These efforts have not affected the incidence of adverse neurological outcome following CPB. Investigations into the use of anti-inflammatory agents to reduce the incidence of adverse neurological events are likely to continue to be forthcoming as are investigations that attempt to identify genetic factors that predispose to a worsened outcome following CPB.

ELECTROLYTES AND CPB

Monitoring of blood gases and electrolytes during CPB is dependent upon institutional protocols. Point-of-care blood gas analyses generally provide information in a timely fashion. Most frequently hyperkalemia secondary to cardioplegia delivery can complicate the restoration of sinus rhythm prior to separation from CPB. Often a potassium concentration between 5 and 6 mEq/L is well tolerated. Patients with elevated potassium concentrations prior to separation from CPB may need to be treated with regular insulin and dextrose to drive potassium intracellularly. Furosemide can be given to augment a potassium losing diuresis. A mild respiratory alkalosis may similarly help to transiently lower elevated potassium concentrations prior to separation from CPB. Patients with renal failure may be acidotic at baseline and may require dialysis immediately postoperatively to eliminate potassium acquired in the cardioplegia solution.

Sodium concentration is usually well maintained during CPB and rarely requires treatment. Serum calcium is often low during bypass secondary to the dilution of albumin. Some blood gas machines measure ionized calcium; however, calcium administration during CPB or as an adjuvant to aid in separation from bypass is controversial. Although ionized calcium concentration may fall at the outset of CPB, this is usually transient. Calcium chloride administration may impair the action of inotropes, and its hemodynamic effects are short lived.[21] Nonetheless, cardiac surgery patients are often administered supplemental calcium chloride in lactated Ringer solution used for fluid maintenance. When a low ionized calcium is thought to contribute to a patient's hemodynamic instability, 200 to 300 mg boluses of $CaCl_2$ can be given. Routine administration of 1000 mg of $CaCl_2$ prior to bypass separation is not recommended.

Occasionally patients develop a low-ionized magnesium concentration. Decreased ionized magnesium may lead to dysrhythmias, and as such, supplemental magnesium (1-2 g) can be given prior to separation from bypass.

Acid-base balance during CPB is largely dependent upon the delivery of suitable amounts of oxygen to the tissues. As discussed previously, what constitutes adequate delivery is predicated upon pump flow, hemoglobin concentration, hemoglobin's release of oxygen to the tissues, and tissue oxygen consumption. If oxygen delivery is not sufficient, the patient will develop a metabolic acidosis. Management of metabolic acidosis on CPB is centered at correcting the underlying cause rather than simply giving the patient sodium bicarbonate. Should profound acidemia occur when the patient is on CPB, it is important to consider not only malignant hyperthermia in the differential diagnosis but also the possibility of ischemic mesenteric organs. Emboli associated with CPB institution can produce multiple areas of organ ischemia. Patients with vascular disease may have inadequate mesenteric perfusion leading also to ischemia, inflammation, and vasodilatory states.

ANTICOAGULATION AND CPB

As mentioned in Chapter 4, anticoagulation is essential to prevent the development of clot as blood is exposed to the non-physiologic surfaces of the bypass machine. Both coagulation and inflammatory cascades are activated by the interface of blood with the bypass circuit.[22] Some bypass circuits have attempted to attenuate the interface between blood and CPB machine by using heparin-bonded materials. Heparin coating of the bypass circuit appears to reduce both coagulation and inflammatory processes. However, heparin bonding to the CPB circuit does not eliminate the need for systemic anticoagulation.

Delivery and confirmation of adequate anticoagulation is essential before initiating CPB.

Generic, unfractionated heparin is most frequently used to achieve anticoagulation for CPB. Unfractionated heparin in the range of 3 to 4 mg/kg is administered intravenously (or by the surgeon directly into the right atrium) when requested. An activated clotting time and a heparin concentration assay are obtained following circulation of the heparin. The activated clotting time (ACT) is obtained by mixing a blood sample with a small amount of kaolin or diatomaceous earth. Contact initiates clotting that is timed. The normal ACT is 110 to 120 seconds. The acceptable ACT adequate for initiation of CPB is debatable but generally is considered to be 400 to 480 seconds. Heparin potentiates the action of antithrombin III more than 1000-fold and inhibits thrombin and factor Xa. Patients who are deficient in antithrombin III may become resistant to the action of heparin. Supplemental antithrombin III can be given through the transfusion of 2 to 4 units of fresh frozen plasma or, if available, an antithrombin III concentrate. If the initial ACT measure is too low, an additional heparin dose (1 mg/kg) may provide for adequate anticoagulation. Heparin can reduce ionized calcium concentration transiently following administration, and, as such, at times patients vasodilate and become relatively hypotensive. This can be occasionally useful because surgeons often request that blood pressure be reduced at the time of aortic cannulation. Once the aortic cannula is placed and its correct position confirmed by the surgeon, the cannula can be a source of rapid fluid transfusion if necessary, to compensate for transient hypotension. Restoration of vascular tone at this point with small amounts of vasoconstrictors such as phenylephrine can also be used.

With the increased use of heparin in the preoperative period, not only do patients present with antithrombin deficiency but from time to time manifest heparin-induced thrombocytopenia.[23,24] Unfractionated, generic heparin, although inexpensive, can induce thrombocytopenia via both immune- and nonimmune-mediated mechanisms. Nonimmunologically mediated heparin-induced thrombocytopenia HIT (type I) occurs secondary to the direct activation of platelets by heparin. Immune-mediated HIT (type II) is far more severe and occurs when primarily IgG antibodies are directed against platelet factor 4 (PF4-heparin) complexes. The binding of heparin to PF4 results in the expression of antigens which result in an immune response. Ultimately, the antibody response destroys and activates the platelets releasing prothrombic particles, placing the patient at risk for systemic thrombocytopenia and thrombosis. HIT usually becomes manifest 5 to 10 days following heparin exposure heralded by an unexpected decrease in platelet count.

Although a declining platelet count can be secondary to hemodilution, immunoassays can be used to detect the presence of immunoglobulins directed at the PF4-heparin complex. Not all patients who are exposed to heparin develop antibodies. Of those that do develop antibodies, not all develop clinical HIT. Treatment for those patients with suspected HIT includes discontinuation of heparin and initiation of alternative anticoagulant therapy, generally a direct thrombin inhibitor.

Management of CPB for the HIT patient requires the use of alternative anticoagulation approaches. Consultation with the patient's hematologist and discussion of these options with the surgeon and the perfusionist should be undertaken in advance of bringing the patient to the operating room. Extensive guidelines are available from the Society of Thoracic Surgeons, the Society of Cardiovascular Anesthesiologists, and the American Society of ExtraCorporeal Technology for the management of the HIT patient in need of cardiac surgery.[25] Recommendations include:

- Performance of a heparin platelet antibody test following a fall in platelet count of 50% or a thrombotic event 5 to 14 days following heparin administration
- Serum tests that include functional testing with serotonin release assay (SRA) or heparin-induced platelet activation (HIPA) when platelet factor 4–heparin antibody testing is inconclusive
- In patients with a diagnosis of HIT and in need of an urgent operation requiring CPB, anticoagulation with bivalirudin is a reasonable option.
- In patients with significant renal dysfunction who are seropositive for HIT and require urgent operation requiring CPB, use of plasmapheresis, argatroban, or heparin with antiplatelet agents (such as tirofiban or iloprost) may be considered, understanding that there are increased risks of bleeding with these interventions.

There are a number of alternatives to heparin to provide for anticoagulation; however, none possesses the simplicity of delivery, ease of monitoring, and swiftness of reversal as done by heparin. Direct thrombin inhibitors such as bivalirudin can be used in the HIT patient. Bivalirudin has a relatively short half-life, but none of the direct thrombin inhibitors have a specific reversal agent similar to protamine. Consequently, patients can have prolonged bleeding following completion of the bypass run. The guidelines suggest that in patients who require bivalirudin who bleed excessively following CPB, a combination of ultrafiltration, hemodialysis, factor VIIa administration and blood product delivery may be considered to improve hemostasis. Cardiac surgery is ideally avoided in patients with acute HIT. Indeed, the development of HIT in cardiac surgery is associated with an increase in mortality and major morbidity.[26,27] All patients with previous or current HIT should be carefully reviewed with the surgeon, perfusionists, and hematologist to outline the best plan for perioperative anticoagulation and the presence or absence of HIT antibodies determined.

Reversal of heparin anticoagulation with protamine was discussed in Chapter 4.

The guidelines suggest that protamine overdosage (e.g., no more than 2.6 mg protamine per 100 units of heparin) should be avoided as it will inhibit platelet function. However, in patients who received greater than 400 IU/kg of heparin there is a risk of heparin rebound which can be attenuated by a protamine infusion of 25 mg/h for up to 6 hours following CPB termination.

SYSTEMIC INFLAMMATION AND CPB

In addition to activating the coagulation cascade, CPB also contributes to the perioperative inflammatory response including complement activation, cytokine release, and leukocyte activation[28] (Figure 17–3). The inflammatory response may contribute to the development of various postoperative complications including respiratory failure, renal dysfunction, neurological injury, and hemodynamic instability.

The contact of blood with the materials of the bypass circuit leads to activation of the inflammatory response. The coagulation, inflammatory, complement, and fibrinolytic systems are all closely linked and activated with CPB. Although anticoagulation inhibits clot formation, the entire cascade is nonetheless active. Complement activation in and of itself can produce tissue injury secondary to neutrophil activation as well as C5a-mediated increases in capillary permeability and loss of vascular tone. CPB may also contribute to inflammation through the release of endotoxin from the patient's gut. Additionally, ischemia and reperfusion injury to the heart following release of the aortic cross clamp may contribute as well to the perioperative inflammatory response in patients managed with CPB.

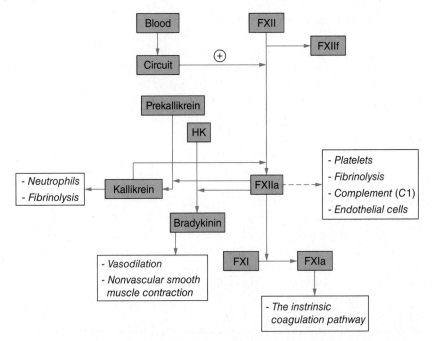

Figure 17–3. Contact of blood with the bypass circuit activates the coagulation and inflammatory systems. When blood contacts the bypass circuit, FXII is cleaved into factors FXIIa and FXIIf. FXIIa activates FXI and the intrinsic coagulation cascade. It likewise activates kininogen (HK) to produce bradykinin. Kallikrein is also activated producing fibrinolysis and neutrophil activation. Contact also indirectly activates platelets and the complement cascade. [Adapted with permission from Warren OJ, Smith AJ, Alexiou C, et al: The inflammatory response to cardiopulmonary bypass: part 1—mechanisms of pathogenesis, *J Cardiothorac Vasc Anesth.* 2009 Apr;23(2):223-231.]

A variety of strategies have been suggested to mitigate the inflammatory response to CPB. Aprotinin, complement inhibitors, phosphodiesterase inhibitors, steroids, statins, levosimendan, and the avoidance of homologous blood products, and others have all been suggested to beneficially affect the inflammatory response to CPB. Landis et al. in a critical review of approaches to attenuate the systemic inflammatory response to CPB concluded "that no single intervention used on its own demonstrates strong evidence for limiting adverse outcomes as a result of the systemic inflammatory response."[29] Landis et al. suggest that those interventions that are "most promising" target multiple inflammatory pathways. It is likely that efforts will be ongoing to further understand the genetic influences that contribute to the inflammatory response to CPB and its consequences. Inflammation associated with CPB may also degrade the endothelial glycocalyx leading to possible damage to vascular endothelial cells resulting in edema, fluid extravasation, and leukocyte adhesion.[30,31]

The systemic inflammatory response contributes to post CPB vasoplegia resulting in hypotension. Vasopressors, vasopressin, and methylene blue restore vascular resistance and blood pressure.

ECHOCARDIOGRAPHY AND CPB

Echocardiography is useful in the CPB patient in two ways. First, echocardiography can help to determine where and if the aorta should be cannulated. Second, echocardiography can assist the surgeon in confirming the placement of various catheters as well as the adequacy of ventricular de-airing.

The risk of stroke during heart surgery with CPB in patients with severely atherosclerotic aortas has been discussed. Both TEE and EAU can be used to assist the surgeon in locating an appropriate site for aortic cannulation and cross clamp. Mobile plaque consistent with a grade V aorta and increased stroke risk can be detected by EAU and avoided (Video 17–2). In patients where the aorta cannot be cannulated, options include off-pump procedures or abandonment of the procedure. TEE can be used to assist the surgeon in determining the adequacy of de-airing of the heart. At times surgeons place a left ventricular vent via one of the pulmonary veins into the left heart (Video 17–3). In doing so, the left heart can be decompressed during the bypass period—particularly if the aortic valve is incompetent. Occasionally this vent disrupts the mitral valve and can appear as newly developed mitral regurgitation.

During the pump run, the heart is decompressed and TEE imagery becomes unclear. When not in use, the echo machine should be deactivated so as to minimize any thermal injury to the esophagus.

EXTRACORPOREAL MEMBRANE OXYGENATION (ECMO)

ECMO is used to treat both cardiac and respiratory failure. ECMO, like CPB, drains deoxygenated blood from the venous system and returns oxygenated blood to the patient. Like CPB, ECMO requires anticoagulation with careful monitoring. Venovenous (VV) ECMO is used to support patients with respiratory failure.

In VV ECMO, oxygenated blood is returned to the venous circulation and the patient's own heart pumps blood to the tissues. In venoarterial extracorporeal membrane oxygenation (VA ECMO), the blood is returned to a peripheral artery (e.g., femoral artery or axillary artery in peripheral VA ECMO) or directly into the ascending aorta (central VA ECMO) and the circuit provides both perfusion and gas exchange. As with partial CPB, any blood that is not drained into the VA ECMO circuit will pass through the heart and lungs and will be ejected to the aorta. Blood from the arterial line of the ECMO circuit and blood from the heart both enter the aorta.[32] Blood from the ECMO circuit is fully oxygenated. Blood that passes through diseased lungs may be inadequately oxygenated. This differential hypoxia leads to the so called "North South syndrome" where poorly oxygenated blood is delivered to the coronary and carotid arteries (after having been ejected by the heart) and highly oxygenated blood is delivered to the viscera (having been pumped by the ECMO circuit).[32] Blood gas sampling from the right radial artery is critical to screen for potential differential tissue oxygenation because blood from the heart would likely perfuse the innominate artery.[32] Monaco et al. in a review of ECMO suggest that use of a veno arterial venous ECMO circuit or cannulation of the subclavian or axillary artery will mitigate differential tissue hypoxemia associated with VA ECMO.[32] Moreover, they compare VV ECMO, VA ECMO, and CPB as well as provide some insights into ECMO management (see Tables 17–1 and 17–2).

Table 17–1. Comparison of Advantages and Disadvantages of Extracorporeal Membrane Oxygenation and Cardiopulmonary Bypass

	VA ECMO	**VV ECMO**	**CPB**
Advantages	• Low anticoagulation requirement (target ACT 180-220 s) • Reduced hemodilution and inflammatory activation • No cardiotomy reservoir → no air-blood surface and no cancer dissemination risk • Can be used to provide postoperative support with no circuit/cannulation changes • Easier patient transportation • Provides full cardiorespiratory support	• Low anticoagulation requirement (target ACT 180-220 s)* • Reduced hemodilution and inflammatory activation • No cardiotomy reservoir → no air-blood surface and no cancer dissemination risk • No risk of differential hypoxia syndrome • No increase in LV afterload • Can be used to provide postoperative support with no circuit/cannulation changes	• Provides full cardio-respiratory support • Cardiotomy reservoir → lower risk of hemodynamic instability due to intraoperative blood loss • Bubble detector/filter → reduced risk of air embolism • Additional pumps for cardioplegic solution venting, suctioning, and selective organ perfusion with controlled flows

(Continued)

Table 17–1. Comparison of Advantages and Disadvantages of Extracorporeal Membrane Oxygenation and Cardiopulmonary Bypass (*Continued*)

	VA ECMO	VV ECMO	CPB
		• Easier patient transportation • Possibility to use single double-lumen cannula • Possibility to mobilize the patient early in case of prolonged support in the ICU	
Disadvantages	• Risk of differential hypoxia syndrome (for peripheral cannulation) • Increase in LV afterload (particularly for peripheral cannulation) → possible need for inotropes/additional MCS to unload left ventricle • No cardiotomy reservoir → higher risk of hemodynamic instability due to intraoperative blood loss • No bubble detector/filter → risk of air embolism	• Provides respiratory support only; no hemodynamic support • Possible blood recirculation with reduced gas exchange efficacy • No cardiotomy reservoir → higher risk of hemodynamic instability due to severe intraoperative blood loss • No bubble detector/filter → risk of air embolism	• High anticoagulation requirement (target ACT > 480 s) • Higher hemodilution and inflammatory activation • Risk of differential hypoxia syndrome (for peripheral cannulation) • Increase in LV afterload (particularly for peripheral cannulation) if no aortic cross clamp and cardioplegic arrest used • Cardiotomy reservoir → air-blood surface and theoretic cancer dissemination risk • Patient transport while under support extremely difficult • Direct transition to postoperative support extremely difficult

Abbreviations: ACT, activated clotting time; CPB, cardiopulmonary bypass; ICU, intensive care unit; LV, left ventricular; MCS, mechanical circulatory support; VA ECMO, venoarterial extracorporeal membrane oxygenation; VV ECMO, venovenous extracorporeal membrane oxygenation.
*Cases of heparin-free VV ECMO in high bleeding risk patients have been described.
Reproduced with permission from Monaco F, Belletti A1, Bove T, et al: Extracorporeal Membrane Oxygenation: Beyond Cardiac Surgery and Intensive Care Unit: Unconventional Uses and Future Perspectives, *J Cardiothorac Vasc Anesth*. 2018 Aug;32(4):1955-1970.

Table 17–2. Tips and Tricks for Peripheral Venoarterial Extracorporeal Membrane Oxygenation Management

Suggestion	Reason
Do not use volatile anesthetics (consider if VV ECMO or if anesthesia depth is monitored)	Lungs are bypassed during VA ECMO
EtCO$_2$ is unreliable and may be abnormally low	Lungs are bypassed during VA ECMO
Blood gas abnormalities are managed by manipulating the ECMO setting (flow and swipe gas) and native cardiac output	Gas exchange is provided largely by ECMO oxygenator
ABG and SpO$_2$ should be monitored on right upper extremity	Oxygenated blood flow is provided by ECMO Risk of differential hypoxia syndrome (Harlequin syndrome)
Two cannulae in plain sight detected the shade of the blood color (arteriosus = bright red; venous = dark red)	Oxygenator/O$_2$ supply failure may occur [due to several causes including human error (e.g., O$_2$ source not connected to ECMO)]
Extra care during patient transport	Massive bleeding in case of cannula disconnection High risk of technical errors in O$_2$ supply
Extra care to avoid air in intravenous line	Air may enter ECMO circuit and cause arterial embolism or pump stop

Abbreviations: ABG, blood gas analysis; ECMO, extracorporeal membrane oxygenation; EtCO$_2$, end-tidal carbon dioxide; O$_2$, oxygen; SpO$_2$, peripheral oxygen saturation; VA, venoarterial.
Reproduced with permission from Monaco F, Belletti A1, Bove T, et al: Extracorporeal Membrane Oxygenation: Beyond Cardiac Surgery and Intensive Care Unit: Unconventional Uses and Future Perspectives, *J Cardiothorac Vasc Anesth.* 2018 Aug;32(4):1955-1970.

REFERENCES

1. Bechtel A, Huffmyer J. Anesthetic management for cardiopulmonary bypass: update for 2014. *Semin Cardiothorac Vasc Anesth.* 2014;18(2):101-116.
2. Murphy G, Hessell II E, Groom R. Optimal perfusion during cardiopulmonary bypass: an evidenced based approach. *Anesth Analg.* 2009;108(5):1394-1417.
3. Gold J, Charlson M, Williams-Russo P, et al. Improvement of outcomes after coronary artery bypass. A randomized trial comparing intraoperative high versus low mean arterial pressure. *J Thorac Cardiovasc Surg.* 1995;110:1302-1311.
4. Sun LY, Chung AM, Farkouh ME, et al. Defining an intraoperative hypotension threshold in association with stroke in cardiac surgery. *Anesthesiology.* 2018;129(3):440-447.
5. Vedel A, Holmgaard F, Rasmussen L, et al. High target versus low target blood pressure management during cardiopulmonary bypass to prevent cerebral injury in cardiac surgery patients: a randomized controlled trial. *Circulation.* 2018;137:1770-1780.
6. Hori D, Brown C, Ono M, et al. Arterial pressure above the upper cerebral autoregulation limit during cardiopulmonary bypass is associated with postoperative delirium. *Br J Anaesth.* 2014;113(6):1009-1017.
7. Licker M, Ellenberger C, Sierra J, et al. Cardioprotective effects of acute normovolemic hemodilution in patients undergoing coronary artery bypass surgery. *Chest.* 2005;128:838-847.
8. Esper S, Subramaniam K, Tanaka K. Pathophysiology of cardiopulmonary bypass: current strategies for the prevention and treatment of anemia, coagulopathy and organ dysfunction. *Semin Cardiothorac Vasc Anesth.* 2014;18(2):161-176.
9. Lindsay A, Xu M, Sessler D, et al. Lactate clearance time and concentration linked to morbidity and death in cardiac surgical patients. *Ann Thorac Surg.* 2013;95(2):486-492.
10. Grigore A, Grocott H, Mathew J, et al. The rewarming rate and increased peak temperature alter neurocognitive outcome after cardiac surgery. *Anesth Analg.* 2002;94:4-10.
11. Hogue C, Palin C, Arrowsmith J. Cardiopulmonary bypass management and neurologic outcomes: an evidence-based appraisal of current practices. *Anesth Analg.* 2006;103(1):21-37.

12. Azis K, Meduoye A. Is pH-stat or alpha-stat the best technique to follow in patients undergoing deep hypothermic circulatory arrest. *Interact Cardiovasc Thorac Surg.* 2010;10:271-282.

13. Jonas R. Technique of circulatory arrest makes a difference. *J Thorac Cadiovasc Surg.* 2018;156(1):40-41.

14. Broderick P, Damberg A, Ziganshin B, et al. Alpha-stat versus pH-stat: we do not pay it much mind. *J Thorac Cadiovasc Surg.* 2018;156(1):40-41.

15. Ali J, Miles L, Abu-Omar Y, et al. Global cardioplegia practices: results from the global cardiopulmonary bypass survey. *J Extra Corpor Technol.* 2018;50(2):83-93.

16. Roach G, Kanchuger M, Mora-Mangano C, et al. Adverse cerebral outcomes after coronary bypass surgery. *NEJM.* 1996;335:1857-1863.

17. Grocott H, White W, Morris R, et al. Genetic polymorphisms and the risk of stroke after cardiac surgery. *Stroke.* 2005;36:1854.

18. Hartman G, Yao F, Bruefach M, et al. Severity of atheromatous disease diagnosed by transesophageal echocardiography predicts stroke and other outcomes associated with coronary artery surgery: a prospective study. *Anesth Analg.* 1996;110:1302-1311.

19. Gold J, Torres K, Maldarelli W, et al. Improving outcomes in coronary surgery: the impact of echo-directed aortic cannulation and hemodynamic management in 500 patients. *Ann Thorac Surg.* 2004;78:1579-1585.

20. Hogue C, Gottesman R, Stearns J. Mechanisms of cerebral injury from cardiac surgery. *Crit Care Clin.* 2008;24(1):83-98.

21. Prielipp R, Butterworth J. Calcium is not routinely indicated during separation from cardiopulmonary bypass. *J Cardiothorac Vasc Anesth.* 1997;11(7):908-912.

22. Warren O, Watret A, deWit K, et al. The inflammatory response to cardiopulmonary bypass: part 2— anti-inflammatory therapeutic strategies. *J Cardiothorac Vasc Anesth.* 2009;23(3):384-393.

23. Murphy G, Marymount J. Alternative anticoagulation management strategies for the patient with heparin induced thrombocytopenia undergoing cardiac surgery. *J Cardiothorac Vasc Anesth.* 2007;21(1):113-126.

24. Trossaert M, Gaillard A, Commin P, et al. High incidence of anti-heparin/platelet 4 antibodies after cardiopulmonary bypass surgery. *Br J Haematol.* 1998;101:653-655.

25. Shore-Lesserson L, Baker R, Ferraris V, et al. The Soceity of Thoracic Surgeons, The Society of Cardiovascular Anesthesiologists, and the American Society of ExtraCorporeal Technology: clinical practice guidelines—anticoagulation during cardiopulmonary bypass. *Ann Thorac Surg.* 2018;105:650-662.

26. Lee G, Arepally G. Diagnosis and management of heparin induced thrombocytopenia. *Hematol Oncol Clin North Am.* 2013;27:541-563.

27. Seigerman M, Cavallaro P, Itagaki S, et al. Incidence and outcomes of heparin induced thrombocytopenia in patients undergoing cardiac surgery in North America: an analysis of the nationwide inpatient sample. *J Cardiothorac Vasc Anesth.* 2014;28(1):98-102.

28. Warren O, Smith A, Alexiou C. The inflammatory response to cardiopulmonary bypass: part 1— mechanisms of pathogenesis. *J Cardiothorac Vasc Anesth.* 2009;23(2):223-231.

29. Landis R, Brown J, Fitzgerald D, et al. Attenuating the systemic inflammatory response to adult cardiopulmonary bypass: a critical reviw of the evidence base. *J Extra Corpor Technol.* 2014;46:197-211.

30. Myers G, Wegner J. Endothelial glycocalyx and cardiopulmonary bypass. *J Extra Corpor Technol.* 2017;49:174-181.

31. Pesonen E, Passov A, Anersson S, et al. Glycocalyx degradation and inflammation in cardiac surgery. *J Cardiothorac Vasc Anesth.* 2019;33(2):341-345.

32. Monaco F, Belletti A, Bove T, et al. Extracorporeal membrane oxygenation: beyond cardiac surgery and intensive care unit: unconventional uses and future perspectives. *J Cardiothorac Vasc Anesth.* 2018;32(4):1955-1970.

REVIEWS

Barry A, Chaney M, London M. Anesthetic management during cardiopulmonary bypass: a systematic review. *Anesth Analg.* 2015;120:749-769.

Engelman R, Baker R, Likosky D, et al. The Society of Thoracic Surgeons, The Society of Cardiovascular Anesthesiologists, and The American Society of ExtraCorporeal Technology: temperature management during cardiopulmonary bypass. *J Extra Corpor Technol.* 2015;47(3):145-154.

Millar J, Fanning J, McDonald C, et al. The inflammatory response to extracorporeal oxygenation (ECMO); a review of the pathophysiology. *Critical Care.* 2016;20:387.

Postoperative Analgesia for Cardiac Surgery

TOPICS

Cardiac surgery is associated with significant postoperative pain. Common sources include surgical incision pain, pain associated with rib retraction, and pain from chest tubes and other perioperative appliances. Other potential causes include incomplete revascularization of the myocardium, sternal wires, epicardial pacing leads, and sternocostal and costovertebral pain from retraction.[1]

The surgical approach has an obvious impact on the severity of postoperative pain. For example, minimally invasive cardiac procedures may produce less overall tissue injury and result in less postoperative pain. Postoperative pain for midline sternotomy has often been described to be moderate, and patients' anticipated pain level tends to be much greater than the actual pain they experience postoperatively.[2] On the other hand, thoracotomy has been associated with a greater degree of both pain and functional limitation, due to the pain associated with breathing and coughing.[3] Endoscopic vein graft harvesting has decreased the severity of postoperative leg pain, as well as the infection and wound dehiscence rate.[4]

Patient risk factors also play a role in the incidence and severity of postcardiac surgical pain, with younger patients (< 60 years old) and those with a higher New York Heart Association (NYHA) class incurring higher pain scores.[5,6]

WHAT ARE THE SYSTEMIC IMPLICATIONS OF PAIN IN THE CARDIAC SURGERY PATIENT?

The Stress Response

In addition to the discomfort and suffering that postoperative pain accords, the central nervous system responds to the barrage of noxious afferent impulses with a cascade of neurohumoral responses that impair healing and recovery and promote poor clinical outcomes. This so-called stress response is an adaptive mechanism that serves to liberate fuel through catabolism for energy-dependent fight-or-flight activities, increase blood pressure and heart rate, and promote coagulopathy, inflammation, and immune suppression. This is initiated both through the trauma of the surgical procedure and, uniquely in the case of cardiac surgery, through the use of cardiopulmonary bypass.

Pathophysiologic changes include increased oxygen consumption and energy expenditure, increased secretion of adrenocorticotrophic hormone, cortisol, epinephrine, norepinephrine, insulin, and growth hormone, and decreased total tri-iodothyronine levels. Quantifiable metabolic consequences of these changes include hyperglycemia, hyperlactatemia, increased free fatty acid concentrations, hypokalemia, increased production of inflammatory cytokines, and increased consumption of complement and adhesion molecules. Cortisol levels can increase to more than 500% of baseline levels and remain elevated for several days.[7] Particularly concerning is the rise in catecholamine levels, as these contribute to postoperative arrythmias.[8]

Effective attenuation of the entire stress response is not practically achievable, as the effect contributed by cardiopulmonary bypass is difficult to mitigate (see Chapter 17). However, management of postoperative pain is a factor within the anesthesiologist's control. Control of pain by any means will aid in reducing the stress response, but because of the robust nature of the afferent impulses and the duration over which they are delivered to the central nervous system, treatment regimens must be aggressive to have an effect. Typically, this has required the use of multimodal therapies or the combination of systemic and regional modalities.

Chronic Pain

As our understanding of postoperative pain improves, it has been recognized that acute pain and chronic pain are no longer two separate elements, but are rather two points on a continuum of a pain experience that begins at the time of surgery. As such, many patients will continue to experience pain well after their surgical procedures, eventually manifesting chronic, neuropathic pain that is present after the incisions have healed. Approximately 30% of cardiac patients will develop chronic sternotomy pain lasting 6 months or longer following surgery, and is usually localized to the arms, shoulder, or legs.[9] For patients undergoing thoracotomy, chronic pain known as the "post-thoracotomy pain syndrome" is present in approximately 50% of patients and can lead to disabling chronic neuropathic pain and disability.[10]

Trauma to peripheral nerves at the time of sternotomy, thoracotomy, or during dissection of the internal mammary artery has been linked to the risk of developing postoperative hyperalgesia or chronic pain; in the latter case, the pain is typically localized to the left sternal border.[11]

Effective pain management following surgery can possibly aid in the prevention of evolution of acute to chronic pain. For example, patients receiving a single-shot paravertebral block (PVB) with bupivacaine versus sham block for mastectomy have been shown to have a significantly reduced incidence of chronic incisional pain at 12 months.[12] The mechanism for this reduction may relate to the prevention of spinal column recruitment of wide-receptive field neurons, or "wind-up," a phenomenon that leads to allodynia and hyperalgesia. Several risk factors have been identified as leading to the development of chronic postoperative pain, including psychologic vulnerability, anxiety, and the degree of postoperative pain, all of which are modifiable by a well-planned and executed analgesic plan.[13] Indeed, thoracic epidural analgesia has been found to reduce depression and post-traumatic stress disorder following cardiac surgery.[14]

WHAT MODALITIES ARE AVAILABLE TO TREAT POSTOPERATIVE PAIN?

Systemic Opioids

Intravenous opioids are one of the mainstays of postcardiac analgesia. Ease of administration, predictable effect, and excellent bioavailability are several of the advantages of this method of pain control. Because most postcardiac surgical patients are transferred to an intensely monitored setting and not awakened immediately after surgery, concerns regarding the respiratory depressive effects of opioids are to a large degree ameliorated, at least for the initial several hours until extubation is planned.

Opioid drugs can be naturally occurring (such as morphine or codeine), synthetic (such as fentanyl or tramadol), or semisynthetic (such as hydromorphone). Following cardiac surgery, opioids are typically delivered via either a nurse-controlled (NCA) or patient-controlled opioid analgesia (PCA) regimen. Clearly, to employ the PCA option a patient must be conscious and able to understand the mechanism of pain medication delivery, and for that reason it may not be practical in the immediate postoperative period. However, in a meta-analysis of randomized trials, PCA led to significantly decreased pain scores after cardiac surgery compared to NCA.[15] In addition, the cumulative morphine dose was significantly higher with PCA at 24 and 48 hours, suggesting that pain is undertreated in this population when NCA is utilized. Side effects such as respiratory depression and sedation, morbidity and mortality, and ICU and hospital length of stay were not shown to be different between regimens. One randomized controlled trial reported that the incidence of nausea was significantly less with PCA compared with NCA, despite using an overall larger dose of morphine.[16] Importantly, the use of a background infusion of morphine when PCA is prescribed increases the total amount of opioid consumed, with little or no clinically relevant improvement in analgesia.[17,18]

Although morphine remains the opioid that most clinicians prescribe following cardiac surgical procedures, other systemic opioids have been investigated for their potential to improve recovery profiles. When compared with PCA morphine, PCA remifentanil was shown to result in significantly reduced pain scores on coughing and movement with remifentanil following coronary artery bypass grafting (CABG).[19] Despite this, the group reported excellent analgesia (numeric rating scale < 3) with either regimen overall. A comparison of PCA morphine, fentanyl, and remifentanil following off-pump coronary bypass grafting (OPCAB) demonstrated that the use of remifentanil PCA resulted in similar pain scores as the other opioids, but with less pruritus than fentanyl, and less nausea and vomiting than morphine.[20] Because of its ultrashort duration, remifentanil may be particularly useful for avoiding serious side effects such as respiratory depression, as a titrated infusion has been shown to be an effective and safe analgesic regimen in extubated patients after cardiac surgery without resulting in respiratory compromise.[21]

Typically, patients will be converted to oral opioid analgesics as early feeding is initiated, based on the usage of parenteral opioids (i.e., PCA morphine). This is often done within the first 24 hours after surgery.[22] The use of sustained-release opioids such as oxycodone or morphine facilitate a background level of analgesia, and immediate-release versions of the same drugs can be used for breakthrough.

Tramadol is a unique drug that acts both as a mu-opioid agonist, as well as a weak inhibitor of the reuptake of norepinephrine and serotonin, which is thought to enhance analgesia without clinically relevant respiratory depression. It has been well validated as a treatment for mild to moderate postoperative pain, and studies have found equivalency to typical NCA doses of opioids following cardiac surgery.[23,24] But et al. demonstrated that a single dose of tramadol administered prior to extubation following CABG was associated with a reduction of up to 25% in morphine consumption, as well as a decrease in the visual analog scale (VAS) scores within the first 4 hours postoperatively.[25] Because of its effect on serotonin, tramadol use is associated with an increase in postoperative nausea and vomiting and should not be administered in epileptics.[26]

With growing concerns related to the opioid crisis multimodal analgesia regimens are preferred to analgesia regimens heavily dependent on narcotic analgesia.

Nonsteroidal Anti-Inflammatory Drugs

NSAIDs have both analgesic and anti-inflammatory properties and are effective in treating mild to moderate pain when used alone. Combined with other modalities such as opioids, NSAIDs can be used as adjuncts to treat more severe pain and are useful in reducing opioid requirements.[27]

NSAIDs inhibit the enzyme cyclooxygenase (COX), thereby decreasing the production of prostaglandins that contribute to inflammation and sensitization of nociceptive fibers. There are two isoforms of the COX enzyme, COX-1 and COX-2. COX-1 is a constitutive enzyme that facilitates the formation of prostaglandins found in blood vessels, stomach, and kidneys and is involved in the preservation of gastric mucosa and maintenance of renal blood flow. In contrast, COX-2 is the inducible isoform, upregulated after tissue injury.

Nonselective NSAIDs have anti-inflammatory and analgesic effects but at the expense of increased gastropathy, decreased renal perfusion, and reduced platelet aggregation.[28] Acetylsalicylic acid (ASA) is an example of a nonselective NSAID that the majority of cardiac surgical patients are prescribed specifically for its antiplatelet effects. Controversy surrounding adverse myocardial outcomes in patients taking COX-2 specific inhibitors has led to a great deal of concern over their use in patients at risk for coronary thrombosis. Data demonstrating an association with coronary and cerebral thrombosis resulted in the withdrawal of both rofecoxib and valdecoxib from the U.S. market.[29] Parecoxib, an intravenous prodrug of valdecoxib, was issued a letter of nonapproval by the FDA in 2005 for similar reasons. Celecoxib, on the other hand, appears to have little effect on coronary thrombosis.[30] However, the use of any COX-2 inhibitor in patients with ischemic heart disease should be approached with caution, as other agents are available.

Rapanos et al. demonstrated that the combination of indomethacin with morphine after cardiac surgery resulted in reduced postoperative pain scores and opioid use without an increase in NSAID-related side effects.[31] Other NSAIDs such as diclofenac and ketoprofen have also been shown to reduce both opioid requirements, opioid-related side effects, and pain scores.[32,33] NSAIDs appear to not significantly increase postoperative bleeding or renal dysfunction in postcardiac surgical patients.[34] An FDA black box warning from 2005 alerted practitioners to a contraindication to ketorolac use following coronary artery bypass graft surgery. However, ketorolac has been suggested as safe for use by some authors.

Acetaminophen

Acetaminophen is a common drug for mild to moderate pain. Its favorable safety profile and lack of interactions with other drugs, and absence of any effect on coagulation make it a useful adjunct, with its principal contraindication being patients with hepatic disease. The intravenous form, paracetamol, is in theory ideal for patients after cardiac surgery, who can remain nil by mouth for a day or more following surgery.

Despite the theoretical benefits, data are mixed regarding the overall efficacy of acetaminophen following cardiac surgery, with groups reporting small or no differences with respect to pain scores compared to placebo.[35,36] Moreover, a meta-analysis of seven randomized trials showed that the addition of acetaminophen to morphine analgesia after cardiac surgery reduced morphine consumption by 20%, but had no effect on morphine-related side effects or patient satisfaction.[37]

Thoracic Epidural Analgesia

Thoracic epidural analgesia (TEA) with local anesthetics has been used in cardiac surgery for decades.[38] Its benefits include superior analgesia,[14] improved pulmonary function,[39,40] reduced time to extubation,[14,41,42] as well as coronary vasodilation and/or cardioprotection.[43-45] It is also the most effective technique by which the stress response is suppressed.[46] Liu et al. published a meta-analysis of 15 randomized trials and 1178 patients undergoing CABG and found significantly reduced pain scores and time to extubation, reduced pulmonary complications, and reduced risk of dysrhythmias.[47] On the other hand, mortality and myocardial infarction rates were not improved with the use of TEA. However, in a more recent and larger meta-analysis (33 trials, 2366 patients), the composite endpoint of mortality and myocardial infarction was significantly reduced from 5.2% to 2.7%.[48] The effect of TEA on incidence of atrial fibrillation is unclear; although it was not shown to be reduced for on-pump cardiac surgery,[49] a significant reduction was found in off-pump coronary surgery (23.7% versus 3%).[50]

The technique's beneficial effects can be explained by the halting of afferent neural input from the surgical site to the spinal cord and higher centers in the central nervous system. This not only provides excellent analgesia, but also prevents the initiation of the stress response, which limits the release of catecholamines and counter-regulatory hormones and attenuates the hypercoagulable state that might otherwise predispose to thrombotic events postoperatively. In addition, sympathetic blockade of spinal levels T1 to T4 by TEA can block cardiac afferent (thereby reducing anginal symptoms) and efferent fibers (promoting coronary vasodilation and reducing heart rate and left ventricular work index). Jakobsen et al. conducted 2-D echocardiograms in patients with ischemic heart disease and found that TEA resulted in improved left ventricular systolic and diastolic function, likely mediated through improved cardiac loading conditions.[51] Note that for the thoracic epidural to be of maximum benefit, it should be placed at the level of T3/T4, to best provide analgesia to the sternal area (T2-T5), as well as provide sympathetic blockade of the cardioaccelerator fibers (T1-T4). The skin overlying the superior aspect of the sternum and manubrium is not covered by thoracic nerves but is instead innervated by the supraclavicular nerve (C3/C4), a branch of the cervical plexus. This is effectively supplemented with a lateral subcutaneous field block at the level of the clavicular heads.

Despite its attractive theoretical benefits, the use of TEA is controversial and is not widespread. The greatest barrier to its implementation is likely the fear of epidural hematoma associated with anticoagulation for cardiopulmonary bypass. Estimation of this risk is approximately 1:12,000 procedures performed, with 95% confidence intervals of 1:2100 to 1:68,000.[52] To reduce the risk of incurring a hematoma, most publications advise placing the epidural the evening prior to surgery. This practice, however, is clearly impractical in an age of same-day admissions. Indeed, there is no evidence that insertion the night before surgery reduces the risk compared to insertion on the day of surgery.[53] Practically speaking, epidural catheters should be placed as early as possible on the morning of surgery (i.e., after the intravenous line is inserted) and only in patients who have a normal coagulation profile at baseline. This ensures at least 1 hour prior to anticoagulation, which is consistent with the recommendations of the American Society of Regional Anesthesia Consensus Conference on Neuraxial Anesthesia and Anticoagulation.[54] The patient should be monitored closely for signs and symptoms of an expanding hematoma. Difficulty arises when a traumatic tap is encountered. The Consensus Conference recommends a delay of 24 hours to ensure that complete clotting of the epidural vein has occurred. Clearly, these issues must be discussed with the patient prior to the procedure during the informed consent. The postoperative local anesthetic infusion should consist of the lowest concentration possible that provides analgesia, but not motor block (e.g., ropivacaine 0.15%-0.2%), to help aid in the possible diagnosis of epidural hematoma, should increasing motor weakness be noted.

Intrathecal Opioids

Another regional analgesic option for postcardiac surgery is intrathecal opioids. Morphine is by far the drug studied best, by virtue of its ability to confer a long (e.g., 24 hours) period of quality analgesia. Various doses (250-4000 µg) have been used, with larger doses likely to prolong the time to extubation due to the respiratory depressive effects.[55] This is usually a consideration only if the patients are to be fast-tracked.

A meta-analysis of 17 trials enrolling 668 patients demonstrated little difference in important outcomes between those randomized to receive intrathecal opioids or not; however, the incidence of pruritus was significantly higher in the intervention group.[47] Moreover, a recent meta-analysis of 1106 patients receiving general anesthesia with or without spinal opioids showed no difference in mortality, myocardial infarction, or length of hospital stay.[56] The addition of 100 µg of clonidine to 500 mg of spinal morphine appears to decrease postoperative pain scores and time to extubation.[57]

Although the risk of epidural hematoma is rare (and probably lower than that of an epidural), the true incidence is unknown, and discussion of the potential for this complication with the patient is warranted. In general, this technique has fallen out of favor due to the lack of substantial benefit and the potential for delaying fast-track extubation.

Regional Blocks and Cardiac Surgery

Concern over epidural hematoma formation with TEA has led some practitioners to consider alternative regional methods for postoperative pain control such as intercostal and paravertebral blocks.

Intercostal nerve (IC) blocks are simple to perform and, if properly performed, result in excellent analgesia of the chest and upper abdominal wall. Typically, these blocks are used for thoracotomy or minithoracotomy incisions. Disadvantages include the potential for pleural, lung parenchymal, or vascular puncture, and the need to perform bilateral blockade if the patient's incision is midline. In addition, IC blocks do not block visceral pleural pain, as the sympathetic nerves are not blocked. Traditionally, IC blocks are performed at the angle of the rib, which is impractical in an intubated postcardiac surgical patient. Instead, bilateral IC blockade with parasternal catheters has been employed by the surgeon effectively after cardiac surgery, reducing morphine requirements and hospital length of stay.[58]

Paravertebral block involves injection of local anesthetic in the paravertebral space immediately lateral to the place from where the spinal nerves emerge from the intervertebral foramina. It is typically performed prior to inducing general anesthesia for cardiac surgery, and excellent analgesia can be achieved with infusion catheters located on either side of the midline. Advantages over the IC block include more complete analgesia of the posterior chest wall, and sympathetic block of the involved levels, which aids in visceral pain and provides cardiac sympathectomy. PVB has been found to be as effective for analgesia as TEA for MIDCAB.[59]

Disadvantages include the potential for needle misadventure and subsequent pneumothorax or neuraxial placement of the needle. Also, 10% of patients exhibit parasympathetic reactions at needle placement resulting in hypotension, bradycardia, and near syncope. This technique may also be a problem in patients with spinal anomalies, trauma, or a history of spine surgery. Recently, an ultrasound-guided technique of continuous PVB using a more lateral intercostal approach has been described to potentially minimize the risk of vascular puncture, nerve injury, and pneumothorax.[60] This technique takes advantage of the continuity that exists between the intercostal and paravertebral spaces to provide a method of continuous paravertebral block PVB that may provide advantages when compared with the classical approach for the continuous paravertebral nerve block.

PVB has been used extensively for thoracotomy and has been shown in a systematic review to be as effective as epidural analgesia for pain management following thoracotomy.[61] However, the side-effect profile appears to favor PVB over TEA for this population. Pulmonary function assessed by peak expiratory flow rate was significantly better preserved in the paravertebral group. In addition, epidural block was associated with a higher incidence of urinary retention, nausea, pruritus, and hypotension. Finally, epidurals were associated with delayed operative start time, and a higher rate of technical failure and displacement.

Efforts have been made to simplify some of these regional approaches by infusing local anesthetic directly into the fascial plane of the sternotomy wound by catheters. Results have been mixed, however, with studies showing both a favorable effect and no effect on pain scores following cardiac surgery.[62,63]

ENHANCED RECOVERY FOLLOWING CARDIAC SURGERY

Increasingly, patients are managed according to enhanced recovery bundles.[64,65] Enhanced recovery incorporates pre-, intra-, and postoperative strategies that improve outcomes following surgery (Figure 18–1 and Table 18–1).

Analgesia regimens include various multimodal interventions including regional anesthesia to facilitate early mobility. Noss et al. provide a summary of analgesia approaches that could contribute to enhanced recovery pathways (Table 18–2).

In addition to the use of multimodal analgesia regimens, enhanced recovery protocols seek to avoid hypothermia and prevent delirium. It is likely that individual institutions will design bundles and over time consensus will coalesce around the effectiveness of certain interventions compared with others.

SUMMARY

Cardiac surgery can lead to a significant degree of postoperative pain that has traditionally been managed with intravenous opioids. The nowadays trends toward fast tracking and enhanced recovery of patients after cardiac surgery have made careful

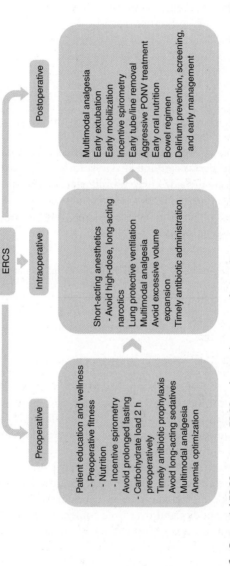

Figure 18–1. Potential ERCS strategy. ERCS, enhanced recovery for cardiac surgery; PONV, postoperative nausea and vomiting. [Reproduced with permission from Noss C, Prusinkiewicz C2, Nelson G, et al: Enhanced Recovery for Cardiac Surgery, *J Cardiothorac Vasc Anesth.* 2018 Dec;32(6): 2760-2770.]

Table 18-1. Detailed Protocol for Enhanced Recovery after Surgery Pathway

Preoperative bundle
- Preoperative assessment, education, and psychological counselling conducted by trained research personnel
- EPO therapy from admission to hospital
- Shorten NPO time and carbohydrate beverage intake at 2 h before anaesthesia
- No preoperative sedative or anticholinergic drug use
- Antibiotic prophylaxis within 1 h of anaesthesia
- PVNB before anaesthesia

Intraoperative bundle
- Fast-track cardiac anaesthesia with short-acting narcotic and sedative agents
- Optimization of CPB: total priming fluid reduction to <1500 mL, retrograde oxygenated blood cardioplegia perfusion, modified ultrafiltration, albumin infusion to maintain a stable plasma colloid osmotic pressure
- Lung protection strategy: low tidal volume (6-7 mL/kg) ventilation, positive end-expiratory pressure (5 mm Hg), lung recruitment maneuver
- Goal-directed fluid management to optimize stroke volume guided by TOE
- Cerebral oxygen saturation monitor and bispectral index monitor
- Blood conservation measures: cell saver, antiplasmin agent and TEG monitor
- Ropivacaine infiltration at incision site

Postoperative bundle
- Multimodal postoperative analgesia (PCA, PVNB, infiltration at incision site)
- PONV prevention (ondansetron)
- EPO therapy
- Early oral intake after tracheal extubation
- Early removal of drainage tube
- Early mobilization as soon as possible

Abbreviations: CPB, cardiopulmonary bypass; EPO, erythropoietin; NPO, nil per os; PCA, patient-controlled analgesia; PONV, postoperative nausea and vomiting; PVNB, paravertebral nerve block; TOE, transoesophageal echocardiography; TEG, thromboelastography.
Reproduced with permission from Li M, Zhang J, Gan TJ, et al: Enhanced recovery after surgery pathway for patients undergoing cardiac surgery: a randomized clinical trial, *Eur J Cardiothorac Surg.* 2018 Sep 1;54(3): 491-497.

planning of postoperative analgesia an even more important concern. Multimodal therapeutic plans using a variety of agents (see Table 18–1) can be customized to meet the needs of a specific patient.

Thoracic epidural analgesia has been shown to improve a variety of important outcomes, including the composite endpoint of mortality and myocardial infarction. Despite this, concern regarding the potential for epidural hematoma has limited its use, regardless of evidence pointing to its overall safety. Alternatively, other regional anesthesia techniques such as pectoralis fascial blocks and paravertebral blocks may be incorporated into enhanced recovery pathways.[66]

Table 18–2. Analgesia Intervention Targets

Intervention	Commonly reported dosing	Mechanism
Preoperative		
Gabapentinoids	Gabapentin 300-1200 mg and pregabalin up to 300 mg	Voltage-gated calcium channel
Steroids	Dexamethasone 0.1-0.2 mg/kg	Anti-inflammatory
Intraoperative		
Ketamine	0.06-0.15 mg/kg/h	NMDA antagonism
Magnesium	32 nmol/kg/h; bolus 5-50 mg/ kg; infusion 6-30 mg/kg/h; median 24-h dose 8.5 g	NMDA antagonism
Lidocaine	1-3 mg/kg/h	Sodium channel blockade— mediated attenuation of central sensitization, anti-inflammatory, inhibition of spontaneous ectopic nerve impulse generation, and selective inhibition of evoked spinal cord C fiber activity
Spinal anesthesia	Intrathecal morphine 4-20 µg/ kg, maximum 2 mg	Intrathecal opioid ± cardiac sympathectomy
Paravertebral block	Variable titrated continuous infusion and boluses of local anesthetic	Anesthesia of the surgical site
Postoperative		
Paravertebral block	Variable titrated continuous infusion and boluses of local anesthetic	Anesthesia of the surgical site
Epidural analgesia	Variable titrated continuous infusion and boluses of local anesthetic	Anesthesia of surgical site
PECS block	30 mL 0.2% ropivacaine	Anesthesia of pectoral nerves
Serratus anterior plane block	30 mL 0.25% levobupivacaine; 5 mL/h 0.125% levobupivacaine	Anesthesia of hemithorax
Continuous prefascial block	4 mL/h 0.25%-0.5% bupivacaine	Anesthesia of the sternal incision
Ketamine	0.06-0.15 mg/kg/h	NMDA antagonism
Lidocaine	2-3 mg/kg/h or 2-3 mg/min	Sodium channel blockade— mediated attenuation of central sensitization, anti-inflammatory, inhibition of spontaneous ectopic nerve impulse generation and selective inhibition of evoked spinal cord C fiber activity
Gabapentinoids	Gabapentin 400-600 3 times/d	Voltage-gated calcium channel

Abbreviations: NMDA, N-methyl-D-aspartate; PECS, pectoralis nerve block.
Reproduced with permission from Noss C, Prusinkiewicz C2, Nelson G, et al: Enhanced Recovery for Cardiac Surgery, *J Cardiothorac Vasc Anesth.* 2018 Dec;32(6):2760-2770.

REFERENCES

1. Alston RP, Pechon P. Dysaesthesia associated with sternotomy for heart surgery. *Br J Anaesth.* 2005;95:153-158.

2. Nay PG, Elliott SM, Harrop-Griffiths AW. Postoperative pain. Expectation and experience after coronary artery bypass grafting. *Anaesthesia.* 1996;51:741-743.

3. Diegeler A, Walther T, Metz S, et al. Comparison of MIDCAP versus conventional CABG surgery regarding pain and quality of life. *Heart Surg Forum.* 1999;2:290-295; discussion 295-296.

4. Andreasen JJ, Nekrasas V, Dethlefsen C. Endoscopic vs open saphenous vein harvest for coronary artery bypass grafting: a prospective randomized trial. *Eur J Cardiothorac Surg.* 2008;34:384-389.

5. Kalso E, Mennander S, Tasmuth T, Nilsson E. Chronic post-sternotomy pain. *Acta Anaesthesiol Scand.* 2001;45:935-939.

6. Mueller XM, Tinguely F, Tevaearai HT, Revelly JP, Chiolero R, von Segesser LK. Pain location, distribution, and intensity after cardiac surgery. *Chest.* 2000;118:391-396.

7. Hoda MR, El-Achkar H, Schmitz E, Scheffold T, Vetter HO, De Simone R. Systemic stress hormone response in patients undergoing open heart surgery with or without cardiopulmonary bypass. *Ann Thorac Surg.* 2006;82:2179-2186.

8. Riles TS, Fisher FS, Schaefer S, Pasternack PF, Baumann FG. Plasma catecholamine concentrations during abdominal aortic aneurysm surgery: the link to perioperative myocardial ischemia. *Ann Vasc Surg.* 1993;7:213-219.

9. Meyerson J, Thelin S, Gordh T, Karlsten R. The incidence of chronic post-sternotomy pain after cardiac surgery—a prospective study. *Acta Anaesthesiol Scand.* 2001;45:940-944.

10. Karmakar MK, Ho AM. Post-thoracotomy pain syndrome. *Thorac Surg Clin.* 2004;14:345-352.

11. Eisenberg E, Pultorak Y, Pud D, Bar-El Y. Prevalence and characteristics of post coronary artery bypass graft surgery pain (PCP). *Pain.* 2001;92:11-17.

12. Kairaluoma PM, Bachmann MS, Rosenberg PH, Pere PJ. Preincisional paravertebral block reduces the prevalence of chronic pain after breast surgery. *Anesth Analg.* 2006;103:703-708.

13. Perkins FM, Kehlet H. Chronic pain as an outcome of surgery. A review of predictive factors. *Anesthesiology.* 2000;93:1123-1133.

14. Royse C, Royse A, Soeding P, Blake D, Pang J. Prospective randomized trial of high thoracic epidural analgesia for coronary artery bypass surgery. *Ann Thorac Surg.* 2003;75:93-100.

15. Bainbridge D, Martin JE, Cheng DC. Patient-controlled versus nurse-controlled analgesia after cardiac surgery—a meta-analysis. *Can J Anaesth.* 2006;53:492-499.

16. O'Halloran P, Brown R. Patient-controlled analgesia compared with nurse-controlled infusion analgesia after heart surgery. *Intensive Crit Care Nurs.* 1997;13:126-129.

17. Dal D, Kanbak M, Caglar M, Aypar U. A background infusion of morphine does not enhance postoperative analgesia after cardiac surgery. *Can J Anaesth.* 2003;50:476-479.

18. Guler T, Unlugenc H, Gundogan Z, Ozalevli M, Balcioglu O, Topcuoglu MS. A background infusion of morphine enhances patient-controlled analgesia after cardiac surgery. *Can J Anaesth.* 2004;51:718-722.

19. Baltali S, Turkoz A, Bozdogan N, et al. The efficacy of intravenous patient-controlled remifentanil versus morphine anesthesia after coronary artery surgery. *J Cardiothorac Vasc Anesth.* 2009;23:170-174.

20. Gurbet A, Goren S, Sahin S, Uckunkaya N, Korfali G. Comparison of analgesic effects of morphine, fentanyl, and remifentanil with intravenous patient-controlled analgesia after cardiac surgery. *J Cardiothorac Vasc Anesth.* 2004;18:755-758.

21. Steinlechner B, Koinig H, Grubhofer G, et al. Postoperative analgesia with remifentanil in patients undergoing cardiac surgery. *Anesth Analg.* 2005;100:1230-1235, table of contents.

22. Kogan A, Medalion B, Raanani E, et al. Early oral analgesia after fast-track cardiac anesthesia. *Can J Anaesth.* 2007;54:254-261.

23. Manji M RC, Jones P, Ariffin S, Faroqui M. Tramadol for postoperative analgesia in coronary artery bypass graft surgery [abstract]. *Br J Anaesth.* 1997;78:A87.

24. Sellin MLV, Sicsic JC. Postoperative pain: tramadol vs morphine after cardiac surgery [abstract]. *Br J Anaesth.* 1998;80:41.

25. But AK, Erdil F, Yucel A, Gedik E, Durmus M, Ersoy MO. The effects of single-dose tramadol on postoperative pain and morphine requirements after coronary artery bypass surgery. *Acta Anaesthesiol Scand.* 2007;51:601-606.

26. Desmeules JA. The tramadol option. *Eur J Pain.* 2000;4 (suppl A):15-21.

27. Tramer MR, Williams JE, Carroll D, Wiffen PJ, Moore RA, McQuay HJ. Comparing analgesic efficacy of non-steroidal anti-inflammatory drugs given by different routes in acute and chronic pain: a qualitative systematic review. *Acta Anaesthesiol Scand.* 1998;42:71-79.

28. Vane JR, Botting RM. Mechanism of action of aspirin-like drugs. *Semin Arthritis Rheum.* 1997;26:2-10.

29. Sanghi S, MacLaughlin EJ, Jewell CW, et al. Cyclooxygenase-2 inhibitors: a painful lesson. *Cardiovasc Hematol Disord Drug Targets.* 2006;6:85-100.

30. Dajani EZ, Islam K. Cardiovascular and gastrointestinal toxicity of selective cyclo-oxygenase-2 inhibitors in man. *J Physiol Pharmacol.* 2008;59 (suppl 2):117-133.

31. Rapanos T, Murphy P, Szalai JP, Burlacoff L, Lam-McCulloch J, Kay J. Rectal indomethacin reduces postoperative pain and morphine use after cardiac surgery. *Can J Anaesth.* 1999;46:725-730.

32. Dhawan N, Das S, Kiran U, Chauhan S, Bisoi AK, Makhija N. Effect of rectal diclofenac in reducing postoperative pain and rescue analgesia requirement after cardiac surgery. *Pain Pract.* 2009;9: 385-393.

33. Hynninen MS, Cheng DC, Hossain I, et al. Non-steroidal anti-inflammatory drugs in treatment of postoperative pain after cardiac surgery. *Can J Anaesth.* 2000;47:1182-1187.

34. Kulik A, Ruel M, Bourke ME, et al. Postoperative naproxen after coronary artery bypass surgery: a double-blind randomized controlled trial. *Eur J Cardiothorac Surg.* 2004;26:694-700.

35. Lahtinen P, Kokki H, Hendolin H, Hakala T, Hynynen M. Propacetamol as adjunctive treatment for postoperative pain after cardiac surgery. *Anesth Analg.* 2002;95:813-819, table of contents.

36. Cattabriga I, Pacini D, Lamazza G, et al. Intravenous paracetamol as adjunctive treatment for postoperative pain after cardiac surgery: a double blind randomized controlled trial. *Eur J Cardiothorac Surg.* 2007;32:527-531.

37. Remy C, Marret E, Bonnet F. Effects of acetaminophen on morphine side-effects and consumption after major surgery: meta-analysis of randomized controlled trials. *Br J Anaesth.* 2005;94:505-513.

38. Robinson RJ, Brister S, Jones E, Quigly M. Epidural meperidine analgesia after cardiac surgery. *Can Anaesth Soc J.* 1986;33:550-555.

39. Scott NB, Turfrey DJ, Ray DA, et al. A prospective randomized study of the potential benefits of thoracic epidural anesthesia and analgesia in patients undergoing coronary artery bypass grafting. *Anesth Analg.* 2001;93:528-535.

40. Groeben H. Epidural anesthesia and pulmonary function. *J Anesth.* 2006;20:290-299.

41. Priestley MC, Cope L, Halliwell R, et al. Thoracic epidural anesthesia for cardiac surgery: the effects on tracheal intubation time and length of hospital stay. *Anesth Analg.* 2002;94:275-282, table of contents.

42. Barrington MJ, Kluger R, Watson R, Scott DA, Harris KJ. Epidural anesthesia for coronary artery bypass surgery compared with general anesthesia alone does not reduce biochemical markers of myocardial damage. *Anesth Analg.* 2005;100:921-928.

43. Berendes E, Schmidt C, Van Aken H, et al. Reversible cardiac sympathectomy by high thoracic epidural anesthesia improves regional left ventricular function in patients undergoing coronary artery bypass grafting: a randomized trial. *Arch Surg.* 2003;138:1283-1290, discussion 1291.

44. Blomberg S, Emanuelsson H, Kvist H, et al. Effects of thoracic epidural anesthesia on coronary arteries and arterioles in patients with coronary artery disease. *Anesthesiology.* 1990;73:840-847.

45. Kock M, Blomberg S, Emanuelsson H, Lomsky M, Stromblad SO, Ricksten SE. Thoracic epidural anesthesia improves global and regional left ventricular function during stress-induced myocardial ischemia in patients with coronary artery disease. *Anesth Analg.* 1990;71:625-630.

46. Loick HM, Schmidt C, Van Aken H, Junker R, Erren M, Berendes E, et al. High thoracic epidural anesthesia, but not clonidine, attenuates the perioperative stress response via sympatholysis and reduces the release of troponin T in patients undergoing coronary artery bypass grafting. *Anesth Analg.* 1999;88:701-709.

47. Liu SS, Block BM, Wu CL. Effects of perioperative central neuraxial analgesia on outcome after coronary artery bypass surgery: a meta-analysis. *Anesthesiology.* 2004;101:153-161.

48. Bignami E, Landoni G, Biondi-Zoccai GG, et al. Epidural analgesia improves outcome in cardiac surgery: a meta-analysis of randomized controlled trials. *J Cardiothorac Vasc Anesth.* 2009;24(4): 586-597.

49. Tenenbein PK, Debrouwere R, Maguire D, et al. Thoracic epidural analgesia improves pulmonary function in patients undergoing cardiac surgery. *Can J Anaesth.* 2008;55:344-350.

50. Bakhtiary F, Therapidis P, Dzemali O, et al. Impact of high thoracic epidural anesthesia on incidence of perioperative atrial fibrillation in off-pump coronary bypass grafting: a prospective randomized study. *J Thorac Cardiovasc Surg.* 2007;134:460-464.

51. Jakobsen CJ, Nygaard E, Norrild K, et al. High thoracic epidural analgesia improves left ventricular function in patients with ischemic heart. *Acta Anaesthesiol Scand.* 2009;53:559-564.

52. Bracco D, Hemmerling T. Epidural analgesia in cardiac surgery: an updated risk assessment. *Heart Surg Forum.* 2007;10:E334-E337.

53. Chaney MA. Intrathecal and epidural anesthesia and analgesia for cardiac surgery. *Anesth Analg.* 2006;102:45-64.

54. Horlocker TT, Wedel DJ, Benzon H, et al. Regional anesthesia in the anticoagulated patient: defining the risks (the second ASRA Consensus Conference on Neuraxial Anesthesia and Anticoagulation). *Reg Anesth Pain Med.* 2003;28:172-197.

55. Konstantatos A, Silvers AJ, Myles PS. Analgesia best practice after cardiac surgery. *Anesthesiol Clin.* 2008;26:591-602.

56. Zangrillo A, Bignami E, Biondi-Zoccai GG, et al. Spinal analgesia in cardiac surgery: a meta-analysis of randomized controlled trials. *J Cardiothorac Vasc Anesth.* 2009;23:813-821.

57. Nader ND, Li CM, Dosluoglu HH, Ignatowski TA, Spengler RN. Adjuvant therapy with intrathecal clonidine improves postoperative pain in patients undergoing coronary artery bypass graft. *Clin J Pain.* 2009;25:101-106.

58. McDonald SB, Jacobsohn E, Kopacz DJ, et al. Parasternal block and local anesthetic infiltration with levobupivacaine after cardiac surgery with desflurane: the effect on postoperative pain, pulmonary function, and tracheal extubation times. *Anesth Analg.* 2005;100:25-32.

59. Dhole S, Mehta Y, Saxena H, Juneja R, Trehan N. Comparison of continuous thoracic epidural and paravertebral blocks for postoperative analgesia after minimally invasive direct coronary artery bypass surgery. *J Cardiothorac Vasc Anesth.* 2001;15:288-292.

60. Ben-Ari A, Moreno M, Chelly JE, Bigeleisen PE. Ultrasound-guided paravertebral block using an intercostal approach. *Anesth Analg.* 2009;109:1691-1694.

61. Scarci M, Joshi A, Attia R. In patients undergoing thoracic surgery is paravertebral block as effective as epidural analgesia for pain management? *Interact Cardiovasc Thorac Surg.* 2010;10:92-96.

62. Magnano D, Montalbano R, Lamarra M, et al. Ineffectiveness of local wound anesthesia to reduce postoperative pain after median sternotomy. *J Card Surg.* 2005;20:314-318.

63. White PF, Rawal S, Latham P, et al. Use of a continuous local anesthetic infusion for pain management after median sternotomy. *Anesthesiology.* 2003;99:918-923.

64. Noss C, Prusinkiewicz C, Nelson G, et al. Enhanced recovery for cardiac surgery. *J CardioThorac Vasc Anesth.* 2018 (epub ahead of print).

65. Li M, Zhang J, Gan T, et al. Enhanced recovery after surgery pathway for patients undergoing cardiac surgery: a randomized clinical trial. *Eur J Cardiothoracic Surg.* 2018; doi:10.1093/ejcts/ezy100.

66. Kumar K, Kayane R, Singh N, et al. Efficacy of bilateral pectoralis nerve block for ultrafast tracking and postoperative pain management in cardiac surgery. *Ann Card Anesth.* 2018;21(3):333-338.

REVIEWS

Bigeleisen P, Goehner N. Novel approaches in pain management in cardiac surgery. *Curr Opin Anesthesiol.* 2015;28:89-94.

Oliveri L, Jerzewski K, Kulik A. Black box warning: is ketorolac safe for use after cardiac surgery? *J. Cardiothorac Vasc Anesth.* 2014;28(2):274-279.

Index

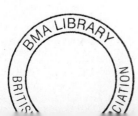